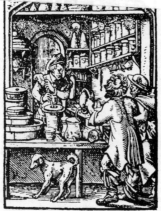

28ᵀᴴ EDITION

"Desire to take medicines ... distinguishes man from animals."
—Sir William Osler

Editor-in-Chief
Richard J. Hamilton, MD, FAAEM, FACMT, FACEP
Professor and Chair, Department of Emergency Medicine
Drexel University College of Medicine
Philadelphia, PA

JONES & BARTLETT
L E A R N I N G

World Headquarters
Jones & Bartlett Learning
5 Wall Street
Burlington, MA 01803
978-443-5000
info@jblearning.com
www.jblearning.com

Jones & Bartlett Learning books and products are available through most bookstores
and online booksellers. To contact Jones & Bartlett Learning directly, call 800-832-
0034, fax 978-443-8000, or visit our website www.jblearning.com.

> Substantial discounts on bulk quantities of Jones & Bartlett Learning publications
> are available to corporations, professional associations, and other qualified
> organizations. For details and specific discount information, contact the special
> sales department at Jones & Bartlett Learning via the above contact information
> or send an email to specialsales@jblearning.com.

The information in the *Pocket Pharmacopoeia* is compiled from sources believed to
be reliable, and exhaustive efforts have been put forth to make the book as accurate
as possible. The *Pocket Pharmacopoeia* is edited by a panel of drug information experts with extensive peer review and input from more than 50 practicing clinicians of
multiple specialties. Our goal is to provide health professionals focused, core prescribing
information in a convenient, organized, and concise fashion. We include FDA-approved
dosing indications and those off-label uses that have a reasonable basis to support their
use. *However, the accuracy and completeness of this work cannot be guaranteed.* Despite
our best efforts this book may contain typographical errors and omissions. The *Pocket
Pharmacopoeia* is intended as a quick and convenient reminder of information you have
already learned elsewhere. The contents are to be used as a guide only, and healthcare
professionals should use sound clinical judgment and individualize therapy to each
specific patient care situation. This book is not meant to be a replacement for training,
experience, continuing medical education, or studying the latest drug prescribing
literature. This book is sold without warranties of any kind, expressed or implied, and
the publisher and editors disclaim any liability, loss, or damage caused by the contents.
Although drug companies purchase and distribute our books as promotional items, the
Tarascon editorial staff alone determines all book content.

ISSN: 1945-9076
ISBN: 978-1-284-02670-2
6048
Printed in the United States of America
17 16 15 14 13   10 9 8 7 6 5 4 3 2 1

Production Credits

Chief Executive Officer: Ty Field
President: James Homer
V.P., Design and Production: Anne Spencer
V.P., Manufacturing and Inventory
    Control: Therese Connell
Manufacturing and Inventory Control
    Supervisor: Amy Bacus
Executive Editor: Nancy
    Anastasi Duffy

Production Editor:
    Daniel Stone
Digital Marketing Manager: Jennifer
    Sharp
Composition: Newgen
Text and Cover Design:
    Anne Spencer/Kristin E. Parker
Printing and Binding: Cenveo
Cover Printing: Cenveo

If you obtained your *Pocket Pharmacopoeia* from a bookstore, please send your address to info@tarascon.com. This allows you to be the first to hear of updates! (We don't sell or distribute our mailing lists, by the way.)

The cover woodcut is *The Apothecary* by Jost Amman, Frankfurt, 1574.

Last year we left you doing a procedure without adequate lighting... you needed to solve the dilemma of the three lights with three unmarked light switches all the way across the room. The best way to do this is to first label the switches 1, 2, and 3. Turn switch 1 on for 1 minute, then shut it off and turn on switch 2. Now walk to the bedside and feel the lights. The warm light is 1, the light that is on is 2, and the cold light is 3. Now get a sharpie and label the lights before you forget!

This year's puzzler centers on a daily frustration – commuting to work. One morning, you are headed to work in heavy traffic and reaching the halfway point, you notice that your average speed was 10 mph. You know that to be on time your average speed was supposed to be 20 mph. How fast would you have to travel over the second half of the commute to bring your average speed up to 16 mph? How fast would you have to travel to be on time for work?

CONTENTS

ANALGESICS 1
Antirheumatic Agents 1
Muscle Relaxants 2
Non-Opioid Analgesic
  Combinations 2
Non-Steroidal Anti-
  Inflammatories 4
Opioid Agonist-
  Antagonists 6
Opioid Agonists 7
Opioid Analgesic
  Combinations 9
Opioid Antagonists 12
Other Analgesics 12
ANESTHESIA 13
Anesthetics and Sedatives 13
Local Anesthetics 13
Myasthenia Gravis 13
Neuromuscular Blockade
  Reversing Agents 14
Neuromuscular Blockers 14
ANTIMICROBIALS 14
Aminoglycosides 14
Antifungal Agents 14
Antimalarials 16
Antimycobacterial Agents 18
Antiparasitics 18
Antiviral Agents 19
Carbapenems 32
Cephalosporins 32
Macrolides 37
Penicillins 38
Quinolones 42
Sulfonamides 42
Tetracyclines 44
Other Antimicrobials 44
CARDIOVASCULAR 46
ACE Inhibitors 46
Aldosterone Antagonists 48
Angiotensin Receptor
  Blockers (ARBs) 49
Anti-Dysrhythmics/
  Cardiac Arrest 49
Anti-Hyperlipidemic
  Agents 53
Antiadrenergic Agents 59
Antihypertensives 60
Antiplatelet Drugs 62
Beta-Blockers 63
Calcium Channel
  Blockers (CCBs) 65

Diuretics 67
Nitrates 68
Pressors/Inotropes 69
Pulmonary Arterial
  Hypertension 70
Thrombolytics 70
Volume Expanders 71
Other 71
CONTRAST MEDIA 72
MRI Contrast 72
Radiography Contrast 73
DERMATOLOGY 73
Acne Preparations 73
Actinic Keratosis
  Preparations 75
Antibacterials (Topical) 75
Antifungals (Topical) 76
Antiparasitics (Topical) 77
Antipsoriatics 78
Antivirals (Topical) 79
Atopic Dermatitis
  Preparations 79
Corticosteroid/
  Antimicrobial
  Combinations 81
Hemorrhoid Care 81
Other Dermatologic
  Agents 81
ENDOCRINE &
METABOLIC 83
Androgens / Anabolic
  Steroids 83
Bisphosphonates 84
Corticosteroids 85
Diabetes-Related 86
Diagnostic Agents 94
Gout-Related 94
Minerals 94
Nutritionals 98
Phosphate Binders 98
Thyroid Agents 98
Vitamins 99
Other 101
ENT 103
Antihistamines 103
Antitussives /
  Expectorants 105
Decongestants 105
Ear Preparations 106
Mouth and Lip
  Preparations 107

Nasal Preparations 107
GASTROENTEROLOGY 109
Antidiarrheals 109
Antiemetics 109
Antiulcer 111
Laxatives 115
Ulcerative Colitis 118
Other GI Agents 118
HEMATOLOGY 120
Anticoagulants 120
Colony-Stimulating
  Factors 124
Other Hematological
  Agents 125
HERBAL & ALTERNATIVE
THERAPIES 126
IMMUNOLOGY 131
Immunizations 131
Immunoglobulins 133
Immunosuppression 134
Other 135
NEUROLOGY 135
Alzheimer's Disease 135
Anticonvulsants 136
Migraine Therapy 140
Multiple Sclerosis 141
Myasthenia Gravis 141
Parkinsonian Agents 142
Other Agents 144
OB/GYN 145
Contraceptives 145
Estrogens 146
Hormone Combinations 147
Labor Induction /
  Cervical Ripening 150
Ovulation Stimulants 150
Progestins 150
Selective Estrogen
  Receptor Modulators 151
Uterotonics 151
Vaginitis Preparations 151
Other OB/GYN Agents 153
ONCOLOGY 154
OPHTHALMOLOGY 155
Antiallergy 155
Antibacterials 156
Antiviral Agents 157
Corticosteroid &
  Antibacterial
  Combinations 157
Corticosteroids 158

Glaucoma Agents 159
Mydriatics &
  Cycloplegics 160
Non-Steroidal
  Anti-Inflammatories 161
Other Ophthalmologic
  Agents 161
PSYCHIATRY 162
Antidepressants 162
Antimanic (Bipolar)
  Agents 166

Antipsychotics 167
Anxiolytics/Hypnotics 171
Combination Drugs 173
Drug-Dependence
  Therapy 173
Stimulants/ADHD/
  Anorexiants 173
PULMONARY 176
Beta Agonists 176
Combinations 178
Inhaled Steroids 179

Leukotriene Inhibitors 180
Other Pulmonary
  Medications 180
TOXICOLOGY 181
UROLOGY 183
Benign Prostatic
  Hyperplasia 183
Bladder Agents 183
Erectile Dysfunction 185
Nephrolithiasis 186
INDEX 187

PAGE INDEX FOR TABLES

GENERAL
Abbreviations ix
Therapeutic drug levels ix
Pediatric drugs x
Pediatric vital signs and
  IV drugs x
Conversions xi
P450 isozymes xii
Inhibitors, inducers,
  and substrates of
  P-Glycoprotein xvi
Drug therapy reference
  websites xvi
Adult emergency
  drugs 208
Cardiac dysrhythmia
  protocols 209
ANALGESICS
NSAIDs 5
Opioid equivalency 8
Fentanyl transdermal 9
ANTIMICROBIALS
Bacterial pathogens 26
Antiviral drugs for
  influenza 29
Cephalosporins 33
Acute otitis media in
  children 34
STDs/vaginitis 35
Penicillins 39

Acute bacterial sinusitis in
  adults and children 40
SBE prophylaxis 41
Quinolones 42
C. difficile infection in
  adults 43
CARDIOVASCULAR
HTN therapy 46
ACE inhibitors 47
QT interval drugs 50
LDL cholesteral goals 54
Lipid reduction by
  class/agent 55
LDL-C reduction by
  statin dose 57
Cardiac parameters 69
Thrombolysis in MI 71
DERMATOLOGY
Topical steroids 80
ENDOCRINE
Corticosteroids 85
A1C Reduction in
  Type 2 Diabetes 89
Diabetes numbers 90
Injectable insulins 91
Fluoride supplementation 95
IV solutions 96
Potassium (oral forms) 97
ENT
ENT combinations 104

GASTROENTEROLOGY
H pylori treatment 113
HEMATOLOGY
Enoxaparin adult
  dosing 122
Heparin dosing for
  ACS 123
Heparin dosing for
  DVT/PE 124
Therapeutic goals for
  anticoagulation 124
IMMUNOLOGY
Child immunizations 134
Tetanus 135
NEUROLOGY
Dermatomes 143
OB/GYN
Emergency
  contraception 147
Oral contraceptives 148
Drugs in pregnancy 153
PSYCHIATRY
Antipsychotics 169
Body mass index 175
PULMONARY
Peak flow 177
Inhaled steroids 178
Inhaler colors 181
TOXICOLOGY
Antidotes 182

*Affiliations are given for information purposes only, and no affiliation sponsorship is claimed.

PREFACE TO THE TARASCON POCKET PHARMACOPOEIA®

The *Tarascon Pocket Pharmacopoeia®* arranges drugs by clinical class with a comprehensive index in the back. Trade names are italicized and CAPITALIZED. Drug doses shown in mg/kg are generally intended for children, while fixed doses represent typical adult recommendations. Brackets indicate currently available formulations, although not all pharmacies stock all formulations. The availability of generic, over-the-counter, and scored formulations is mentioned. We have set the disease or indication in red for the pharmaceutical agent. It is meant to function as an aid to find information quickly. Codes are as follows:

▶ **METABOLISM & EXCRETION:** L = primarily liver, K = primarily kidney, LK = both, but liver > kidney, KL = both, but kidney > liver.

♀ **SAFETY IN PREGNANCY:** A = Safety established using human studies, B = Presumed safety based on animal studies, C = Uncertain safety; no human studies and animal studies show an adverse effect, D = Unsafe - evidence of risk that may in certain clinical circumstances be justifiable, X = Highly unsafe - risk of use outweighs any possible benefit. For drugs that have not been assigned a category: + Generally accepted as safe, ? Safety unknown or controversial, – Generally regarded as unsafe.

▶ **SAFETY IN LACTATION:** + Generally accepted as safe, ? Safety unknown or controversial, – Generally regarded as unsafe. Many of our "+" listings are from the AAP policy "The Transfer of Drugs and Other Chemicals Into Human Milk" (see www.aap.org) and may differ from those recommended by the manufacturer.

© **DEA CONTROLLED SUBSTANCES:** I = High abuse potential, no accepted use (eg, heroin, marijuana), II = High abuse potential and severe dependence liability (eg, morphine, codeine, hydromorphone, cocaine, amphetamines, methylphenidate, secobarbital). Some states require triplicates. III = Moderate dependence liability (eg, *Tylenol #3, Vicodin*), IV = Limited dependence liability (benzodiazepines, propoxyphene, phentermine), V = Limited abuse potential (eg, *Lomotil*).

$ **RELATIVE COST:** Cost codes used are "per month" of maintenance therapy (eg, antihypertensives) or "per course" of short-term therapy (eg, antibiotics). Codes are calculated using average wholesale prices (at press time in US dollars) for the most common indication and route of each drug at a typical adult dosage. For maintenance therapy, costs are calculated based upon a 30-day supply or the quantity that might typically be used in a given month. For short-term therapy (ie, 10 days or less), costs are calculated on a single treatment course. When multiple forms are available

Code	Cost
$	< $25
$$	$25 to $49
$$$	$50 to $99
$$$$	$100 to $199
$$$$$	≥ $200

(eg, generics), these codes reflect the least expensive generally available product. When drugs don't neatly fit into the classification scheme above, we have assigned codes based upon the relative cost of other similar drugs. *These codes should be used as a rough guide only*, as (1) they reflect cost, not charges, (2) pricing often varies substantially from location to location and time to time, and (3) HMOs, Medicaid, and buying groups often negotiate quite different pricing. Check with your local pharmacy if you have any questions.

🍁 **CANADIAN TRADE NAMES:** Unique common Canadian trade names not used in the US are listed after a maple leaf symbol. Trade names used in both nations or only in the US are displayed without such notation.

■ **BLACK BOX WARNINGS:** This icon indicates that there is a black box warning associated with this drug. Note that the warning itself is not listed.

ABBREVIATIONS IN TEXT

AAP – American Academy of Pediatrics
ACCP – American College of Chest Physicians
ACT – activated clotting time
ADHD – attention deficit hyperactivity disorder
AHA – American Heart Association
Al – aluminum
ANC – absolute neutrophil count
ASA – aspirin
BP – blood pressure
BPH – benign prostatic hyperplasia
BUN – blood urea nitrogen
Ca – calcium
CAD – coronary artery disease
cap – capsule
cm – centimeter
CMV – cytomegalovirus
CNS – central nervous system
COPD – chronic obstructive pulmonary disease
CrCl – creatinine clearance
CVA – stroke
CYP – cytochrome P450

D5W – 5% dextrose
dL – deciliter
DM – diabetes mellitus
DPI – dry powder inhaler
DRESS – drug rash eosinophilia and systemic symptoms
ECG – electrocardiogram
EPS – extrapyramidal symptoms
ET – endotracheal
g – gram
GERD – gastroesophageal reflux disease
gtts – drops
GU – genitourinary
h – hour
HAART – highly active antiretroviral therapy
Hb – hemoglobin
HCTZ – hydrochlorothiazide
HIT – heparin-induced thrombocytopenia
HSV – herpes simplex virus
HTN – hypertension
IM – intramuscular
INR – international normalized ratio
IU – international units
IV – intravenous
JRA – juvenile rheumatoid arthritis

kg – kilogram
lbs – pounds
LFT – liver function test
LV – left ventricular
LVEF – left ventricular ejection fraction
m^2 – square meters
MAOI – monoamine oxidase inhibitor
mcg – microgram
MDI – metered dose inhaler
mEq – milliequivalent
mg – milligram
Mg – magnesium
MI – myocardial infarction
min – minute
mL – milliliter
mm – millimeter
mo – months old
MRSA – methicillin-resistant *Staphylococcus aureus*
ng – nanogram
NHLBI – National Heart, Lung, and Blood Institute
NPH – neutral protamine hagedorn
NS – normal saline
N/V – nausea/vomiting
NYHA – New York Heart Association

OA – osteoarthritis
oz – ounces
pc – after meals
PO – by mouth
PR – by rectum
prn – as needed
PTT – partial thromboplastin time
q – every
RA – rheumatoid arthritis
RSV – respiratory syncytial virus
SC – subcutaneous
sec – second
soln – solution
supp – suppository
susp – suspension
tab – tablet
TB – tuberculosis
TCA – tricyclic antidepressant
TNF – tumor necrosis factor
TPN – total parenteral nutrition
UTI – urinary tract infection
wt – weight
y – year
yo – years old

THERAPEUTIC DRUG LEVELS

Drug	Level	Optimal Timing
amikacin peak	20–35 mcg/mL	30 minutes after infusion
amikacin trough	<5 mcg/mL	Just prior to next dose
carbamazepine trough	4–12 mcg/mL	Just prior to next dose
cyclosporine trough	50–300 ng/mL	Just prior to next dose
digoxin	0.8–2.0 ng/mL	Just prior to next dose
ethosuximide trough	40–100 mcg/mL	Just prior to next dose
gentamicin peak	5–10 mcg/mL	30 minutes after infusion
gentamicin trough	<2 mcg/mL	Just prior to next dose
lidocaine	1.5–5 mcg/mL	12–24 hours after start of infusion
lithium trough	0.6–1.2 meq/l	Just prior to first morning dose
NAPA	10–30 mcg/mL	Just prior to next procainamide dose
phenobarbital trough	15–40 mcg/mL	Just prior to next dose
phenytoin trough	10–20 mcg/mL	Just prior to next dose
primidone trough	5–12 mcg/mL	Just prior to next dose
procainamide	4–10 mcg/mL	Just prior to next dose
quinidine	2–5 mcg/mL	Just prior to next dose
theophylline	5–15 mcg/mL	8–12 hours after once daily dose
tobramycin peak	5–10 mcg/mL	30 minutes after infusion
tobramycin trough	<2 mcg/mL	Just prior to next dose
valproate trough (epilepsy)	50–100 mcg/mL	Just prior to next dose
valproate trough (mania)	45–125 mcg/mL	Just prior to next dose
vancomycin trough[1]	10–20 mg/L	Just prior to next dose
zonisamide[2]	10–40 mcg/mL	Just prior to dose

[1]Maintain trough >10 mg/L to avoid resistance; optimal trough for complicated infections is 15–20 mg/L
[2]Ranges not firmly established but supported by clinical trial results

PEDIATRIC DRUGS		*Age*	*2mo*	*4mo*	*6mo*	*9mo*	*12mo*	*15mo*	*2yo*	*3yo*	*5yo*
		Kg	5	6½	8	9	10	11	13	15	19
		lbs	11	15	17	20	22	24	28	33	42
med	***strength***	***freq***	***teaspoons of liquid per dose*** *(1 tsp = 5 mL)*								
Tylenol (mg)		q4h	80	80	120	120	160	160	200	240	280
Tvlenol (tsp)	160/t	q4h	½	½	¾	¾	1	1	1¼	1½	1¾
ibuprofen (mg)		q6h	--	--	75[†]	75[†]	100	100	125	150	175
ibuorofen (tsp)	100/t	q6h	--	--	¾t	¾t	1	1	1¼	1½	1¾
amoxicillin or	125/t	bid	1	1¼	1½	1¾	1¾	2	2¼	2¾	3½
Augmentin	200/t	bid	½	¾	1	1	1¼	1¼	1½	1¾	2¼
(not otitis media)	250/t	bid	½	½	¾	¾	1	1	1¼	1¼	1¾
	400/t	bid	¼	½	½	½	¾	¾	¾	1	1
amoxicillin,	200/t	bid	1	1¼	1¾	2	2	2¼	2¾	3	4
(otitis media)‡	250/t	bid	¾	1¼	1½	1½	1¾	1¾	2¼	2½	3¼
	400/t	bid	½	¾	¾	1	1	1¼	1½	1½	2
Auamentin ES‡	600/t	bid	?	½	½	¾	¾	¾	1	1¼	1½
azithromycin*§	100/t	qd	¼[†]	½[†]	½	½	½	½	¾	¾	1
(5-day Rx)	200/t	qd	--	¼[†]	¼	¼	¼	¼	½	½	½
Bactrim/Septra	---	bid	½	¾	1	1	1	1¼	1½	1½	2
cefaclor*	125/t	bid	1	1	1¼	1½	1½	1¾	2	2½	3
*	250/t	bid	½	½	¾	¾	¾	1	1	1¼	1½
cefadroxil	125/t	bid	½	¾	1	1	1¼	1¼	1½	1¾	2¼
*	250/t	bid	¼	½	½	½	¾	¾	¾	1	1
cefdinir	125/t	qd	--	¾[†]	1	1	1	1¼	1½	1¾	2
Cefixime	100/t	qd	½	½	¾	¾	¾	1	1	1¼	1½
cefprozil*	125/t	bid	--	¾[†]	1	1	1¼	1½	1½	2	2¼
*	250/t	bid	--	½[†]	½	½	¾	¾	¾	1	1¼
cefuroxime	125/t	bid	--	¾	¾	1	1	1	1½	1¾	2¼
cephalexin	125/t	qid	--	½	¾	¾	1	1	1¼	1½	1¾
*	250/t	qid	--	¼	¼	½	½	½	¾	¾	1
clarithromycin	125/t	bid	½[†]	½	½	½	¾	¾	¾	1	1¼
*	250/t	bid	--	--	--	¼	½	½	½	½	¾
dicloxacillin	62½/t	qid	½	¾	1	1	1¼	1¼	1½	1¾	2
nitrofurantoin	25/t	qid	¼	½	½	½	½	¾	¾	¾	1
Pediazole	---	tid	½	½	¾	¾	1	1	1	1¼	1½
penicillin V**	250/t	bid-tid	--	1	1	1	1	1	1	1	1
cetirizine	5/t	qd	--	--	½	½	½	½	½	½	½
Benadryl	12.5/t	q6h	½	½	¾	¾	1	1	1¼	1½	2
prednisolone	15/t	qd	¼	½	½	¾	¾	¾	1	1	1¼
prednisone	5/t	qd	1	1¼	1½	1¾	2	2¼	2½	3	3¾
Robitussin	---	q4h	--	--	¼[†]	¼[†]	½	½	¾	¾	1
Tylenol w/ codeine		q4h	--	--	--	--	--	--	--	1	1

* Dose shown is for otitis media only; see dosing in text for alternative indications.

† Dosing at this age/weight not recommended by manufacturer.

‡ AAP now recommends high dose (80-90 mg/kg/d) for all otitis media in children; with Augmentin used as ES only.

§ Give a double dose of azithromycin the first day.

**AHA dosing for streptococcal pharyngitis. Treat for 10 days.

tsp/t = teaspoon; q = every; h = hour; kg = kilogram; Lbs = pounds; ml = mililiter; bid = two times per day; qd = every day; qid = four times per day; tid =three times per day

PEDIATRIC VITAL SIGNS AND INTRAVENOUS DRUGS

Age		Pre-matr	New-born	2m	4m	6m	9m	12m	15m	2y	3y	5y
Weight	(kg)	2	3½	5	6½	8	9	10	11	13	15	19
	(lbs)	4¼	7½	11	15	17	20	22	24	28	33	42
Maint fluids	(mL/h)	8	14	20	26	32	36	40	42	46	50	58
ET tube	(mm)	2½	3/3½	3½	3½	3½	4	4	4½	4½	4½	5
Defib	(Joules)	4	7	10	13	16	18	20	22	26	30	38
Systolic BP	(high)	70	80	85	90	95	100	103	104	106	109	114
	(low)	40	60	70	70	70	70	70	70	75	75	80
Pulse rate	(high)	145	145	180	180	180	160	160	160	150	150	135
	(low)	100	100	110	110	110	100	100	100	90	90	65
Resp rate	(high)	60	60	50	50	50	46	46	30	30	25	25
	(low)	35	30	30	30	24	24	20	20	20	20	20
adenosine	(mg)	0.2	0.3	0.5	0.6	0.8	0.9	1	1.1	1.3	1.5	1.9
atropine	(mg)	0.1	0.1	0.1	0.13	0.16	0.18	0.2	0.22	0.26	0.30	0.38
Benadryl	(mg)	-	-	5	6½	8	9	10	11	13	15	19
bicarbonate	(meq)	2	3½	5	6½	8	9	10	11	13	15	19
dextrose	(g)	1	2	5	6½	8	9	10	11	13	15	19
epinephrine	(mg)	.02	.04	.05	.07	.08	.09	0.1	0.11	0.13	0.15	0.19
lidocaine	(mg)	2	3½	5	6½	8	9	10	11	13	15	19
morphine	(mg)	0.2	0.3	0.5	0.6	0.8	0.9	1	1.1	1.3	1.5	1.9
mannitol	(g)	2	3½	5	6½	8	9	10	11	13	15	19
naloxone	(mg)	.02	.04	.05	.07	.08	.09	0.1	0.11	0.13	0.15	0.19
diazepam	(mg)	0.6	1	1.5	2	2.5	2.7	3	3.3	3.9	4.5	5
fosphenytoin*	(PE)	40	70	100	130	160	180	200	220	260	300	380
lorazepam	(mg)	0.1	0.2	0.3	0.35	0.4	0.5	0.5	0.6	0.7	0.8	1.0
phenobarb	(mg)	30	60	75	100	125	125	150	175	200	225	275
phenytoin*	(mg)	40	70	100	130	160	180	200	220	260	300	380
ampicillin	(mg)	100	175	250	325	400	450	500	550	650	750	1000
ceftriaxone	(mg)	-	-	250	325	400	450	500	550	650	750	1000
cefotaxime	(mg)	100	175	250	325	400	450	500	550	650	750	1000
gentamicin	(mg)	5	8	12	16	20	22	25	27	32	37	47

*Loading doses; fosphenytoin dosed in "phenytoin equivalents."

CONVERSIONS	Liquid:	Weight:
Temperature:	1 fluid ounce = 30 mL	1 kilogram = 2.2 lbs
F = (1.8) C + 32	1 teaspoon = 5 mL	1 ounce = 30 g
C = (F − 32)/1.8	1 tablespoon = 15 mL	1 grain = 65 mg

INHIBITORS, INDUCERS, AND SUBSTRATES OF CYTOCHROME P450 ISOZYMES

The cytochrome P450 (CYP) inhibitors and inducers below do not necessarily cause clinically important interactions with substrates listed. We exclude in vitro data which can be inaccurate. Refer to the *Tarascon Pocket Pharmacopoeia* drug interactions database (PDA edition) or other resources for more information if an interaction is suspected based on this chart. A drug that inhibits CYP subfamily activity can block the metabolism of substrates of that enzyme and substrate accumulation and toxicity may result. CYP inhibitors are classified by how much they increase the area-under-the-curve (AUC) of a substrate: weak (1.25-2 fold), moderate (2–5 fold), or strong (≥5 fold). A drug that induces CYP subfamily activity increases substrate metabolism and reduced substrate efficacy may result. CYP inducers are classified by how much they decrease the AUC of a substrate: weak (20-50%), moderate (50-80%) or strong (≥80%). A drug is considered a sensitive substrate if a CYP inhibitor increases the AUC of that drug by ≥5-fold. While AUC increases of >50% often do not affect patient response, smaller increases can be important if the therapeutic range is narrow (eg, theophylline, warfarin, cyclosporine). This table may be incomplete since new evidence about drug interactions is continually being identified.

CYP1A2

Inhibitors. *Strong*: ciprofloxacin, fluvoxamine. *Moderate*: methoxalan, mexiletine, oral contraceptives, phenylpropanolamine, vemurafenib, zileuton. *Weak*: acyclovir, allopurinol, caffeine, cimetidine, disulfiram, echinacea, famotidine, norfloxacin, propafenone, propranolol, terbinafine, ticlopidine, verapamil. *Unclassified*: amiodarone, atazanavir, citalopram, clarithromycin, deferasirox, erythromycin, estradiol, isoniazid, peginterferon alfa-2a.
Inducers. *Moderate*: montelukast, phenytoin, smoking. *Weak*: omeprazole, phenobarbital. *Unclassified*: carbamazepine, charcoal-broiled foods, rifampin, ritonavir, tipranavir/ritonavir.
Substrates. *Sensitive*: caffeine, duloxetine, melatonin, rameltion, tacrine, tizanidine. *Unclassified*: acetaminophen, amitriptyline, asenapine, bendamustine, cinacalcet, clomipramine, clozapine, cyclobenzaprine, estradiol, fluvoxamine, haloperidol, imipramine, loxapine, mexiletine, mirtazapine, naproxen, olanzapine, ondansetron, pomalidomide, propranolol, rasagiline, riluzole, roflumilast, ropinirole, ropivacaine, R-warfarin, theophylline, zileuton, zolmitriptan.

CYP2B6

Inhibitors: *Weak*: clopidogrel, prasugrel, ticlopidine.
Inducers: *Moderate*: efavirenz, rifampin. *Weak*: nevirapine. *Unclassified*: baicalin (ingredient of Limbrel).
Substrates: *Sensitive*: bupropion, efavirenz. *Unclassified*: cyclophosphamide, ketamine, methadone, nevirapine, prasugrel.

CYP2C8

Inhibitors. *Strong*: gemfibrozil. *Moderate*: deferasirox. *Weak*: fluvoxamine, ketoconazole, trimethoprim.
Inducers: *Moderate*: rifampin. *Unclassified*: barbiturates, carbamazepine, rifabutin.
Substrates. *Sensitive*: repaglinide. *Unclassified*: amiodarone, carbamazepine, dabrafenib, ibuprofen, isotretinoin, loperamide, montelukast, paclitaxel, pioglitazone, rosiglitazone, treprostanil.

CYP2C9

Inhibitors. *Moderate*: amiodarone, fluconazole, miconazole, oxandrolone. *Weak*: capecitabine, cotrimoxazole, etravirine, fluvastatin, fluvoxamine, metronidazole, sulfinpyrazone, tigecycline, voriconazole, zafirlukast. *Unclassified*: cimetidine, fenofibrate, fenofibric acid, fluorouracil, imatinib, isoniazid, leflunomide.
Inducers: *Moderate*: carbamazepine, rifampin. *Weak*: aprepitant, bosentan, elvitegravir (in *Stribild*), phenobarbital, St John's wort. *Unclassified*: rifapentine.
Substrates. *Sensitive*: celecoxib. *Unclassified*: azilsartan, bosentan, chlorpropamide, diclofenac, etravirine, fluoxetine, flurbiprofen, fluvastatin, formoterol, glimepiride, glipizide, glyburide, ibuprofen, irbesartan, losartan, mefenamic acid, meloxicam, montelukast, naproxen, nateglinide, ospemifene, phenytoin, piroxicam, ramelteon, sildenafil, tolbutamide, torsemide, vardenafil, voriconazole, S-warfarin, zafirlukast, zileuton.

CYP2C19

Inhibitors. *Strong*: fluconazole, fluvoxamine, ticlopidine. *Moderate*: esomeprazole, fluoxetine, moclobemide, omeprazole, voriconazole. *Weak*: armodafinil, carbamazepine, cimetidine, etravirine, felbamate, human growth hormone, ketoconazole, oral contraceptives. *Unclassified*: chloramphenicol, isoniazid, modafinil, oxcarbazepine .
Inducers. *Moderate*: rifampin. *Unclassified*: efavirenz, St John's wort.
Substrates. *Sensitive*: lansoprazole, omeprazole. *Unclassified*: amitriptyline, bortezomib, carisoprodol, cilostazol, citalopram, clobazam, clomipramine, clopidogrel, clozapine, cyclophosphamide, desipramine, dexlansoprazole, diazepam, escitalopram, esomeprazole, etravirine, formoterol, imipramine, lacosamide, methadone, moclobamide, nelfinavir, pantoprazole, phenytoin, progesterone, proguanil, propranolol, rabeprazole, sertraline, voriconazole, R-warfarin.

CYP2D6

Inhibitors. *Strong*: bupropion, fluoxetine, paroxetine, quinidine.
Moderate: cinacalcet, dronedarone, duloxetine, mirabegron, terbinafine.
Weak: amiodarone, asenapine, celecoxib, cimetidine, desvenlafaxine, diltiazem, diphenhydramine, echinacea, escitalopram, febuxostat, gefitinib, hydralazine, hydroxychloroquine, imitinib, methadone, oral contraceptives, propafenone, ranitidine, ritonavir, sertraline, telithromycin, venlafaxine, vemurafenib, verapamil. *Unclassified*: abiraterone, chloroquine, clobazam, clomipramine,

cobicistat (in *Stribild*), fluphenazine, haloperidol, lorcaserin, lumefantrine, metoclopramide, moclobamide, perphenazine, quinine, ranolazine, thioridazine.
Inducers: None known.
Substrates. *Sensitive:* atomoxetine, desipramine, dextromethorphan, metoprolol, nebivolol, perphenazine, tolterodine, venlafaxine. ***Unclassified:*** amitriptyline, aripiprazole, carvedilol, cevimeline, chlorpheniramine, chlorpromazine, cinacalcet, clomipramine, codeine*, darifenacin, dihydrocodeine, dolasetron, donepezil, doxepin, duloxetine, fesoterodine, flecainide, fluoxetine, formoterol, galantamine, haloperidol, hydrocodone, iloperidone, imipramine, loratadine, loxapine, maprotiline, methadone, methamphetamine, metoclopramide, meclizine, mexiletine, mirtazapine, morphine, nortriptyline, ondansetron, paroxetine, promethazine, propafenone, propranolol, quetiapine, risperidone, ritonavir, tamoxifen, tetrabenazine, thioridazine, timolol, tramadol*, trazodone.
* Metabolism by CYP2D6 required to convert to active analgesic metabolite; analgesia may be impaired by CYP2D6 inhibitors.

CYP3A4

Inhibitors. *Strong:* boceprevir, clarithromycin, cobicistat (in *Stribild*), conivaptan, indinavir, itraconazole, ketoconazole, lopinavir-ritonavir, nefazodone, nelfinavir, posaconazole, ritonavir, saquinavir, telaprevir, telithromycin, voriconazole. ***Moderate:*** aprepitant, atazanavir, crizotinib, darunavir-ritonavir, diltiazem, dronedarone, erythromycin, fluconazole, fosamprenavir, grapefruit juice (variable), imatinib, verapamil. ***Weak:*** alprazolam, amiodarone, amlodipine, atorvastatin, bicalutamide, cilostazol, cimetidine, cyclosporine, fluoxetine, fluvoxamine, ginko, goldenseal, isoniazid, ivacaftor, lapatinib, nilotinib, oral contraceptives, ranitidine, ranolazine, ticagrelor, tipranavir-ritonavir, zileuton. ***Unclassified:*** danazol, miconazole, quinine, quinupristin/dalfopristin, sertraline.
Inducers. *Strong:* carbamazepine, phenytoin, rifampin, rifapentine, St Johns wort. ***Moderate:*** bosentan, efavirenz, etravirine, modafinil, nafcillin. ***Weak:*** aprepitant, armodafinil, clobazam, echinacea, fosamprenavir, pioglitazone, rufinamide. ***Unclassified:*** artemether, barbiturates, dexamethasone, ethosuximide, griseovulvin, nevirapine, oxcarbazepine, primidone, rifabutin, ritonavir vemurafenib.
Substrates. *Sensitive:* alfentanil, aprepitant, budesonide, buspirone, conivaptan, darifenacin, darunavir, dasatinib, dronedarone, eletriptan, eplerenone, everolimus, felodipine, fluticasone, indinavir, ivacaftor, lomitapide, lopinavir, lovastatin, lurasidone, maraviroc, midazolam, nisoldipine, quetiapine, saquinavir, sildenafil, simvastatin, sirolimus, tipranavir, tolvaptan, triazolam, vardenafil. ***Unclassified:*** alfuzosin, aliskiren, almotriptan, alprazolam, amiodarone, amlodipine, apixaban, aripiprazole, armodafinil, artemether (in *Coartem*), atazanavir, atorvastatin, avanafil, axitinib, bedaquiline, boceprevir, bortezomib, bosentan, bosutinib, brentuximab, bromocriptine, buprenorphine, cabozantinib, carbamazepine, cevimeline, cilostazol, cinacalcet, cisapride, citalopram, clarithromycin, clomipramine, clonazepam, clopidogrel, clobazam, clozapine, cobicistat

(in *Stribild*), colchicine, corticosteroids, crizotinib, cyclophosphamide, cyclosporine, dabrafenib, dapsone, desogestrel, desvenlafaxine, dexamethasone, dexlansoprazole, diazepam, dihydroergotamine, diltiazem, disopyramide, docetaxel, dofetilide, dolasetron, domperidone, donepezil, doxorubicin, dutasteride, efavirenz, elvitegravir (in *Stribild*), ergotamine, erlotinib, erythromycin, escitalopram, esomeprazole, eszopiclone, ethinyl estradiol, etoposide, etravirine, fentanyl, fesoterodine, finasteride, fosamprenavir, fosaprepitant, galantamine, gefitinib, guanfacine, haloperidol, hydrocodone, ifosfamide, iloperidone, imatinib, imipramine, irinotecan, isradipine, itraconazole, ixabepilone, ketamine, ketoconazole, lansoprazole, lapatinib, letrozole, lidocaine, loratadine, loxapine, lumefantrine (in *Coartem*), methylergonovine, mifepristone, mirtazapine, modafinil, mometasone, nateglinide, nefazodone, nelfinavir, nevirapine, nicardipine, nifedipine, nilotinib, nimodipine, ondansetron, ospemifene, oxybutynin, oxycodone, paclitaxel, pantoprazole, pazopanib, pimozide, pioglitazone, pomalidomide, ponatinib, prasugrel, praziquantel, quinidine, quinine, rabeprazole, ramelteon, ranolazine, regorafenib, repaglinide, rifabutin, rifampin, ritonavir, rivaroxaban, roflumilast, romidepsin, ruxolitinib, saxagliptin, sertraline, silodosin, solifenacin, sufentanil, sunitinib, tacrolimus, tadalafil, tamoxifen, telaprevir, telithromycin, temsirolimus, testosterone, tiagabine, ticagrelor, tinidazole, tofacitinib, tolterodine, tramadol, trazodone, verapamil, vilazodone, vinblastine, vincristine, vinorelbine, voriconazole, R-warfarin, zaleplon, ziprasidone, zolpidem, zonisamide.

INHIBITORS, INDUCERS, AND SUBSTRATES OF P-GLYCOPROTEIN

The p-glycoprotein (P-gp) inhibitors and inducers below do not necessarily cause clinically important interactions with substrates listed. We attempt to exclude in vitro data which can be inaccurate. Refer to the Tarascon Pocket Pharmacopoeia drug interactions database (PDA edition) or other resources for more information if an interaction is suspected based on this chart. P-gp is an efflux transporter that pumps drugs out of cells. In the gut P-gp, reduces drug absorption by pumping drugs into the gut lumen. In the kidney, it increases drug excretion by pumping drugs into urine. P-gp inhibitors can increase exposure to P-gp substrates, potentially increasing their risk of toxicity. P-gp inducers can reduce exposure to P-gp substrates, increasing their risk of treatment failure. Some drugs are dual inhibitors of P-gp and CYP 3A4 (e.g. clarithromycin, dronedarone, erythromycin, itraconazole, ketoconazole, verapamil), while others are dual inducers of P-gp and CYP 3A4 (e.g. carbamazepine, phenytoin, rifampin, St John's wort).

Inhibitors: Amiodarone, atorvastatin, azithromycin, captopril, carvedilol clarithromycin, cobicistat (in *Stribild*), conivaptan, cyclosporine, darunavir-ritonavir, dipyridamole, dronedarone, erythromycin, etravirine, everolimus, felodipine ,indinavir, isradipine, itraconazole, ketoconazole, lapatinib, lomitapide, lopinavir-ritonavir, nifedipine, nilotinib, posaconazole, quinidine, ranolazine, ritonavir, saquinavir-ritonavir, telaprevir, ticagrelor, verapamil.

Inducers: Carbamazepine, fosamprenavir, phenytoin, rifampin, St John's wort, tipranavir-ritonavir.

Substrates: Aliskiren, ambrisentan, apixaban, boceprevir, clobazam, colchicine, cyclosporine, dabigatran, digoxin, diltiazem, docetaxel, etoposide, everolimus, fexofenadine, fosamprenavir, imatinib, indinavir, lapatinib, linagliptin, loperamide, lovastatin, maraviroc, morphine, nadolol, nilotinib, paclitaxel, pomalidomide, posaconazole, pravastatin, propranolol, ranolazine, rivaroxaban, romidepsin, saquinavir, saxagliptin, silodosin, sirolimus, sitagliptin, tacrolimus, telaprevir, tolvaptan, topotecan, vinblastine, vincristine.

DRUG THERAPY REFERENCE WEBSITES (selected)

Professional societies or governmental agencies with drug therapy guidelines

AAP	American Academy of Pediatrics	www.aap.org
ACC	American College of Cardiology	www.acc.org
ACCP	American College of Chest Physicians	www.chestnet.org
ACCP	American College of Clinical Pharmacy	www.accp.com
ADA	American Diabetes Association	www.diabetes.org
AHA	American Heart Association	www.heart.org
AHRQ	Agency for Healthcare Research and Quality	www.ahcpr.gov
AIDSinfo	HIV Treatment, Prevention, and Research	www.aidsinfo.nih.gov
AMA	American Medical Association	www.ama-assn.org
APA	American Psychiatric Association	www.psych.org
APA	American Psychological Association	www.apa.org
ASHP	Amer. Society Health-Systems Pharmacists	
	Drug Shortages Resource Center	www.ashp.org/shortages
ATS	American Thoracic Society	www.thoracic.org
CDC	Centers for Disease Control and Prevention	www.cdc.gov
CDC	CDC bioterrorism and radiation exposures	www.bt.cdc.gov
IDSA	Infectious Diseases Society of America	www.idsociety.org
MHA	Malignant Hyperthermia Association	www.mhaus.org

Other therapy reference sites

Cochrane library	www.cochrane.org
Emergency Contraception Website	www.not-2-late.com
Immunization Action Coalition	www.immunize.org
QTDrug lists	www.crediblemeds.org/
Managing Contraception	www.managingcontraception.com

ANALGESICS

Antirheumatic Agents—Biologic Response Modifiers

NOTE: *Death, sepsis, and serious infections (eg, TB and invasive fungal infections) have been reported.*

ADALIMUMAB (*Humira*) RA, psoriatic arthritis, ankylosing spondylitis: 40 mg SC q 2 weeks, alone or in combination with methotrexate or other disease-modifying antirheumatic drugs (DMARDs). May increase frequency to once a week if not on methotrexate. Crohn's disease: 160 mg SC at week 0, 80 mg at week 2, then 40 mg every other week starting with week 4. [Trade only: 40 mg prefilled glass syringes or vials with needles, 2 per pack. 20 mg vial with needles, 2 per pack.] ▶Serum ♀B ▶– $$$$$ ■

ANAKINRA (*Kineret*) RA: 100 mg SC daily. [Trade only: 100 mg prefilled graduated glass syringes with needles, 7 or 28 per box.] ▶K ♀B ▶? $$$$$ ■

ETANERCEPT (*Enbrel*) RA, psoriatic arthritis, ankylosing spondylitis: 50 mg SC once a week. Plaque psoriasis: 50 mg SC 2 times per week for 3 months, then 50 mg SC once a week. JRA: age 4 to 17 yo: 0.8 mg/kg SC once a week, to max single dose of 50 mg. Max dose per injection site is 25 mg. [Trade only: 25, 50 mg prefilled syringes in cartons of 4] ▶Serum ♀B ▶– $$$$$ ■

GOLIMUMAB (*Simponi*) RA, psoriatic arthritis, ankylosing spondylitis: 50 mg SC q month, alone (ankylosing spondylitis, psoriatic arthritis) or in combination with methotrexate (rheumatoid arthritis, psoriatic arthritis). Ulcerative colitis: 200 mg SC at week 0, 100 mg at week 2, then 100 mg every 4 weeks. [Trade only: 50 mg and 100 mg prefilled syringes with or without autoinjector.] ▶Serum ♀B ▶? $$$$$ ■

INFLIXIMAB (*Remicade*) RA: 3 mg/kg IV in combination with methotrexate at 0, 2, and 6 weeks. Ankylosing spondylitis: 5 mg/kg IV at 0, 2, and 6 weeks. Plaque psoriasis, psoriatic arthritis, moderately to severely active Crohn's disease, ulcerative colitis, or fistulizing disease: 5 mg/kg IV infusion at 0, 2, and 6 weeks, then q 8 weeks. ▶Serum ♀B ▶? $$$$$ ■

Antirheumatic Agents—Disease Modifying Antirheumatic Drugs (DMARDs)

AZATHIOPRINE (*Azasan, Imuran*) RA: Initial dose 1 mg/kg (50 to 100 mg) PO daily or divided two times per day. Increase after 6 to 8 weeks. [Generic/Trade: Tabs 50 mg, scored. Trade only (Azasan): 75, 100 mg, scored.] ▶LK ♀D ▶– $$$ ■

HYDROXYCHLOROQUINE (*Plaquenil*) RA: Start 400 to 600 mg PO daily, then taper to 200 to 400 mg daily. SLE: 400 mg PO one to two times per day to start, then taper to 200 to 400 mg daily. [Generic/Trade: Tabs 200 mg, scored.] ▶K ♀C ▶+ $ ■

LEFLUNOMIDE (*Arava*) RA: Loading dose: 100 mg PO daily for 3 days. Maintenance dose: 10 to 20 mg PO daily. [Generic/Trade: Tabs 10, 20 mg. Trade only: Tabs 100 mg.] ▶LK ♀X ▶– $$$$$ ■

METHOTREXATE—RHEUMATOLOGY (*Rheumatrex, Trexall*) RA, psoriasis: Start with 7.5 mg PO single dose once a week or 2.5 mg PO q 12 h for 3 doses given once a week. Max dose 20 mg/week. Supplement with 1 mg/day of folic acid. Chemotherapy doses vary by indication. [Trade only (Trexall): Tabs 5, 7.5, 10, 15 mg. Dose Pak (Rheumatrex) 2.5 mg (# 8, 12, 16, 20, 24). Generic/Trade: Tabs 2.5 mg, scored.] ▶LK ♀X ▶– $$ ■

Muscle Relaxants

BACLOFEN (*Lioresal,* ✦ *Lioresal, Lioresal D.S.*) Spasticity related to MS or spinal cord disease/injury: Start 5 mg PO three times per day, then increase by 5 mg/dose q 3 days until 20 mg PO three times per day. Max dose 20 mg four times per day. [Generic only: Tabs 10, 20 mg.] ▶K ♀C ▶+ $

CARISOPRODOL (*Soma*) Acute musculoskeletal pain: 350 mg PO three to four times per day. Abuse potential. [Generic/Trade: Tabs 350 mg. Trade only: Tabs 250 mg.] ▶LK ♀? ▶–©IV $

CHLORZOXAZONE (*Parafon Forte DSC, Lorzone, Remular-S*) Musculoskeletal pain: 500 to 750 mg PO three to four times per day to start. Decrease to 250 mg three to four times per day. [Generic/Trade: Tabs 500 mg (Parafon Forte DSC 500 mg tabs, scored). Trade only: Tabs 250 mg (Remular-S), Tabs 375, 750 mg (Lorzone)] ▶LK ♀C ▶? $

CYCLOBENZAPRINE (*Amrix, Flexeril, Fexmid*) Musculoskeletal pain: Start 5 to 10 mg PO three times per day, max 30 mg/day or 15 to 30 mg (extended-release) PO daily. Not recommended in elderly. [Generic/Trade: Tab 5, 7.5, 10 mg. Extended-release caps 15, 30 mg ($$$$$).] ▶LK ♀B ▶? $

DANTROLENE (*Dantrium*) Chronic spasticity related to spinal cord injury, CVA, cerebral palsy, MS: 25 mg PO daily to start, up to max of 100 mg two to four times per day if necessary. Malignant hyperthermia: 2.5 mg/kg rapid IV push q 5 to 10 min continuing until symptoms subside or to a maximum total dose of 10 mg/kg. [Generic/Trade: Caps 25, 50, 100 mg.] ▶LK ♀C ▶– $$$$ ■

METAXALONE (*Skelaxin*) Musculoskeletal pain: 800 mg PO three to four times per day. [Generic/Trade: Tabs 800 mg, scored.] ▶LK ♀? ▶? $$$$

METHOCARBAMOL (*Robaxin, Robaxin-750*) Acute musculoskeletal pain: 1500 mg PO four times per day or 1000 mg IM/IV three times per day for 48 to 72 h. Maintenance: 1000 mg PO four times per day, 750 mg PO q 4 h, or 1500 mg PO three times per day. Tetanus: Specialized dosing. [Generic/Trade: Tabs 500 and 750 mg. OTC in Canada.] ▶LK ♀C ▶? $

ORPHENADRINE (*Norflex,* ✦ *Orphenace,*) Musculoskeletal pain: 100 mg PO two times per day. 60 mg IV/IM two times per day. [Generic only: 100 mg extended-release. OTC in Canada.] ▶LK ♀C ▶? $$

TIZANIDINE (*Zanaflex*) Muscle spasticity due to MS or spinal cord injury: 4 to 8 mg PO q 6 to 8 h prn, max 36 mg/day. [Generic/Trade: Tabs 4 mg, scored. Caps 2, 4, 6 mg. Generic only: Tabs 2 mg.] ▶LK ♀C ▶? $$$$

Non-Opioid Analgesic Combinations

ASCRIPTIN (acetylsalicylic acid + aluminum hydroxide + magnesium hydroxide + calcium carbonate, *Aspir-Mox*) Multiple strengths. 1 to 2 tabs PO q 4 h. [OTC Trade only: Tabs 325 mg aspirin/50 mg magnesium hydroxide/50 mg Al hydroxide/50 mg Ca carbonate (Ascriptin and Aspir-Mox). 500 mg aspirin/33 mg magnesium hydroxide/33 mg Al hydroxide/237 mg Ca carbonate (Ascriptin Maximum Strength).] ▶K ♀D ▶? $

BUFFERIN (acetylsalicylic acid + calcium carbonate + magnesium oxide + magnesium carbonate) 1 to 2 tabs/caps PO q 4 h. Max 12 in 24 h. [OTC Trade only: Tabs/caps 325 mg aspirin/158 mg Ca carbonate/63 mg of magnesium oxide/34 mg of magnesium carbonate. Bufferin ES: 500 mg aspirin/222.3 mg Ca carbonate/88.9 mg of magnesium oxide/55.6 mg of Mg carbonate.] ▶K ♀D ▶? $

ESGIC (acetaminophen + butalbital + caffeine) 1 to 2 tabs or caps PO q 4 h. Max 6 in 24 h. [Generic only: Tabs/caps, 325 mg acetaminophen/50 mg butalbital/40 mg caffeine. Oral soln 325/50/40 mg per 15 mL. Generic/Trade: Tabs, Esgic Plus is 500/50/40 mg.] ▶LK ♀C ▶? $

EXCEDRIN MIGRAINE (acetaminophen + acetylsalicylic acid + caffeine) 2 tabs/caps/geltabs PO q 6 h while symptoms persist. Max 8 tabs/caps/geltabs in 24 h. [OTC Generic/Trade: Tabs/caps/geltabs 250 mg acetaminophen/250 mg aspirin/65 mg caffeine.] ▶LK ♀D ▶? $

FIORICET (acetaminophen + butalbital + caffeine) 1 to 2 caps PO q 4 h. Max 6 caps in 24 h. [Generic/Trade: Tabs 325 mg acetaminophen/50 mg butalbital/40 mg caffeine.] ▶LK ♀C ▶? $

FIORINAL (acetylsalicylic acid + butalbital + caffeine, ✦ Trianal) 1 to 2 tabs PO q 4 h. Max 6 tabs in 24 h. [Generic/Trade: Caps 325 mg aspirin/50 mg butalbital/40 mg caffeine.] ▶KL ♀D ▶—◎III $

GOODY'S EXTRA STRENGTH HEADACHE POWDER (acetaminophen + acetylsalicylic acid + caffeine) 1 powder PO followed with liquid, or stir powder into a glass of water or other liquid. Repeat in 4 to 6 h prn. Max 4 powders in 24 h. [OTC trade only: 260 mg acetaminophen/520 mg aspirin/32.5 mg caffeine per powder paper.] ▶LK ♀D ▶? $

NORGESIC (orphenadrine + acetylsalicylic acid + caffeine) Multiple strengths; write specific product on Rx. Norgesic: 1 to 2 tabs PO three to four times per day. Norgesic Forte: 1 tab PO three to four times per day. [Generic only: Tabs 25 mg orphenadrine/385 mg aspirin/30 mg caffeine (Norgesic). Tabs 50/770/60 mg (Norgesic Forte).] ▶KL ♀D ▶? $$$

PHRENILIN (acetaminophen + butalbital) Tension or muscle contraction headache: 1 to 2 tabs PO q 4 h. Max 6 in 24 h. [Generic/Trade: Tabs, 325 mg acetaminophen/50 mg butalbital (Phrenilin). Caps, 650/50 mg (Phrenilin Forte).] ▶LK ♀C ▶? $

SEDAPAP (acetaminophen + butalbital) 1 to 2 tabs PO q 4 h. Max 6 tabs in 24 h. [Generic only: Tabs 650 mg acetaminophen/50 mg butalbital.] ▶LK ♀C ▶? $

SOMA COMPOUND (carisoprodol + acetylsalicylic acid) 1 to 2 tabs PO four times per day. Abuse potential. [Generic Only: Tabs 200 mg carisoprodol/325 mg aspirin.] ▶KL ♀D ▶—◎IV $$$

ULTRACET (tramadol + acetaminophen, ✦ Tramacet) Acute pain: 2 tabs PO q 4 to 6 h prn, (up to 8 tabs/day for no more than 5 days). Adjust dose in elderly and renal dysfunction. Avoid in opioid-dependent patients. Seizures may occur if concurrent antidepressants or seizure disorder. [Generic/Trade: Tabs 37.5 mg tramadol/325 mg acetaminophen.] ▶KL ♀C ▶— $$

Non-Steroidal Anti-Inflammatories—COX-2 Inhibitors

CELECOXIB (*Celebrex*) OA, ankylosing spondylitis: 200 mg PO daily or 100 mg PO two times per day. RA: 100 to 200 mg PO two times per day. Familial adenomatous polyposis: 400 mg PO two times per day with food. Acute pain, dysmenorrhea: 400 mg single dose, then 200 mg two times per day prn. An additional 200 mg dose may be given on day 1 if needed. JRA: Give 50 mg PO two times per day for age 2 to 17 yo and wt 10 to 25 kg, give 100 mg PO two times per day for wt greater than 25 kg. Contraindicated in sulfonamide allergy. [Trade only: Caps 50, 100, 200, 400 mg.] ▶L ♀C (D in 3rd trimester) ▶? $$$$$ ■

Non-Steroidal Anti-Inflammatories—Salicylic Acid Derivatives

ACETYLSALICYLIC ACID (*Ecotrin, Empirin, Halfprin, Bayer, Anacin, ZORprin, Aspirin,* ✦*Asaphen, Entrophen, Novasen*) Analgesia: 325 to 650 mg PO/ PR q 4 to 6 h. Platelet aggregation inhibition: 81 to 325 mg PO daily. [Generic/ Trade (OTC): Tabs, 325, 500 mg; chewable 81 mg; enteric-coated 81, 162 mg (Halfprin), 81, 325, 500 mg (Ecotrin), 650, 975 mg. Trade only: Tabs, controlled-release 650, 800 mg (ZORprin, Rx). Generic only (OTC): Supps 60, 120, 200, 300, 600 mg.] ▶K ♀D ▶? $
CHOLINE MAGNESIUM TRISALICYLATE (*Trilisate*) RA/OA: 1500 mg PO two times per day. [Generic only: Tabs 500, 750, 1000 mg. Soln 500 mg/5 mL.] ▶K ♀C (D in 3rd trimester) ▶? $$
DIFLUNISAL (*Dolobid*) Pain: 500 to 1000 mg initially, then 250 to 500 mg PO q 8 to 12 h. RA/OA: 500 mg to 1 g PO divided two times per day. [Generic only: Tabs 500 mg.] ▶K ♀C (D in 3rd trimester) ▶— $$$ ■
SALSALATE (*Salflex, Disalcid, Amigesic*) RA/OA: 3000 mg/day PO divided q 8 to 12 h. [Generic only: Tabs 500, 750 mg, scored.] ▶K ♀C (D in 3rd trimester) ▶? $$ ■

Non-Steroidal Anti-Inflammatories—Other

ARTHROTEC (diclofenac + misoprostol) OA: One 50/200 tab PO three times per day. RA: One 50/200 tab PO three to four times per day. If intolerant, may use 50/200 or 75/200 PO two times per day. Misoprostol is an abortifacient. [Generic/Trade: Tabs 50 mg/200 mcg, 75 mg/200 mcg, diclofenac/ misoprostol.] ▶LK ♀X ▶— $$$$$ ■
DICLOFENAC (*Voltaren, Voltaren XR, Cataflam, Flector, Zipsor, Cambia,* ✦*Voltaren Rapide,* ✦*Voltaren SR,* ✦*Voltaren Ophtha [eye drops], Pennsaid [topical product] Voltaren Emulgel [topical product]*) Multiple strengths; write specific product on Rx. Immediate- or delayed-release: 50 mg PO two to three times per day or 75 mg PO two times per day. Extended-release (Voltaren XR): 100 to 200 mg PO daily. Patch (Flector): Apply 1 patch to painful area two times per day. Gel: 2 to 4 g to affected area four times per day. Acute migraine with or without aura: 50 mg single dose (Cambia). [Generic/Trade: Tabs, immediate-release (Cataflam) 50 mg, extended-release (Voltaren XR)

(cont.)

100 mg. Generic only: Tabs, delayed-release 25, 50, 75 mg. Trade only: Patch (Flector) 1.3% diclofenac epolamine. Topical gel (Voltaren) 1% 100 g tube. Trade only: Caps, liquid-filled (Zipsor) 25 mg. Trade only: Powder for oral soln (Cambia) 50 mg.] ▶L ♀C (D in 3rd trimester) ▶– $$$ ■

ETODOLAC Multiple strengths; write specific product on Rx. Immediate-release: 200 to 400 mg PO two to three times per day. Extended-release: 400 to 1200 mg PO daily. [Generic only: Caps immediate-release: 200, 300 mg, Tabs immediate-release: 400, 500 mg, Tabs extended-release: 400, 500, 600 mg.] ▶L ♀C (D in 3rd trimester) ▶– $ ■

FLURBIPROFEN (*Ansaid, ✦Froben, Froben SR*) 200 to 300 mg/day PO divided two to four times per day. [Generic/Trade: Tabs immediate-release 50, 100 mg.] ▶L ♀B (D in 3rd trimester) ▶+ $$$ ■

IBUPROFEN (*Motrin, Advil, Nuprin, Rufen, NeoProfen, Caldolor*) 200 to 800 mg PO three to four times per day. Peds older than 6 mo: 5 to 10 mg/kg PO q 6 to 8 h. GI perforation and necrotizing enterocolitis have been reported with NeoProfen. [OTC: Caps/Liqui-Gel Caps 200 mg. Tabs 100, 200 mg. Chewable tabs 100 mg. Susp (infant gtts) 50 mg/1.25 mL (with calibrated dropper), 100 mg/5 mL. Rx Generic/Trade: Tabs 400, 600, 800 mg.] ▶L ♀B (D in 3rd trimester) ▶+ $ ■

INDOMETHACIN (*Indocin, Indocin SR, Indocin IV, ✦Indocid-P.D.A.*) Multiple strengths; write specific product on Rx. Immediate-release preparations: 25 to 50 mg PO three times per day. Sustained-release: 75 mg cap PO one to two times per day. [Generic Only: Caps, immediate-release 25, 50mg. Caps, sustained-release 75 mg. Trade only: Suppository 50 mg. Oral susp 25 mg/5 mL (237 mL).] ▶L ♀B (D in 3rd trimester) ▶+ $ ■

KETOPROFEN (*Orudis, Orudis KT, Actron, Oruvail*) Immediate-release: 25 to 75 mg PO three to four times per day. Extended-release: 100 to 200 mg cap PO daily. [Rx Generic only: Caps, extended-release 200 mg. Caps, immediate-release 50, 75 mg.] ▶L ♀B (D in 3rd trimester) ▶– $$$ ■

KETOROLAC (*Toradol*) Moderately severe acute pain 15 to 30 mg IV/IM q 6 h or 10 mg PO q 4 to 6 h prn. Combined duration IV/IM and PO is not to exceed 5 days. [Generic only: Tabs 10 mg.] ▶L ♀C (D in 3rd trimester) ▶+ $ ■

Analgesics—NSAIDs

Salicylic acid derivatives	ASA, diflunisal, salsalate, Trilisate
Propionic acids	flurbiprofen, ibuprofen, ketoprofen, naproxen, oxaprozin
Acetic acids	diclofenac, etodolac, indomethacin, ketorolac, nabumetone, sulindac, tolmetin
Fenamates	meclofenamate
Oxicams	meloxicam, piroxicam
COX-2 inhibitors	celecoxib

Note: If one class fails, consider another.

MECLOFENAMATE Mild to moderate pain: 50 mg PO q 4 to 6 h prn. Max dose 400 mg/day. Menorrhagia and primary dysmenorrhea: 100 mg PO three times per day for up to 6 days. RA/OA: 200 to 400 mg/day PO divided three to four times per day. [Generic only: Caps 50, 100 mg.] ▶L ♀B (D in 3rd trimester) ▶– $$$ ■

MEFENAMIC ACID (*Ponstel*, ✦*Ponstan*) Mild to moderate pain, primary dysmenorrhea: 500 mg PO initially, then 250 mg PO q 6 h prn for no more than 1 week. [Generic/Trade: Caps 250 mg.] ▶L ♀D ▶– $$$$$ ■

MELOXICAM (*Mobic*, ✦*Mobicox*) RA/OA: 7.5 mg PO daily. JRA age 2 yo or older: 0.125 mg/kg PO daily. [Generic/Trade: Tabs 7.5, 15 mg. Susp 7.5 mg/5 mL (1.5 mg/mL).] ▶L ♀C (D in 3rd trimester) ▶? $ ■

NABUMETONE (*Relafen*) RA/OA: Initial: Two 500 mg tabs (1000 mg) PO daily. May increase to 1500 to 2000 mg PO daily or divided two times per day. [Generic only: Tabs 500, 750 mg.] ▶L ♀C (D in 3rd trimester) ▶– $$ ■

NAPROXEN (*Naprosyn, Aleve, Anaprox, EC-Naprosyn, Naprelan, Prevacid NapraPac*) Immediate-release: 250 to 500 mg PO two times per day. Delayed-release: 375 to 500 mg PO two times per day (do not crush or chew). Controlled-release: 750 to 1000 mg PO daily. JRA: Give 2.5 mL PO two times per day for wt 13 kg or less, give 5 mL PO two times per day for 14 to 25 kg, give 7.5 mL PO two times per day for 26 to 38 kg. 500 mg naproxen equivalent to 550 mg naproxen sodium. [OTC Generic/Trade (Aleve): Tabs immediate-release 200 mg. OTC Trade only (Aleve): Caps, Gelcaps immediate-release 200 mg. Rx Generic/Trade: Tabs immediate-release (Naprosyn) 250, 375, 500 mg, (Anaprox) 275, 550 mg. Tabs delayed-release enteric coated (EC-Naprosyn) 375, 500 mg. Tabs, controlled-release (Naprelan) 375, 500, 750 mg. Susp (Naprosyn) 125 mg/5 mL. Prevacid NapraPac: 7 lansoprazole 15 mg caps packaged with 14 naproxen tabs 375 mg or 500 mg.] ▶L ♀B (D in 3rd trimester) ▶+ $$$ ■

OXAPROZIN (*Daypro*) 1200 mg PO daily. [Generic/Trade: Tabs 600 mg, trade scored.] ▶L ♀C (D in 3rd trimester) ▶– $$$ ■

PIROXICAM (*Feldene, Fexicam*) 20 mg PO daily. [Generic/Trade: Caps 10, 20 mg.] ▶L ♀B (D in 3rd trimester) ▶+ $$$ ■

SULINDAC (*Clinoril*) 150 to 200 mg PO two times per day. [Generic/Trade: Tabs 200 mg. Generic only: Tabs 150 mg.] ▶L ♀B (D in 3rd trimester) ▶– $ ■

TOLMETIN (*Tolectin*) 200 to 600 mg PO three times per day. [Generic only: Tabs 200 (scored), 600 mg. Caps 400 mg.] ▶L ♀C (D in 3rd trimester) ▶+ $$$ ■

Opioid Agonist-Antagonists

BUPRENORPHINE (*Buprenex, Butrans, Subutex*) Analgesia: 0.3 to 0.6 mg IV/IM q 6 h prn. Treatment of opioid dependence (must undergo special training and be registered to prescribe for this indication): Induction: 8 mg SL on day 1, 16 mg SL on day 2. Maintenance: 16 mg SL daily. Can individualize to range of 4 to 24 mg SL daily. Moderate to severe chronic pain: 5 to 20 mcg/h patch changed q 7 days. [Generic Only: SL Tabs 2, 8 mg. Trade only (Butrans): transdermal patches 5, 10, 20 mcg/h.] ▶L ♀C ▶–©III ₹ IV, $$$$$ SL ■

BUTORPHANOL (*Stadol, Stadol NS*) 0.5 to 2 mg IV or 1 to 4 mg IM q 3 to 4 h prn. Nasal spray (Stadol NS): 1 spray (1 mg) in 1 nostril q 3 to 4 h. Abuse potential. [Generic only: Nasal spray 1 mg/spray, 2.5 mL bottle (14 to 15 doses/bottle).] ▶LK ♀C ▶+©IV $$$ ■

NALBUPHINE (*Nubain*) 10 to 20 mg IV/IM/SC q 3 to 6 h prn. ▶LK ♀? ▶? $

PENTAZOCINE (*Talwin NX*) 30 mg IV/IM q 3 to 4 h prn (Talwin). 1 tab PO q 3 to 4 h. (Talwin NX = 50 mg pentazocine/0.5 mg naloxone). [Generic/Trade: Tabs 50 mg with 0.5 mg naloxone, trade scored.] ▶LK ♀C ▶?©IV $$$ ■

Opioid Agonists

CODEINE 0.5 to 1 mg/kg up to 15 to 60 mg PO/IM/IV/SC q 4 to 6 h. Do not use IV in children. [Generic only: Tabs 15, 30, 60 mg. Oral soln: 30 mg/5 mL.] ▶LK ♀C ▶–©II $ ■

FENTANYL (*Duragesic, Actiq, Fentora, Sublimaze, Abstral, Subsys, Lazanda, Onsolis*) Transdermal (Duragesic): 1 patch q 72 h (some with chronic pain may require q 48 h dosing). May wear more than 1 patch to achieve the correct analgesic effect. Transmucosal lozenge (Actiq) for breakthrough cancer pain: 200 to 1600 mcg; goal is 4 lozenges on a stick per day in conjunction with long-acting opioid. Buccal tab (Fentora) for breakthrough cancer pain: 100 to 800 mcg, titrated to pain relief. Buccal soluble film (Onsolis) for breakthrough cancer pain: 200 to 1200 mcg, titrated to pain relief. Sublingual tab (Abstral) for breakthrough cancer pain: 100 mcg, may repeat once after 30 minutes. Sublingual spray (Subsys) for breakthrough cancer pain: 100 mcg, may repeat once after 30 minutes. Nasal spray (Lazanda) for breakthrough cancer pain: 100 mcg. Adult analgesia/procedural sedation: 50 to 100 mcg slow IV over 1 to 2 min; carefully titrate to effect. Analgesia: 50 to 100 mcg IM q 1 to 2 h prn. [Generic/Trade: Transdermal patches 12, 25, 50, 75, 100 mcg/h. Actiq lozenges on a stick, berry flavored 200, 400, 600, 800, 1200, 1600 mcg. Trade only: (Fentora) buccal tab 100, 200, 400, 600, 800 mcg, packs of 4 or 28 tabs. Trade only: (Onsolis) buccal soluble film 200, 400, 600, 800 and 1200 mcg in child-resistant, protective foil, packs of 30 films. Trade only: (Abstral) sublingual tab: 100, 200, 300, 400, 600, 800 mcg, packs of 4 or 32 tabs. Trade only: (Subsys) sublingual spray: 100, 200, 400, 600, 800, 1200, 1600 mcg blister packs in cartons of 10 and 30 (30 only for for 1200 and 1600 mcg). Trade only: (Lazanda) nasal spray: 100, 400 mcg/spray, 8 sprays/bottle.] ▶L ♀C ▶+©II $ - varies by therapy ■

HYDROMORPHONE (*Dilaudid, Exalgo, ✦ Hydromorph Contin, Jurnista*) Adults: 2 to 4 mg PO q 4 to 6 h. 0.5 to 2 mg IM/SC or slow IV q 4 to 6 h. 3 mg PR q 6 to 8 h. Titrate dose as high as necessary to relieve cancer or nonmalignant pain where chronic opioids are necessary. Peds age 12 yo or younger: 0.03 to 0.08 mg/kg PO q 4 to 6 h prn or give 0.015 mg/kg/dose IV q 4 to 6 h prn. Controlled-release tabs: 8 to 64 mg daily. [Generic/Trade: Tabs 2, 4, 8 mg (8 mg trade scored). Oral soln 5 mg/5 mL. Trade only: Controlled-release tabs (Exalgo): 8, 12, 16, 32 mg.] ▶L ♀C ▶?©II $$ ■

LEVORPHANOL (*Levo-Dromoran*) 2 mg PO q 6 to 8 h prn. [Generic only: Tabs 2 mg, scored.] ▶L ♀C ▶?©II $$$$

OPIOID EQUIVALENCY*

Opioid	PO	IV/SC/IM	Opioid	PO	IV/SC/IM
buprenorphine	n/a	0.3–0.4 mg	meperidine	300 mg	75 mg
butorphanol	n/a	2 mg	methadone	5–15 mg	2.5–10 mg
codeine	130 mg	75 mg	morphine	30 mg	10 mg
fentanyl	?	0.1 mg	nalbuphine	n/a	10 mg
hydrocodone	20 mg	n/a	oxycodone	20 mg	n/a
hydromorphone	7.5 mg	1.5 mg	oxymorphone	10 mg	1 mg
levorphanol	4 mg	2 mg	pentazocine	50 mg	30 mg

*Approximate equianalgesic doses as adapted from the 2003 American Pain Society (www.ampainsoc.org) guidelines and the 1992 AHCPR guidelines. Not available = "n/a." See drug entries themselves for starting doses. Many recommend initially using lower than equivalent doses when switching between different opioids. IV doses should be titrated slowly with appropriate monitoring. All PO dosing is with immediate-release preparations. Individualize all dosing, especially in the elderly, children, and in those with chronic pain, opioid naive, or hepatic/renal insufficiency.

MEPERIDINE (*Demerol,* pethidine) 1 to 1.8 mg/kg up to 150 mg IM/SC/PO or slow IV q 3 to 4 h. 75 mg meperidine IV/IM/SC is equivalent to 300 mg meperidine PO. [Generic/Trade: Tabs 50 (trade scored), 100 mg. Generic only: Syrup 50 mg/5 mL.] ▶LK ♀C but + ▶+⊙‖ $$

METHADONE (*Diskets, Dolophine, Methadose,* ✦*Metadol*) Severe pain in opioid-tolerant patient: Initial dose is 2.5 mg IM/SC/PO q 8 to 12 h prn. Titrate up by 2.5 mg per dose q 5 to 7 days as necessary to relieve cancer or nonmalignant pain where chronic opioids are necessary. May start as high as 10 mg per dose if opioid-dependent patient and dosing is managed by experienced practitioner using an opioid conversion formula. Opioid dependence: Typical dose to prevent withdrawal is 20 mg PO daily but must be managed by an experienced practitioner. Treatment longer than 3 weeks is maintenance and only permitted in approved treatment programs. Opioid-naive patients: Not recommended in opioid-naive patients as first-line treatment of acute pain, mild chronic pain, postoperative pain, or as a prn medication. [Generic/Trade: Tabs 5, 10 mg. Dispersible tabs 40 mg (for opioid dependence only). Oral concentrate (Intensol): 10 mg/mL. Generic only: Oral soln 5, 10 mg/5 mL.] ▶L ♀C ▶?⊙‖ $ ■

MORPHINE (*MS Contin, Kadian, Avinza, Roxanol, Oramorph SR, MSIR, DepoDur,* ✦*Statex, M.O.S., Doloral, M-Eslon*) Controlled-release tabs (MS Contin, Oramorph SR): Start at 30 mg PO q 8 to 12 h. Controlled-release caps (Kadian): 20 mg PO q 12 to 24 h. Extended-release caps (Avinza): Start at 30 mg PO daily. Do not break, chew, or crush MS Contin or Oramorph SR. Kadian and Avinza caps may be opened and sprinkled in applesauce for easier administration; however, the pellets should not be crushed or chewed. Give 0.1 to 0.2 mg/kg up to 15 mg IM/SC or slow IV q 4 h. Titrate dose as high as necessary to relieve cancer or nonmalignant pain where chronic opioids are necessary. [Generic only: Tabs, immediate-release 15, 30 mg ($). Oral soln: 10 mg/5 mL, 20 mg/5 mL, 20 mg/mL (concentrate). Rectal supps 5, 10, 20, 30 mg. Generic/Trade: Controlled-release tabs (MS Contin) 15, 30, 60, 100,

(cont.)

FENTANYL TRANSDERMALDOSE (Dosing based on ongoing morphine requirement.)

Morphine (IV/IM)	Morphine (PO)	Transdermal fentanyl
10–22 mg/day	60–134 mg/day	25 mcg/h
23–37 mg/day	135–224 mg/day	50 mcg/h
38–52 mg/day	225–314 mg/day	75 mcg/h
53–67 mg/day	315–404 mg/day	100 mcg/h

For higher morphine doses, see product insert for transdermal fentanyl equivalencies.

200 mg ($$$$). Controlled-release caps (Kadian) 20, 30, 50, 60, 80, 100 mg ($$$$$). Trade only: Controlled-release caps (Kadian) 10, 40, 70, 130, 150, 200 mg. Extended-release caps (Avinza) 30, 45, 60, 75, 90, 120 mg.] ▶LK ♀C ▶+⊙II $ – varies by therapy ■

OXYCODONE (*Roxicodone, OxyContin, Percolone, OxyIR, OxyFAST, Oxecta, ✦ Endocodone, Supeudol, OxyNEO, Targin*) Immediate-release preparations: 5 mg PO q 4 to 6 h prn. Controlled-release (OxyContin): 10 to 40 mg PO q 12 h (no supporting data for shorter dosing intervals for controlled-release tabs). Titrate dose as high as necessary to relieve cancer or nonmalignant pain where chronic opioids are necessary. Do not break, chew, or crush controlled-release preparations or Oxecta. [Generic only: Immediate-release: Tabs 5, 10, 20 mg. Caps 5 mg. Oral soln 5 mg/5 mL. Generic/Trade: Tab 15, 30 mg. Oral concentrate 20 mg/mL. Trade only: Immediate-release abuse-deterrent tabs (Oxecta): 5, 7.5 mg. Controlled-release tabs: 10, 15, 20, 30, 40, 60, 80 mg ($$$$$).] ▶L ♀B ▶–⊙II $ – varies by therapy ■

OXYMORPHONE (*Opana, Opana ER*) 10 to 20 mg PO q 4 to 6 h (immediate-release) or 5 mg q 12 h (extended-release) in opioid-naive patients, 1 h before or 2 h after meals. 1 to 1.5 mg IM/SC q 4 to 6 h prn. 0.5 mg IV q 4 to 6 h prn, increase dose until pain adequately controlled. [Generic/Trade: immediate-release (IR) tabs 5,10mg. Extended-release tabs (ER) 7.5 mg, 15 mg. Trade only: Extended-release tabs (Opana ER) 5, 10, 20, 30, 40 mg. Injection 1 mg/ml. Generic only: Extended-release tabs 5, 10, 20, 30, 40 mg.] ▶L ♀C ▶?⊙II $$$$$ ■

Opioid Analgesic Combinations

NOTE: *Refer to individual components for further information. May cause drowsiness and/or sedation, which may be enhanced by alcohol and other CNS depressants. Opioids, carisoprodol, and butalbital may be habit forming. Avoid exceeding 4 g/day of acetaminophen in combination products. Caution people who drink 3 or more alcoholic drinks/day to limit acetaminophen use to 2.5 g/ day due to additive liver toxicity. Opioids commonly cause constipation; concurrent laxatives are recommended. All opioids are pregnancy class D if used for prolonged periods or in high doses at term.*

ANEXIA (hydrocodone + acetaminophen) Multiple strengths; write specific product on Rx. 1 tab PO q 4 to 6 h prn. [Generic only: Tabs 5/325, 5/500, 7.5/325, 7.5/650, 10/750 mg hydrocodone/mg acetaminophen, scored.] ▶LK ♀C ▶–⊙III $

CAPITAL WITH CODEINE SUSPENSION (acetaminophen + codeine) 15 mL PO q 4 h prn. Give 5 mL q 4 to 6 h prn for age 3 to 6 yo, give 10 mL PO q 4 to 6 h prn for age 7 to 12 yo, use adult dose for age older than 12 yo. [Generic only: Solution, 120 mg/5 mL and 12 mg/5 mL (APAP/Codeine).Trade only: Suspension, 120 mg/5 mL and 12 mg/5 mL (APAP/Codeine).] ▶LK ♀C ▶?©V $

COMBUNOX (oxycodone + ibuprofen) 1 tab PO q 6 h prn for no more than 7 days. Max 4 tabs per day. [Generic only: Tabs 5 mg oxycodone/ 400 mg ibuprofen.] ▶L ♀C (D in 3rd trimester) ▶?©II $$$$

EMPIRIN WITH CODEINE (acetylsalicylic acid + codeine, ✦ *292 tab*) Multiple strengths; write specific product on Rx. 1 to 2 tabs PO q 4 h prn. [Generic/Trade: No US formulation available. Tabs 325/30, 325/60 mg aspirin/mg codeine.] ▶LK ♀D ▶—©III $

FIORICET WITH CODEINE (acetaminophen + butalbital + caffeine + codeine) 1 to 2 caps PO q 4 h prn. Max 6 caps per day. [Generic/Trade: Caps 325 mg acetaminophen/50 mg butalbital/40 mg caffeine/30 mg codeine.] ▶LK ♀C ▶—©III $$$

FIORINAL WITH CODEINE (acetylsalicylic acid + butalbital + caffeine + codeine, ✦ *Fiorinal C-1/4, Fiorinal C-1/2, Trianal C-1/4, Trianal C-1/2*) 1 to 2 caps PO q 4 h prn. Max 6 caps/24 h. [Generic/Trade: Caps 325 mg aspirin/50 mg butalbital/40 mg caffeine/30 mg codeine.] ▶LK ♀D ▶—©III $$$

IBUDONE (hydrocodone + ibuprofen) 1 tab PO q 4 to 6 h prn, max dose 5 tabs/day. [Generic/Trade: Tabs 5/200 mg and 10/200 mg hydrocodone/ ibuprofen.] ▶LK ♀— ▶?©III $$

LORCET (hydrocodone + acetaminophen) 1 to 2 caps (5/500) PO q 4 to 6 h prn, max dose 8 caps/day. 1 tab PO q 4 to 6 h prn (7.5/650 and 10/650), max dose 6 tabs/day. [Generic/Trade: Tabs 7.5/ 650, 10/650 mg hydrocodone/ acetaminophen. Generic only: Caps 5/500 mg.] ▶LK ♀C ▶—©III $$

LORTAB (hydrocodone + acetaminophen) 1 to 2 tabs (2.5/500 and 5/500) PO q 4 to 6 h prn, max dose 8 tabs/day. 1 tab (7.5/500 and 10/500 PO) q 4 to 6 h prn, max dose 5 tabs/day. Elixir 15 mL PO q 4 to 6 h prn, max 6 doses/day. [Generic/Trade: Lortab 5/500 (scored), Lortab 7.5/500 (trade scored), Lortab 10/500 mg hydrocodone/mg acetaminophen. Elixir: 7.5/500 mg hydrocodone/mg acetaminophen/15 mL. Generic only: Tabs 2.5/500 mg.] ▶LK ♀C ▶—©III $

MAXIDONE (hydrocodone + acetaminophen) 1 tab PO q 4 to 6 h prn, max dose 5 tabs/day. [Trade only: Tabs 10/750 mg hydrocodone/mg acetaminophen.] ▶LK ♀C ▶—©III $$$$

MERSYNDOL WITH CODEINE (acetaminophen + codeine + doxylamine) Canada only. 1 to 2 tabs PO q 4 to 6 h prn. Max 12 tabs per day. [Canada Trade only: OTC tab 325 mg acetaminophen/8 mg codeine phosphate/5 mg doxylamine.] ▶LK ♀C ▶? $

NORCO (hydrocodone + acetaminophen) 1 to 2 tabs PO q 4 to 6 h prn (5/325), max dose 12 tabs/day. 1 tab (7.5/325 and 10/325) PO q 4 to 6 h prn, max dose 8 and 6 tabs/day, respectively. [Generic/Trade: Tabs 5/325, 7.5/325, 10/325 mg hydrocodone/acetaminophen, scored. Generic only: solution 7.5/325 mg per 15 mL.] ▶LK ♀C ▶?©III $$

PERCOCET (oxycodone + acetaminophen, *Endocet, Primalev, ◆Percocet-demi, Oxycocet, Endocet*) Multiple strengths; write specific product on Rx. 1 to 2 tabs PO q 4 to 6 h prn (2.5/325 and 5/325). 1 tab PO q 4 to 6 h prn (7.5/500 and 10/650). [Generic/trade: oxycodone/acetaminophen Tabs 2.5/325, 5/325, 7.5/325, 7.5/500, 10/325, 10/650 mg. Trade only: (Primalev) tabs 2.5/300, 5/300, 7.5/300, 10/300 Generic Only: 10/500 mg.] ▶L ♀C ▶–©II $

PERCODAN (oxycodone + acetylsalicylic acid, *Endodan, ◆Oxycodan*) 1 tab PO q 6 h prn. [Generic/Trade: Tabs 4.88/325 mg oxycodone/aspirin (trade scored).] ▶LK ♀D ▶–©III $$

ROXICET (oxycodone + acetaminophen) Multiple strengths; write specific product on Rx. 1 tab PO q 6 h prn. Soln: 5 mL PO q 6 h prn. [Generic/Trade: Tabs 5/325 mg. Caps/Caplets 5/500 mg. Soln 5/325 per 5 mL, mg oxycodone/ acetaminophen.] ▶L ♀C ▶–©II $

SOMA COMPOUND WITH CODEINE (carisoprodol + acetylsalicylic acid + codeine) Moderate to severe musculoskeletal pain: 1 to 2 tabs PO four times per day prn. [Generic Only: Tabs 200 mg carisoprodol/ 325 mg aspirin/16 mg codeine.] ▶L ♀D ▶–©III $$$$

SYNALGOS-DC (dihydrocodeine + acetylsalicylic acid + caffeine) 2 caps PO q 4 h prn. [Generic/Trade: Caps 16 mg dihydrocodeine/356.4 mg aspirin/30 mg caffeine.] ▶L ♀C ▶–©III $$$

TALACEN (pentazocine + acetaminophen) 1 tab PO q 4 h prn. [Generic only: Tabs 25 mg pentazocine/ 650 mg acetaminophen, scored.] ▶L ♀C ▶?©IV $$$

TYLENOL WITH CODEINE (codeine + acetaminophen, *◆Tylenol #1, Tylenol # 2, Tylenol # 3, Tylenol # 4, Atasol 8, Atasol 15, Atasol 30*) Multiple strengths; write specific product on Rx. Give 1 to 2 tabs PO q 4 h prn. Elixir: give 5 mL q 4 to 6 h prn for age 3 to 6 yo; give 10 mL q 4 to 6 h prn for age 7 to 12 yo. [Generic only: Tabs Tylenol #2 (15/300). Tylenol with Codeine Elixir/Susp/Soln 12/120 per 5 mL, mg codeine/mg acetaminophen. Generic/Trade: Tabs Tylenol #3 (30/300), Tylenol #4 (60/300).] ▶LK ♀C ▶?©III $

TYLOX (oxycodone + acetaminophen) 1 cap PO q 6 h prn. [Generic only: Caps 5 mg oxycodone/500 mg acetaminophen.] ▶L ♀C ▶–©II $

VICODIN (hydrocodone + acetaminophen) 5/500 (max dose 8 tabs/day) and 7.5/750 (max dose of 5 tabs/day): 1 to 2 tabs PO q 4 to 6 h prn. 10/660: 1 tab PO q 4 to 6 h prn (max of 6 tabs/day). [Generic/Trade: Tabs Vicodin (5/300), Vicodin ES (7.5/300), Vicodin HP (10/300), scored, mg hydrocodone/ mg acetaminophen.] ▶LK ♀C ▶?©III $$$

VICOPROFEN (hydrocodone + ibuprofen) 1 tab PO q 4 to 6 h prn, max dose 5 tabs/day. [Generic/Trade: Tabs 7.5/200 mg hydrocodone/ibuprofen. Generic only: Tabs 2.5/200, 5/200, 10/200 mg.] ▶LK ♀– ▶?©III $$

WYGESIC (propoxyphene + acetaminophen) 1 tab PO q 4 h prn. [Generic only: Tabs 65 mg propoxyphene/650 mg acetaminophen.] ▶L ♀C ▶?©IV $

XODOL (hydrocodone + acetaminophen) 1 tab PO q 4 to 6 h prn, max 6 doses/day. [Generic/Trade: Tabs 5/300, 7.5/300, 10/300 mg hydrocodone/ acetaminophen.] ▶LK ♀C ▶–©III $$$

ZYDONE (hydrocodone + acetaminophen) 1 to 2 tabs (5/400) PO q 4 to 6 h prn, max dose 8 tabs/day. 1 tab (7.5/400, 10/400) q 4 to 6 h prn, max dose 6 tabs/day. [Trade only: Tabs 5/400, 7.5/400, 10/400 mg hydrocodone/ mg acetaminophen.] ▶LK ♀C ▶?⊙III $$

Opioid Antagonists

NALOXONE (*Narcan*) Adult opioid overdose: 0.4 to 2 mg q 2 to 3 min prn. Adult postop reversal: 0.1 to 0.2 mg q 2 to 3 min prn. Peds opioid overdose: 0.01 mg/kg IV; may give 0.1 mg/kg if inadequate response. Peds postop reversal: 0.005 to 0.01 mg q 2 to 3 min prn. May use IM/SC/ET if IV not available. ▶LK ♀B ▶? $

Other Analgesics

ACETAMINOPHEN (*Tylenol, Panadol, Tempra, Ofirmev,* paracetamol, ✦ *Abenol, Atasol, Pediatrix*) 325 to 650 mg PO/PR q 4 to 6 h prn. Max 4 g/day, possibly changing to 3 g/day in near future. Adults and adolescents wt less than 50 kg, give 15 mg/kg IV q 6 h or 12.5 mg/kg IV q 4 h. Max dose 75 mg/kg/day. Adults and adolescents wt 50 kg or greater, give 1000 mg IV q 6 h or 650 mg IV q 4 h. Max dose 4 g/day. OA: 2 extended-release caplets (ie, 1300 mg) PO q 8 h around the clock. Peds: 10 to 15 mg/kg/dose PO/PR q 4 to 6 h prn. Children age 2 to 12 yo, give 15 mg/kg IV q 6 h or 12.5 mg/kg q 4 h. Max dose 75 mg/kg/day. [OTC: Tabs 325, 500, 650 mg. Chewable Tabs 80 mg. Oral disintegrating Tabs 80, 160 mg. Caps/Gelcaps 500 mg. Extended-release caplets 650 mg. Liquid 160 mg/5 mL, 500 mg/15 mL. Supps 80, 120, 325, 650 mg.] ▶LK ♀B ▶+ $

MIDOL TEEN FORMULA (acetaminophen + pamabrom) 2 caps PO q 4 to 6 h. [Generic/Trade: Caps 325 mg acetaminophen/25 mg pamabrom (diuretic).] ▶LK ♀B ▶+ $

TAPENTADOL (*Nucynta, Nucynta ER,* ✦ *Nucynta IR, Nucynta CR*) Moderate to severe acute pain: Immediate-release: 50 to 100 mg PO q 4 to 6 h prn, max 600 mg/day. Moderate to severe chronic pain: Extended-release: 50 to 250 mg PO twice daily. Adjust dose in elderly, renal, and hepatic dysfunction. Avoid in opioid-dependent patients. Seizures may occur with concurrent antidepressants or seizure disorder. [Trade only: Immediate-release ($$$$): Tabs 50, 75, 100 mg. Extended-release ($$$$$): Tabs 50, 100, 150, 200, 250 mg.] ▶LK ♀C ▶–©III $$$$

TRAMADOL (*Ultram, Ultram ER, Ryzolt, Conzip, Rybix ODT,* ✦ *Zytram XL, Tridural, Ralivia, Durela*) Moderate to moderately severe pain: 50 to 100 mg PO q 4 to 6 h prn, max 400 mg/day. Chronic pain, extended-release: 100 to 300 mg PO daily. Adjust dose in elderly, renal, and hepatic dysfunction. Avoid in opioid-dependent patients. Seizures may occur with concurrent serotonergic agents or seizure disorder. [Generic/Trade: Tabs, immediate-release 50 mg. Extended-release tabs 100, 200, 300 mg Trade only: (Conzip) Extended-release caps 100, 150, 200, 300 mg. (Rybix) ODT 50 mg.] ▶KL ♀C ▶– $$$

ANESTHESIA

Anesthetics and Sedatives

DEXMEDETOMIDINE (*Precedex*) ICU sedation less than 24 h: Load 1 mcg/kg over 10 min followed by infusion 0.2 to 0.7 mcg/kg/h titrated to desired sedation endpoint. Beware of bradycardia and hypotension. ▶LK ♀C ▶? $$$$$

ETOMIDATE (*Amidate*) Induction: give 0.3 mg/kg IV. ▶L ♀C ▶? $

KETAMINE (*Ketalar*) 1 to 2 mg/kg IV over 1 to 2 min or 4 mg/kg IM induces 10 to 20 min dissociative state. Concurrent atropine minimizes hypersalivation. [Brand/Generic: 10 mg/mL, 50 mg/mL, 100 mg/mL] ▶L ♀? ▶?©III $

METHOHEXITAL (*Brevital*) Induction: Give 1 to 1.5 mg/kg IV, duration 5 min. ▶L ♀B ▶?©IV $$

MIDAZOLAM (*Versed*) Adult sedation/anxiolysis: 5 mg or 0.07 mg/kg IM; or 1 mg IV slowly q 2 to 3 min up to 5 mg. Peds: 0.25 to 1 mg/kg to max of 20 mg PO, or 0.1 to 0.15 mg/kg IM. IV route (6 mo to 5 yo): Initial dose 0.05 to 0.1 mg/kg IV, then titrated to max 0.6 mg/kg. IV route (6 to 12 yo): Initial dose 0.025 to 0.05 mg/kg IV, then titrated to max 0.4 mg/kg. Monitor for respiratory depression. [Generic only: Injection: 1 mg/mL, 5 mg/mL, Oral liquid 2 mg/mL.] ▶LK ♀D ▶–©IV $

PENTOBARBITAL (*Nembutal*) Pediatric sedation: 1 to 6 mg/kg IV, adjusted in increments of 1 to 2 mg/kg to desired effect, or 2 to 6 mg/kg IM, max 100 mg. ▶LK ♀D ▶?©II $$$$$

PROPOFOL (*Diprivan*) Induction dose: 40 mg IV q 10 sec until induction (2 to 2.5 mg/kg). ICU ventilator sedation: Infusion 5 to 50 mcg/kg/min. Deep sedation: 1 mg/kg IV over 20 to 30 seconds. Repeat 0.5 mg/kg IV prn. ▶L ♀B ▶– $

Local Anesthetics

NOTE: *Risk of chondrolysis in patients receiving intra-articular infusions of local anesthetics following arthroscopic and other surgical procedures.*

ARTICAINE (*Septocaine, Zorcaine*) 4% injection (includes epinephrine). [4% (includes epinephrine 1:100,000).] ▶LK ♀C ▶? $

BUPIVACAINE (*Marcaine, Sensorcaine*) Local and regional anesthesia. [0.25%, 0.5%, 0.75%, all with or without epinephrine.] ▶LK ♀C ▶? $

LIDOCAINE—LOCAL ANESTHETIC (*Xylocaine*) 0.5 to 1% injection with and without epinephrine. Without epinephrine: max dose 4.5 mg/kg not to exceed 300 mg. With epinephrine: max dose 7 mg/kg not exceed 500 mg. Dose for regional block varies by region. Peds: varies by age and weight but max dose 4.5 mg/kg not to exceed 300 mg. [0.5, 1, 1.5, 2%. With epi: 0.5, 1, 1.5, 2%.] ▶LK ♀B ▶? $

MEPIVACAINE (*Carbocaine, Polocaine*) 1 to 2% injection. [1, 1.5, 2, 3%.] ▶LK ♀C ▶? $

Myasthenia Gravis

NEOSTIGMINE (*Bloxiverz*) 0.03 to 0.07 mg/kg slow IV (preceded by atropine or glycopyrrolate). Max 0.07 mg/kg or 5 mg whichever is less. ▶L ♀C ▶? $$$$

Neuromuscular Blockade Reversing Agents

NEOSTIGMINE (*Bloxiverz*) 0.03 to 0.07 mg/kg slow IV (preceded by atropine or glycopyrrolate). Max 0.07 mg/kg or 5 mg whichever is less. ▶L ♀C ▶? $$$$

Neuromuscular Blockers

CISATRACURIUM (*Nimbex*) Paralysis: 0.15 to 0.2 mg/kg IV. Peds: 0.1 mg/kg. Duration 30 to 60 min. ▶Plasma ♀B ▶: $
ROCURONIUM (*Zemuron*) Paralysis: 0.6 mg/kg IV. Duration 30 min. Rapid sequence intubation: 0.6 to 1.2 mg/kg IV ▶L ♀B ▶? $$
SUCCINYLCHOLINE (*Anectine, Quelicin*) Paralysis: 0.6 to 1.1 mg/kg IV. Peds: 2 mg/kg IV. ▶Plasma ♀C ▶: $
VECURONIUM (*Norcuron*) Paralysis: 0.08 to 0.1 mg/kg IV. Duration 15 to 30 min. ▶LK ♀C ▶: $

ANTIMICROBIALS

Aminoglycosides

NOTE: *See also Dermatology and Ophthalmology. Can cause nephrotoxicity, ototoxicity.*

AMIKACIN 15 mg/kg/day (up to 1500 mg/day) IM/IV divided q 8 to 12 h. Peak 20 to 35 mcg/mL, trough less than 5 mcg/mL. Alternative 15 mg/kg IV q 24 h. ▶K ♀D ▶? $$ ■
GENTAMICIN Adults: 3 to 5 mg/kg/day IM/IV divided q 8 h. Peak 5 to 10 mcg/mL, trough less than 2 mcg/mL. Alternative 5 to 7 mg/kg IV q 24 h. Peds: 2 to 2.5 mg/kg q 8 h. ▶K ♀D ▶+ $$ ■
STREPTOMYCIN Combo therapy for TB: 15 mg/kg (up to 1 g) IM daily. 10 mg/kg (up to 750 mg) for age 60 yo or older. Peds: 20 to 40 mg/kg (up to 1 g) IM daily. ▶K ♀D ▶+ $$$$$ ■
TOBRAMYCIN (*Tobi, Bethkis*) Adults: 3 to 5 mg/kg/day IM/IV divided q 8 h. Peak 5 to 10 mcg/mL, trough less than 2 mcg/mL. Alternative 5 to 7 mg/kg IV q 24 h. Peds: 2 to 2.5 mg/kg q 8 h. Cystic fibrosis , age 6 yo to adult: 300 mg nebulized (Tobi, Bethkis) or 4 caps inhaled (Tobi Podhaler) two times per day 28 days, on, then 28 days off. [Trade only: Tobi 300 mg/5mL ampules for nebulizer ($$$$$). Bethkis 300 mg/4 mL ampules for nebulizer ($$$$$). Tobi Podhaler 28 mg caps for inhalation ($$$$$).] ▶K ♀D ▶: $$ ■ = parenteral administration)

Antifungal Agents—Azoles

CLOTRIMAZOLE (✦ *Canesten, Clotrimaderm*) Oral troches 5 times per day for 14 days. [Generic only: Oral troches 10 mg.] ▶L ♀C ▶? $$$$
FLUCONAZOLE (*Diflucan*, ✦ *CanesOral*) Vaginal candidiasis: 150 mg PO single dose ($). All other dosing regimens IV/PO. Oropharyngeal candidiasis: 100 to 200 mg daily for 7 to 14 days. Esophageal candidiasis: 200 to 400 mg

(cont.)

daily for 14 to 21 days. Candidemia: 800 mg on first day, then 400 mg daily. Cryptococcal meningitis (per IDSA guideline): Amphotericin B preferably in combo with flucytosine for at least 2 weeks (induction), followed by fluconazole 400 mg PO once daily for 8 weeks (consolidation), then chronic suppression with fluconazole 200 mg PO once daily until immune system reconstitution. Peds. Oropharyngeal candidiasis: 6 mg/kg on first day, then 3 mg/kg daily for 7 to 14 days. Esophageal candidiasis: 12 mg/kg on first day, then 6 mg/kg daily for 14 to 21 days. Systemic candidiasis, cryptococcal meningitis in AIDS: 12 mg/kg on first day, then 6 to 12 mg/kg daily. [Generic/Trade: Tabs 50, 100, 150, 200 mg. 150 mg tab in single-dose blister pack. Susp 10, 40 mg/mL (35 mL).] ▶K ♀C for single-dose treatment of vaginal candidiasis, D for all other indications ▶+ $$$$

ITRACONAZOLE (*Onmel, Sporanox*) Oral caps for onychomycosis "pulse dosing": 200 mg PO two times per day for 1st week of month for 2 months (fingernails) or 3 to 4 months (toenails). Standard regimen, toenail onychomycosis: 200 mg PO daily with full meal for 12 weeks. Fluconazole-refractory oropharyngeal or esophageal candidiasis: Oral soln 200 mg PO daily for 14 to 21 days. CYP3A4 inhibitor. Contraindicated with dofetilide, ergot alkaloids, lovastatin, PO midazolam, pimozide, quinidine, simvastatin, triazolam. Negative inotrope; do not use for onychomycosis if ventricular dysfunction. [Trade: Tabs 200 mg (Onmel). Oral soln 10 mg/mL (Sporanox-150 mL). Generic/Trade: Caps 100 mg.] ▶L ♀C ▶– $$$$$ ■

MICONAZOLE—BUCCAL (*Oravig*) Oropharyngeal candidiasis: Apply 50 mg buccal tab to gums once daily for 14 days. Increased INR with warfarin. [Trade only: Buccal tabs 50 mg.] ▶L ♀C ▶? $$$$$

POSACONAZOLE (*Noxafil, ✚ Posanol*) Prevention of invasive *Aspergillus* or *Candida* infection, age 13 yo or older: 200 mg (5 mL) PO three times per day. Oropharyngeal candidiasis, age 13 yo or older: 100 mg (2.5 mL) PO two times on day 1, then 100 mg PO once daily for 13 days. Oropharyngeal candidiasis resistant to itraconazole/fluconazole, age 13 yo or older: 400 mg (10 mL) PO two times per day. Take with full meal or liquid nutritional supplement. CYP3A4 inhibitor. [Trade only: Oral susp 40 mg/mL (105 mL).] ▶Glucuronidation ♀C ▶– $$$$$

VORICONAZOLE (*Vfend*) Aspergillosis, systemic *Candida* infections: 6 mg/kg IV q 12 h for 2 doses, then 3 to 4 mg/kg IV q 12 h (use 4 mg/kg for aspergillosis). Esophageal candidiasis or maintenance therapy of aspergillosis/candidiasis: 200 mg PO two times per day. For wt less than 40 kg, reduce to 100 mg PO two times per day. Dosage adjustment for efavirenz: Voriconazole 400 mg PO two times per day with efavirenz 300 mg PO once daily (use caps). Peds younger than 12 yo: 7 mg/kg IV q 12 h. Infuse IV over 2 h. Take tabs or susp 1 h before or after meals. CYP3A4 inhibitor. Many drug interactions. [Generic/Trade: Tabs 50, 200 (contains lactose). Trade only: Susp 40 mg/mL (75 mL).] ▶L ♀D ▶? $$$$$

Antifungal Agents—Echinocandins

ANIDULAFUNGIN (*Eraxis*) Candidemia: 200 mg IV load on day 1, then 100 mg IV once daily. Esophageal candidiasis: 100 mg IV load on day 1, then 50 mg IV once daily. Max infusion rate of 1.1 mg/min to prevent histamine reactions. ▶Degraded chemically ♀C ▶? $$$$$

CASPOFUNGIN (*Cancidas*) Infuse over 1 h. Give 70 mg IV loading dose on day 1, then 50 mg once daily. Peds: 70 mg/m² IV loading dose on day 1, then 50 mg/m² once daily (max of 70 mg/day). ▶KL ♀C ▶? $$$$$

MICAFUNGIN (*Mycamine*) Esophageal candidiasis: 3 mg/kg IV once daily for wt 30 kg or less; 2.5 mg/kg IV up to 150 mg once daily for wt greater than 30 kg. Candidemia, acute disseminated candidiasis, *Candida* peritonitis/abscess, age 4 mo and older: 2 mg/kg up to 100 mg IV once daily. Prevention of candidal infections in bone marrow transplant patients, age 4 mo and older: 1 mg/kg up to 50 mg IV once daily. Infuse over 1 h. Histamine-mediated reactions possible with more rapid infusion. For peds, infuse concentrations greater than 1.5 mg/mL by central catheter. Flush existing IV lines with NS before micafungin infusion. ▶L, feces ♀C ▶? $$$$$

Antifungal Agents—Polyenes

AMPHOTERICIN B DEOXYCHOLATE Test dose 0.1 mg/kg up to 1 mg slow IV. Wait 2 to 4 h, and if tolerated then begin 0.25 mg/kg IV daily and advance to 0.5 to 1.5 mg/kg/day depending on fungal type. Maximum dose 1.5 mg/kg/day. ▶Tissues ♀B ▶? $$$$$ ■

AMPHOTERICIN B LIPID FORMULATIONS (*Amphotec, Abelcet, AmBisome*) Abelcet: 5 mg/kg/day IV over 2 h. AmBisome: 3 to 5 mg/kg/day IV over 2 h. Amphotec: Test dose of 10 mL over 15 to 30 min, observe for 30 min, then 3 to 4 mg/kg/day IV at 1 mg/kg/h. ▶? ♀B ▶? $$$$$

Antifungal Agents—Other

FLUCYTOSINE (*Ancobon*) 50 to 150 mg/kg/day PO divided four times per day. Myelosuppression. [Generic/Trade: Caps 250, 500 mg.] ▶K ♀C ▶– $$$$$ ■

GRISEOFULVIN (*Grifulvin V, ♣ Fulvicin*) Tinea capitis: 500 mg PO daily in adults; 15 to 20 mg/kg (up to 1 g) PO daily in peds. Treat for 4 to 6 weeks, continuing for 2 weeks past symptom resolution. [Generic/Trade: Susp 125 mg/5 mL (120 mL). Tabs 500 mg. Generic only: 250 mg tab.] ▶Skin ♀C ▶? $$$$

NYSTATIN Thrush: 4 to 6 mL PO, swish and swallow four times per day. Infants: 2 mL/dose with 1 mL in each cheek four times per day. Non-esophageal mucus membrane gastrointestinal candidiasis: 1 to 2 tabs PO three times per day. [Generic only: Susp 100,000 units/mL (60, 480 mL). Film-coated tabs: 500,000 units.] ▶Not absorbed ♀B ▶? $

TERBINAFINE (*Lamisil*) Onychomycosis: 250 mg PO daily for 6 weeks to treat fingernails, for 12 weeks to treat toenails. Tinea capitis, age 4 yo or older: Give granules PO once daily with food for 6 weeks: 125 mg for wt less than 25 kg, 187.5 mg for wt 25 to 35 kg, 250 mg for wt more than 35 kg. [Generic/Trade: Tabs 250 mg. Trade only: Oral granules 125, 187.5 mg/packet.] ▶LK ♀B ▶– $$$$$

Antimalarials

NOTE: *For help treating malaria or getting antimalarials, see www.cdc.gov/ malaria or call the CDC "malaria hotline" (770) 488-7788 Monday–Friday 9 am*

(cont.)

to 5 pm EST; after hours/weekend (770) 488-7100. Pediatric doses of antimalarials should never exceed adult doses.

CHLOROQUINE (*Aralen*) Malaria prophylaxis, chloroquine-sensitive areas: 8 mg/kg up to 500 mg PO q week starting 1 to 2 weeks before exposure to 4 weeks after exposure. Chloroquine resistance is widespread. Can prolong QT interval and cause torsades. [Generic only: Tabs 250 mg. Generic/Trade: Tabs 500 mg (500 mg phosphate equivalent to 300 mg base).] ▶KL ♀C but + ▶+ $ ■

COARTEM (**artemether + lumefantrine, coartemether**) Uncomplicated malaria: Take PO with food two times per day for 3 days. On day 1, give 2nd dose 8 h after 1st dose. Dose based on wt: 1 tab for 5 to 14 kg; 2 tabs for 15 to 24 kg; 3 tabs for 25 to 34 kg; 4 tabs for 35 kg or greater. Repeat dose if vomiting occurs within 1 to 2 h. Can prolong QT interval. [Trade only: Tabs, artemether 20 mg + lumefantrine 120 mg.] ▶L ♀C ▶? $$$$

MALARONE (**atovaquone + proguanil**) Prevention of malaria: Give the following dose PO once daily from 1 to 2 days before exposure until 7 days after. Dose based on wt: ½ ped tab for wt 5 to 8 kg; ¾ ped tab for wt 9 to 10 kg; 1 ped tab for wt 11 to 20 kg; 2 ped tabs for 21 to 30 kg; 3 ped tabs for 31 to 40 kg; 1 adult tab for all patients wt greater than 40 kg. Treatment of malaria: Give the following dose PO once daily for 3 days. Dose based on wt: 2 ped tabs for 5 to 8 kg; 3 ped tabs for 9 to 10 kg; 1 adult tab for 11 to 20 kg; 2 adult tabs for 21 to 30 kg; 3 adult tabs for 31 to 40 kg; 4 adult tabs for all patients wt greater than 40 kg. Take with food or milky drink. [Generic/Trade: Adult tabs atovaquone 250 mg + proguanil 100 mg. Pediatric tabs 62.5 mg + 25 mg.] ▶Fecal excretion; LK ♀C ▶? $$$$$

MEFLOQUINE (*Lariam*) Malaria prophylaxis for chloroquine-resistant areas: 250 mg PO once a week from at least 2 weeks before exposure to 4 weeks after. Malaria treatment: 1250 mg PO single dose. Peds malaria prophylaxis: Give the following dose PO once a week starting at least 2 weeks before exposure to 4 weeks after. Dose based on wt: 5 mg/kg (prepared by pharmacist) for wt 9 kg or less; ¼ tab for wt greater than 9 kg to 19 kg; ½ tab for wt greater than 19 kg to 30 kg; ¾ tab for wt greater than 30 to 45 kg; 1 tab for wt greater than 45 kg. Peds malaria treatment: 20 to 25 mg/kg PO single dose or divided in 2 doses given 6 to 8 h apart. Take on full stomach. Neuropsychiatric adverse effects that may persist. [Generic only: Tabs 250 mg.] ▶L ♀B ▶? $$ ■

PRIMAQUINE Prevention of relapse, *P. vivax/ovale* malaria: 0.5 mg/kg (up to 30 mg) base PO daily for 14 days. Do not use unless normal G6PD level. [Generic only: Tabs 26.3 mg (equiv to 15 mg base).] ▶L ♀− ▶− $$$ ■

QUININE (*Qualaquin*) Malaria: 648 mg PO three times per day. Peds: 25 to 30 mg/kg/day (up to 2 g/day) PO divided q 8 h. Treat for 3 days (Africa/South America) or 7 days (Southeast Asia). Also give 7-day course of doxycycline, tetracycline, or clindamycin. Nocturnal leg cramps: 325 mg PO at bedtime. FDA warns that risks exceed potential benefit for this indication. Can cause life-threatening adverse effects: Cinchonism with overdose; hemolysis with G6PD deficiency; hypersensitivity; thrombocytopenia; HUS/TTP; QT interval prolongation; many drug interactions. [Generic/Trade: Caps 324 mg.] ▶L ♀C ▶+ $$$$$ ■

ANTIMICROBIALS

Antimycobacterial Agents

NOTE: *Treat active mycobacterial infection with at least 2 drugs. See guidelines at www.thoracic.org/statements/index.php and www.aidsinfo.nih.gov.*

DAPSONE (*Aczone*) Pneumocystis pneumonia prophylaxis, leprosy: 100 mg PO daily. Pneumocystis pneumonia treatment: 100 mg PO daily with trimethoprim 5 mg/kg PO three times per day for 21 days. Acne (Aczone; $$$$): Apply two times per day. [Generic only: Tabs 25, 100 mg. Trade only (Aczone): Topical gel 5% 30, 60, 90 g.] ▶LK ♀C ▶– $$$$

ETHAMBUTOL (*Myambutol*, ✦ *Etibi*) 15 to 20 mg/kg PO daily. Dose with whole tabs: Give 800 mg PO daily for wt 40 to 55 kg, 1200 mg for wt 56 to 75 kg, 1600 mg for wt 76 to 90 kg. Base dose on estimated lean body wt. Peds: 15 to 20 mg/kg (up to 1 g) PO daily. [Generic/Trade: Tabs 100, 400 mg.] ▶LK ♀C but + $$$$

ISONIAZID (*INH*, ✦ *Isotamine*) Adults: 5 mg/kg (up to 300 mg) PO daily. Peds: 10 to 15 mg/kg (up to 300 mg) PO daily. Hepatotoxicity. Consider supplemental pyridoxine up to 50 mg per day to prevent neuropathy. [Generic only: Tabs 100, 300 mg. Syrup 50 mg/5 mL.] ▶LK ♀C but + ▶+ $ ■

PYRAZINAMIDE (*PZA*, ✦ *Tebrazid*) 20 to 25 mg/kg (up to 2000 mg) PO daily. Dose with whole tabs: Give 750 mg PO daily for wt 40 to 55 kg, 1500 mg for wt 56 to 75 kg, 2000 mg for wt 76 to 90 kg. Base dose on estimated lean body wt. Peds: 15 to 30 mg/kg (up to 2000 mg) PO daily. Hepatotoxicity. [Generic only: Tabs 500 mg.] ▶LK ♀C ▶? $$$$ ■

RIFABUTIN (*Mycobutin*) 300 mg PO daily or 150 mg PO two times per day. Dosage reduction required with protease inhibitors. [Trade only: Caps 150 mg.] ▶L ♀B ▶? $$$$

RIFAMATE (isoniazid + rifampin) 2 caps PO daily on empty stomach. [Trade Only: Caps isoniazid 150 mg + rifampin 300 mg.] ▶LK ♀C but + ▶+ $$$$$ ■

RIFAMPIN (*Rifadin*, ✦ *Rofact*) TB: 10 mg/kg (up to 600 mg) PO/IV daily. Peds: 10 to 20 mg/kg (up to 600 mg) PO/IV daily. *Neisseria meningitidis* carriers: 600 mg PO two times per day for 2 days. Peds: Age younger than 1 mo: 5 mg/kg PO two times per day for 2 days. Age 1 mo or older: 10 mg/kg (up to 600 mg) PO two times per day for 2 days. IV and PO doses are the same. Take oral doses on empty stomach. [Generic/Trade: Caps 150, 300 mg. Pharmacists can make oral susp.] ▶L ♀C but + ▶+ $$$$ ■

RIFAPENTINE (*Priftin, RPT*) TB: 600 mg PO twice a week for 2 months, then once a week for 4 months. Use for continuation therapy only in selected HIV-negative patients. [Trade only: Tabs 150 mg.] ▶Esterases, fecal ♀C ▶? $$$$

RIFATER (isoniazid + rifampin + pyrazinamide) TB, initial 2 months of treatment: 4 tabs PO daily for wt less than 45 kg, 5 tabs daily for wt 45 to 54 kg, 6 tabs daily for wt 55 kg or greater. Take PO on empty stomach. [Trade only: Tabs isoniazid 50 mg + rifampin 120 mg + pyrazinamide 300 mg.] ▶LK ♀C ▶? $$$$$ ■

Antiparasitics

ALBENDAZOLE (*Albenza*) Hydatid disease, neurocysticercosis: 15 mg/kg/day (up to 800 mg/day) for wt less than 60 kg, 400 mg PO two times per day for wt 60 kg or greater. [Trade only: Tabs 200 mg.] ▶L ♀C ▶? $$$$$

ATOVAQUONE (*Mepron*) Pneumocystis pneumonia. Treatment: 750 mg PO two times per day for 21 days. Prevention: 1500 mg PO daily. Take with meals. [Trade only: Susp 750 mg/5 mL (210 mL), foil pouch 750 mg/5 mL (5, 10 mL).] ▶Fecal ♀C ▶? $$$$$

IVERMECTIN (*Stromectol*) Single PO dose of 200 mcg/kg for strongyloidiasis, 200 mcg/kg for scabies (may need to repeat dose in 10 to 14 days), 150 mcg/kg for onchocerciasis. Peds head lice: 200 to 400 mcg/kg PO single dose; repeat in 7 days. Not for children less than 15 kg. Take on empty stomach with water. [Trade only: Tabs 3 mg.] ▶L ♀C ▶+ $$

NITAZOXANIDE (*Alinia*) Cryptosporidial or giardial diarrhea: 100 mg two times per day for age 1 to 3 yo, 200 mg two times per day for 4 to 11 yo, 500 mg two times per day for adults and children 12 yo or older. Give PO with food for 3 days. Use susp if younger than 12 yo. [Trade only: Oral susp 100 mg/5 mL (60 mL). Tabs 500 mg.] ▶L ♀B ▶? $$$$

PAROMOMYCIN (✦ *Humatin*) 25 to 35 mg/kg/day PO divided three times per day with or after meals. [Generic only: Caps 250 mg.] ▶Not absorbed ♀C ▶– $$$$$

PRAZIQUANTEL (*Biltricide*) Schistosomiasis: 20 mg/kg PO q 4 to 6 h for 3 doses. [Trade only: Tabs 600 mg.] ▶LK ♀B ▶– $$$$

PYRANTEL (*Pin-X, Pinworm,* ✦ *Combantrin*) Pinworm, roundworm: 11 mg/kg (up to 1 g) PO single dose. Repeat in 2 weeks for pinworm. [OTC Trade only (Pin-X): Susp 144 mg/mL (equivalent to 50 mg/mL of pyrantel base) 30, 60 mL. Tabs 720.5 mg (equivalent to 250 mg of pyrantel base). OTC Generic only: Caps 180 mg (equivalent to 62.5 mg of pyrantel base).] ▶Not absorbed ♀– ▶? $

TINIDAZOLE (*Tindamax*) Adults: 2 g PO daily for 1 day for trichomoniasis or giardiasis, for 3 days for amebiasis. Bacterial vaginosis: 2 g PO once daily for 2 days or 1 g PO once daily for 5 days. Peds, age older than 3 yo: 50 mg/kg (up to 2 g) PO daily for 1 day for giardiasis, for 3 days for amebiasis. Take with food. [Generic/Trade: Tabs 250, 500 mg. Pharmacists can compound oral susp.] ▶KL ♀C ▶– $$ ∎

Antiviral Agents—Anti-CMV

CIDOFOVIR (*Vistide*) CMV retinitis in AIDS: 5 mg/kg IV once a week for 2 weeks, then 5 mg/kg every other week. Severe nephrotoxicity. ▶K ♀C ▶– $$$$$

FOSCARNET (*Foscavir*) CMV retinitis: 60 mg/kg IV (over 1 h) q 8 h or 90 mg/kg IV (over 1.5 to 2 h) q 12 h for 2 to 3 weeks, then 90 to 120 mg/kg IV daily over 2 h. HSV infection: 40 mg/kg IV (over 1 h) q 8 to 12 h. Nephrotoxicity, seizures. ▶K ♀C ▶? $$$$$ ∎

GANCICLOVIR (*Cytovene*) CMV retinitis: Induction 5 mg/kg IV q 12 h for 14 to 21 days. Maintenance 6 mg/kg IV daily for 5 days per week. Myelosuppression. Potential carcinogen, teratogen. May impair fertility. ▶K ♀C ▶– $$$$$ ∎

VALGANCICLOVIR (*Valcyte*) CMV retinitis: 900 mg PO two times per day for 21 days, then 900 mg PO daily. Prevention of CMV disease in high-risk

(cont.)

ANTIMICROBIALS

transplant patients: 900 mg PO daily given within 10 days post-transplant until 100 days post-transplant for heart or kidney/pancreas or 200 days for kidney transplant. See prescribing information for peds dose. Give with food. Impaired fertility, myelosuppression, potential carcinogen and teratogen. [Trade only: Tabs 450 mg. Oral soln 50 mg/mL.] ▶K ♀C ▶– $$$$$

Antiviral Agents—Anti-Herpetic

ACYCLOVIR *(Zovirax, Sitavig)* Genital herpes: 400 mg PO three times per day for 7 to 10 days for 1st episode, or for 5 days for recurrent episodes. Chronic suppression of genital herpes: 400 mg PO two times per day; in HIV infection use 400 to 800 mg PO two to three times per day. Zoster: 800 mg PO five times per day for 7 to 10 days. Chickenpox: 20 mg/kg (up to 800 mg) PO four times per day for 5 days. Adult IV: 5 to 10 mg/kg IV q 8 h, each dose over 1 h. Herpes encephalitis: 20 mg/kg IV q 8 h for 10 days for age 3 mo to 12 yo; 10 mg/kg IV q 8 h for 10 days for age 12 yo or older. Neonatal herpes: 20 mg/kg IV q 8 h for 21 days for disseminated/CNS disease, for 14 days for skin/mucous membrane infections. Sitavig for recurrent herpes labialis in immunocompetent adults: Apply buccal tab once to upper gum above incisor within 1 h of prodromal symptom onset; put slight pressure on upper lip for 30 seconds to ensure adhesion. Apply to side of mouth with herpes symptoms. [Generic/Trade: Caps 200 mg. Tabs 400, 800 mg. Susp 200 mg/5 mL. Buccal tab (Sitavig): Trade only: 50 mg.] ▶K ♀B ▶+ $

FAMCICLOVIR *(Famvir)* First episode genital herpes: 250 mg PO three times per day for 7 to 10 days. Recurrent genital herpes: 1000 mg PO two times per day for 2 days; give 500 mg two times per day for 7 days if HIV infected. Chronic suppression of genital herpes: 250 mg PO two times per day; 500 mg PO two times per day if HIV infected. Recurrent herpes labialis: 1500 mg PO single dose; 500 mg two times per day for 7 days if HIV infected. Zoster: 500 mg PO three times per day for 7 days. [Generic/Trade: Tabs 125, 250, 500 mg.] ▶K ♀B ▶? $$

VALACYCLOVIR *(Valtrex)* First episode genital herpes: 1 g PO two times per day for 10 days. Recurrent genital herpes: 500 mg PO two times per day for 3 days; if HIV infected give 1 g PO two times per day for 5 to 10 days. Chronic suppression of genital herpes: 500 to 1000 mg PO daily; if HIV infected give 500 mg PO two times per day. Reduction of herpes transmission in immunocompetent patients with no more than 9 recurrences per year: 500 mg PO daily for source partner, in conjunction with safer sex practices. Herpes labialis, age 12 yo or older: 2 g PO q 12 h for 2 doses. Zoster: 1000 mg PO three times per day for 7 days. Chickenpox, age 2 to 18 yo: 20 mg/kg (max of 1 g) PO three times per day for 5 days. [Generic/Trade: Tabs 500, 1000 mg.] ▶K ♀B ▶+ $$$$

Antiviral Agents—Anti-HIV—CCR5 Antagonists

MARAVIROC *(Selzentry, MVC, ✦ Celsentri)* 150 mg PO two times per day with strong CYP3A4 inhibitors (most protease inhibitors including

(cont.)

ritonavir-boosted fosamprenavir, ketoconazole, itraconazole, clarithromycin); 300 mg PO two times per day with drugs that are not strong CYP3A4 inducers/inhibitors (NRTIs, tipranavir-ritonavir, nevirapine, raltegravir; rifabutin without a strong CYP3A4 inhibitor or inducer); 600 mg PO two times per day with strong CYP3A4 inducers (efavirenz, etravirine, rifampin, carbamazepine, phenobarbital, phenytoin). Do not give maraviroc with unboosted fosamprenavir. Tropism test before treatment; not for dual/mixed or CXCR4-tropic HIV infection. Hepatotoxicity with allergic features. [Trade only: Tabs 150, 300 mg.] ▶LK ♀D ▶– $$$$$

Antiviral Agents—Anti-HIV—Combinations

ATRIPLA (efavirenz + emtricitabine + tenofovir) 1 tab PO once daily on empty stomach, preferably at bedtime. [Trade only: Tabs efavirenz 600 mg + emtricitabine 200 mg + tenofovir 300 mg.] ▶LK ♀D ▶– $$$$$ ■

COMBIVIR (lamivudine + zidovudine) 1 tab PO bid for wt 30 kg or greater. [Generic/Trade: Tabs lamivudine 150 mg + zidovudine 300 mg.] ▶LK ♀C ▶– $$$$$ ■

COMPLERA (emtricitabine + rilpivirine + tenofovir) Combination therapy of HIV, treatment-naive adults with baseline HIV RNA ≤100,000 copies/mL or less: 1 tab PO once daily with food. [Trade only: Tabs emtricitabine 200 mg + rilpivirine 25 mg + tenofovir 300 mg.] ▶KL ♀B ▶– $$$$$ ■

EPZICOM (abacavir + lamivudine, ✦ Kivexa) 1 tab PO daily. [Trade only: Tabs abacavir 600 mg + lamivudine 300 mg.] ▶LK ♀C ▶– $$$$$ ■

STRIBILD (elvitegravir + cobicistat + emtricitabine + tenofovir) 1 tab PO once daily with food. Do not use Stribild with other antiretroviral drugs. [Trade only: Tabs elvitegravir 150 mg + cobicistat 150 mg + emtricitibine 200 mg + tenofovir 300 mg.] ▶KL ♀B ▶– $$$$$ ■

TRIZIVIR (abacavir + lamivudine + zidovudine) 1 tab PO two times per day. [Trade only: Tabs abacavir 300 mg + lamivudine 150 mg + zidovudine 300 mg.] ▶LK ♀C ▶– $$$$$ ■

TRUVADA (emtricitabine + tenofovir) Combination therapy for HIV infection: 1 tab PO once daily in combination with other antiretroviral drugs. Pre-exposure prophylaxis (PrEP) of HIV in adults at high risk for sexually acquired HIV or injecting drug users: 1 tab PO once daily. Screen for HIV q 3 months in patients taking it for PrEP. [Trade only: Tabs emtricitabine 200 mg + tenofovir 300 mg.] ▶K ♀B ▶– $$$$$

Antiviral Agents—Anti-HIV—Integrase Strand Transfer Inhibitor

RALTEGRAVIR (*Isentress, RAL*) 400 mg PO two times per day. Increase to 800 mg PO two times per day if given with rifampin. Peds: Film-coated tabs, age 6 yo and older and wt 25 kg or greater: 400 mg PO two times per day. Chew tabs, 2 to 11 yo: Give PO two times per day at a dose of 75 mg for 10 kg to less than 14 kg; 100 mg for 14 kg to less than 20 kg; 150 mg for 20 kg to less than 28 kg; 200 mg for 28 kg to less than 40 kg; 300 mg for 40 kg or more. [Trade only: Film-coated tabs 400 mg. Chewable tabs (contain phenylalanine): 25 mg, 100 mg.] ▶Glucuronidation ♀C ▶– $$$$$

Antiviral Agents—Anti-HIV—Non-Nucleoside Reverse Transcriptase Inhibitors

EFAVIRENZ (*Sustiva, EFV*) Adults and children wt 40 kg or greater: 600 mg PO once daily on an empty stomach, preferably at bedtime. With voriconazole: Use voriconazole 400 mg PO two times per day and efavirenz 300 mg PO once daily. With rifampin: Increase efavirenz to 800 mg PO if wt is 50 kg or greater. Peds, age 3 mo or older and wt 3.5 kg to 40 kg: Consider antihistamine prophylaxis to prevent rash before starting. Give PO once daily at a dose of 100 mg for 3.5 kg to less than 5 kg; 150 mg for 5 kg to less than 7.5 kg; 200 mg for 7.5 kg to less than 15 kg; 250 mg for 15 kg to less than 20 kg; 300 mg for 20 kg to less than 25 kg; 350 mg for 25 kg to less than 32.5 kg; 400 mg for 32.5 kg to less than 40 kg. Take on empty stomach, preferably at bedtime. Capsule contents can be sprinkled on 1 to 2 teaspoons of food; do not give additional food for 2 h. [Trade only: Caps 50, 200 mg. Tabs 600 mg.] ▶L ♀D ▶– $$$$$

ETRAVIRINE (*Intelence, ETR*) Combination therapy for treatment-resistant HIV infection. Adults: 200 mg PO two times per day after meals. Peds, age 6 yo and older: Give two times per day after meals at 100 mg per dose for 16 kg to less than 20 kg; 125 mg per dose for 20 kg to less than 25 kg; 150 mg per dose for 25 kg to less than 30 kg; 200 mg per dose for 30 kg or greater. [Trade only: Tabs 25, 100, 200 mg.] ▶L ♀B ▶– $$$$$

NEVIRAPINE (*Viramune, Viramune XR, NVP*) 200 mg PO daily for 14 days initially. If tolerated, increase to 200 mg PO two times per day or Viramune XR 400 mg PO once daily. Patients maintained on immediate-release tabs can switch directly to Viramune XR. Peds, age 15 days or older: 150 mg/m² PO once daily for 14 days, then 150 mg/m² two times per day (max dose 200 mg two times per day). Viramune XR, age 6 yo and older: 200 mg PO once daily for BSA 0.58 to 0.83 m²; 300 mg PO once daily for BSA 0.84 to 1.16 m²; 400 mg PO once daily for BSA 1.17 m² or greater. To reduce risk of rash, patients should receive immediate-release nevirapine 150 mg/m² once daily (max 200 mg/day) for at least 14 days before conversion to Viramune XR. Patients already maintained on twice daily immediate-release nevirapine can switch directly to Viramune XR. Severe skin reactions and hepatotoxicity. [Generic/Trade: Tabs 200 mg. Trade only: Susp 50 mg/5 mL (240 mL), extended-release tabs (Viramune XR) 100 mg, 400 mg.] ▶LK ♀C ▶– $$$$$ ■

RILPIVIRINE (*Edurant, RPV*) Combination therapy of HIV infection, treatment-naive adults with HIV RNA 100,000 copies/mL or fewer: 25 mg PO once daily with a meal. [Trade only: Tabs 25 mg.] ▶L ♀B ▶– $$$$$

Antiviral Agents—Anti-HIV—Nucleoside/Nucleotide Reverse Transcriptase Inhibitors

ABACAVIR (*Ziagen, ABC*) Adult: 300 mg PO two times per day or 600 mg PO daily. Peds. Oral soln, age 3 mo or older: 8 mg/kg (up to 300 mg) PO two times

(cont.)

per day. Peds, tabs: 150 mg PO two times per day for wt 14 to 21 kg; 150 mg PO q am and 300 mg PO q pm for wt 22 to 29 kg, 300 mg PO two times per day for wt 30 kg or greater. Potentially fatal hypersensitivity. HLA-B*5701 predisposes to hypersensitivity; screen before starting and avoid if positive test. Never rechallenge with abacavir after suspected reaction. [Generic/Trade: Tabs 300 mg scored. Trade only: soln 20 mg/mL (240 mL).] ▶L ♀C ▶– $$$$$ ■

DIDANOSINE (*Videx, Videx EC, DDI*) Videx EC: Give 200 mg PO once daily for wt 20 to 24 kg; 250 mg PO once daily for wt 25 to 59 kg; 400 mg PO once daily for wt 60 kg or greater. Dosage reduction of Videx EC with tenofovir in adults: 200 mg for wt less than 60 kg, 250 mg for wt 60 kg or greater. Dosage reduction unclear with tenofovir if CrCl is less than 60 mL/min. Buffered powder, peds: 100 mg/m² PO two times per day for age 2 weeks to 8 mo; 120 mg/m² PO two times per day for age older than 8 mo (do not exceed adult dose). All formulations usually taken on empty stomach. [Generic/Trade: Delayed-release caps (Videx EC): 125, 200, 250, 400 mg. Pediatric powder for oral soln (buffered with antacid) 10 mg/mL. Generic only: Tabs for oral susp (buffered with antacid) 100, 150, 200 mg.] ▶LK ♀B ▶– $$$$$ ■

EMTRICITABINE (*Emtriva, FTC*) 200 mg cap or 240 mg oral soln PO once daily. Peds, oral soln: 3 mg/kg PO once daily for age 3 mo or younger; 6 mg/kg PO once daily (up to 240 mg) for age older than 3 mo. Can give 200 mg cap PO once daily if wt greater than 33 kg. [Trade only: Caps 200 mg. Oral soln 10 mg/mL (170 mL).] ▶K ♀B ▶– $$$$$ ■

LAMIVUDINE (*Epivir, Epivir-HBV, 3TC,* ✦ *Heptovir*) Epivir for HIV infection. Adults and teens older than 16 yo: 150 mg PO two times per day or 300 mg PO daily. Peds: 4 mg/kg (up to 150 mg) PO two times per day. Can use tabs if wt 14 kg or greater. Epivir-HBV for hepatitis B: Adults: 100 mg PO daily. Peds: 3 mg/kg (up to 100 mg) PO daily. [Generic/Trade: Tabs 150 (scored), 300 mg. Trade only (Epivir): Oral soln 10 mg/mL. Trade only (Epivir-HBV, Heptovir): Tabs 100 mg, oral soln 5 mg/mL.] ▶K ♀C ▶– $$$$$ ■

TENOFOVIR (*Viread, TDF*) Combo therapy for HIV. Adults and adolescents: 300 mg PO daily. Peds, 2 yo and older: 8 mg/kg PO once daily (max 300 mg/day) as oral powder. Tabs for peds, wt 17 kg or greater: Give PO once daily at dose of 150 mg for wt 17 kg to less than 22 kg; 200 mg for wt 22 kg to less than 28 kg; 250 mg for wt 28 kg to less than 35 kg; 300 mg for wt 35 kg or greater. Chronic hepatitis B, adults and peds (age 12 yo and older and wt 35 kg or greater): 300 mg PO daily without regard to meals. For patients who cannot swallow tabs, use 7.5 scoops of oral powder once daily. [Trade only: Tabs 150, 200, 250, 300 mg. Oral powder 40 mg tenofovir/g.] ▶K ♀B ▶– $$$$$ ■

ZIDOVUDINE (*Retrovir, AZT, ZDV*) 600 mg/day PO divided two or three times per day for wt 30 kg or greater. Peds dose based on wt: Give 24 mg/kg/day PO divided two or three times per day for wt 4 to 8 kg, 18 mg/kg/day PO divided two or three times per day for wt 9 to 29 kg. [Generic/Trade: Caps 100 mg. Syrup 50 mg/5 mL (240 mL). Generic only: Tabs 300 mg.] ▶LK ♀C ▶– $$$$$ ■

ANTIMICROBIALS

Antiviral Agents—Anti-HIV—Protease Inhibitors

NOTE: *Many serious drug interactions: Always check before prescribing. Protease inhibitors inhibit CYP3A4. Contraindicated with most antiarrhythmics, alfuzosin, ergot alkaloids, lovastatin, pimozide, rifampin, rifapentine, salmeterol, high-dose sildenafil for pulmonary hypertension, simvastatin, St. John's wort, triazolam. Midazolam contraindicated in labeling; but can use single dose IV cautiously with monitoring for procedural sedation. Monitor INR with warfarin. Avoid inhaled/nasal budesonide/fluticasone with ritonavir if possible; increased corticosteroid levels can cause Cushing's syndrome/adrenal suppression. Other protease inhibitors may increase budesonide/fluticasone levels; find alternatives for long-term use. Reduce colchicine dose; do not coadminister colchicine and protease inhibitors in patients with renal or hepatic dysfunction. Adjust dose of bosentan or tadalafil for pulmonary hypertension. Erectile dysfunction: Single dose of sildenafil 25 mg q 48 h, tadalafil 5 mg (not more than 10 mg) q 72 h, or vardenafil initially 2.5 mg q 72 h. Adverse effects include spontaneous bleeding in hemophiliacs, hyperglycemia, hyperlipidemia, immune reconstitution syndrome, and fat redistribution. Coinfection with hepatitis C or other liver disease increases the risk of hepatotoxicity with protease inhibitors; monitor LFTs at least twice in 1st month of therapy, then q 3 months.*

ATAZANAVIR (*Reyataz, ATV*) Adults, therapy-naive: 400 mg PO once daily (without ritonavir if ritonavir-intolerant) OR 300 mg + ritonavir 100 mg PO both once daily. With tenofovir, therapy-naive: 300 mg + ritonavir 100 mg PO both once daily. With efavirenz, therapy-naive: 400 mg + ritonavir 100 mg PO both once daily. Do not give atazanavir with efavirenz in therapy-experienced patients. Adults, therapy-experienced: 300 mg + ritonavir 100 mg PO both once daily. Peds, age 6 yo or older: Atazanavir/ritonavir PO once daily 150/100 mg for wt 15 to less than 20 kg; 200/100 mg for wt 20 to less than 40 kg; 300/100 mg for 40 kg or greater. Peds, therapy-naive, ritonavir-intolerant, age 13 yo or older and wt 39 kg or greater: 400 mg PO once daily. Give caps with food. Give atazanavir 2 h before or 1 h after buffered didanosine. [Trade only: Caps 100, 150, 200, 300 mg.] ▶L ♀B ▶– $$$$$

DARUNAVIR (*Prezista, DRV*) Therapy-naive or -experienced adults with no darunavir resistance substitutions: 800 mg + ritonavir 100 mg both once daily. Therapy-experienced adults with at least 1 darunavir resistance substitution: 600 mg + ritonavir 100 mg both two times per day. Peds, Treatment-naïve or treatment-experienced without resistance substitutions, age 3 yo or older: Give darunavir + ritonavir both once daily according to wt: Darunavir 35 mg/kg + ritonavir 7 mg/kg for wt 10 kg to less than 15 kg; darunavir 600 mg + ritonavir 100 mg for wt 15 kg to less than 30 kg; darunavir 675 mg + ritonavir 100 mg for wt 30 kg to less than 40 kg; darunavir 800 mg + ritonavir 100 mg for wt 40 kg or greater. Treatment-experienced with at least 1 resistance substitution, age 3 yo or older. Give darunavir + ritonavir both two times per day according to wt: Darunavir 20 mg/kg + ritonavir 7 mg/kg for wt 10 kg to

(cont.)

less than 15 kg; darunavir 375 mg + ritonavir 48 mg for wt 15 to less than 30 kg; darunavir 450 mg + ritonavir 60 mg for wt 30 kg to less than 40 kg; darunavir 600 mg + ritonavir 100 mg for wt 40 kg or greater. Take PO with food. [Trade only: Tabs 75, 150, 600, 800 mg. Susp 100 mg/mL (200 mL).] ▶L ♀B ▶– $$$$$

FOSAMPRENAVIR (*Lexiva, FPV*, ✦*Telzir*) Therapy-naive adults: 1400 mg PO two times per day (without ritonavir) OR 1400 mg + ritonavir 100/200 mg PO both once daily OR 700 mg + ritonavir 100 mg PO both two times per day. *Protease inhibitor–experienced adults:* 700 mg + ritonavir 100 mg PO both two times per day. Peds. Fosamprenavir/ritonavir for *protease inhibitor-naive patients* 4 weeks of age or older, or protease inhibitor-experienced patients, 6 mo or older: Give PO two times per day according to wt: Fosamprenavir 45 mg/kg plus ritonavir 7 mg/kg for wt less than 11 kg; fosamprenavir 30 mg/kg plus ritonavir 3 mg/kg for wt 11 kg to less than 15 kg; fosamprenavir 23 mg/kg plus ritonavir 3 mg/kg for wt 15 kg to less than 20 kg; fosamprenavir 18 mg/kg plus ritonavir 3 mg/kg for wt 20 kg or greater. Do not exceed adult dose of fosamprenavir 700 mg plus ritonavir 100 mg both PO two times per day. For fosamprenavir/ritonavir, can use fosamprenavir tabs if wt 39 kg or greater and ritonavir caps if wt 33 kg or greater. *Fosamprenavir monotherapy for protease inhibitor-naïve patients,* 2 yo or older: 30 mg/kg PO two times per day; can give 1400 mg as tabs PO two times per day if wt 47 kg or greater. Fosamprenavir is only for infants born at 38 weeks' gestation or more who have attained post-natal age of 28 days. Do not use once-daily dosing of fosamprenavir in children. Take tabs without regard to meals. Adults should take susp without food; children should take with food. [Trade only: Tabs 700 mg. Susp 50 mg/mL.] ▶L ♀C ▶– $$$$$

LOPINAVIR-RITONAVIR (*Kaletra, LPV/r*) Adults: 400/100 mg PO two times per day (tabs or oral soln). Can use 800/200 mg PO once daily in patients with less than 3 lopinavir resistance-associated substitutions. Coadministration with efavirenz, nevirapine, fosamprenavir, or nelfinavir: 500/125 mg tabs (use two 200/50 mg + one 100/25 mg tab) or 533/133 mg oral soln (6.5 mL) PO two times per day. Infants, age 14 days to 6 mo: Lopinavir 16 mg/kg PO two times per day. Peds, age 6 mo to 12 yo: Lopinavir 12 mg/kg PO two times per day for wt less than 15 kg, use 10 mg/kg PO two times per day for wt 15 to 40 kg. Coadministration with efavirenz, nevirapine, fosamprenavir, or nelfinavir: Lopinavir 13 mg/kg PO two times per day for wt less than 15 kg, 11 mg/kg PO two times per day for wt 15 to 45 kg. Do not exceed adult dose in children. No once-daily dosing for pediatric or pregnant patients; coadministration with carbamazepine, phenobarbital, phenytoin, efavirenz, nevirapine, fosamprenavir, or nelfinavir; or in patients with 3 or more lopinavir resistance-associated substitutions. Give tabs without regard to meals; give oral soln with food. [Trade only (lopinavir-ritonavir): Tabs 200/50 mg, 100/25 mg. Oral soln 80/20 mg/mL (160 mL).] ▶L ♀C ▶– $$$$$

RITONAVIR (*Norvir, RTV*) Adult doses of 100 mg PO daily to 400 mg PO two times per day used to boost levels of other protease inhibitors. Full-dose

(cont.)

OVERVIEW OF BACTERIAL PATHOGENS (Selected)

By bacterial class
Gram-positive aerobic cocci: _Staph epidermidis_ (coagulase negative), _Staph aureus_ (coagulase positive); Streptococci: _S. pneumoniae_ (_pneumococcus_), _S. pyogenes_ (Group A), _S. agalactiae_ (Group B), _enterococcus_
Gram-positive aerobic/facultatively anaerobic bacilli: _Bacillus, Corynebacterium diphtheriae, Erysipelothrix rhusiopathiae, Listeria monocytogenes, Nocardia_
Gram-negative aerobic diplococci: _Moraxella catarrhalis, Neisseria gonorrhoeae, Neisseria meningitidis_
Gram-negative aerobic coccobacilli: _Haemophilus ducreyi, influenzae_
Gram-negative aerobic bacilli: _Acinetobacter, Bartonella_ species, _Bordetella pertussis, Brucella, Burkholderia cepacia, Campylobacter, Francisella tularensis, Helicobacter pylori, Legionella pneumophila, Pseudomonas aeruginosa, Stenotrophomonas maltophilia, Vibrio cholerae, Yersinia_
Gram-negative facultatively anaerobic bacilli: _Aeromonas hydrophila, Eikenella corrodens, Pasteurella multocida;_ Enterobacteriaceae: _E. coli, Citrobacter, Shigella, Salmonella, Klebsiella, Enterobacter, Hafnia, Serratia, Proteus, Providencia_
Anaerobes: _Actinomyces, Bacteroides fragilis, Clostridium botulinum, Clostridium difficile, Clostridium perfringens, Clostridium tetani, Fusobacterium, Lactobacillus, Peptostreptococcus_
Defective Cell Wall Bacteria: _Chlamydia pneumoniae, Chlamydia psittaci, Chlamydia trachomatis, Coxiella burnetii, Mycoplasma pneumoniae, Rickettsia prowazekii, Rickettsia rickettsii, Rickettsia typhi, Ureaplasma urealyticum_
Spirochetes: _Borrelia burgdorferi, Leptospira, Treponema pallidum_
Mycobacteria: _M. avium_ complex, _M. kansasii, M. leprae, M. tuberculosis_

By bacterial name
Acinetobacter **Gram-negative aerobic bacilli**
Actinomyces **Anaerobes**
Aeromonas hydrophila **Gram-negative facultatively anaerobic bacilli**
Bacillus **Gram-positive aerobic/facultatively anaerobic bacilli**
Bacteroides fragilis **Anaerobes**
Bartonella species **Gram-negative aerobic bacilli**
Bordetella pertussis **Gram-negative aerobic bacilli**
Borrelia burgdorferi **Spirochetes**
Brucella **Gram-negative aerobic bacilli**
Burkholderia cepacia **Gram-negative aerobic bacilli**
Campylobacter **Gram-negative aerobic bacilli**
Chlamydia pneumoniae **Defective cell wall bacteria**
Chlamydia psittaci **Defective cell wall bacteria**
Chlamydia trachomatis **Defective cell wall bacteria**
Citrobacter **Gram-negative facultatively anaerobic bacilli**
Clostridium botulinum **Anaerobes**
Clostridium difficile **Anaerobes**
Clostridium perfringens **Anaerobes**
Clostridium tetani **Anaerobes**
Corynebacterium diphtheriae **Gram-positive aerobic/facultatively anaerobic bacilli**
Coxiella burnetii **Defective cell wall bacteria**

(cont.)

E. coli Gram-negative facultatively anaerobic bacilli
Eikenella corrodens Gram-negative facultatively anaerobic bacilli
Enterobacter Gram-negative facultatively anaerobic bacilli
Enterobacteriaceae Gram-negative facultatively anaerobic bacilli
Enterococcus Gram-positive aerobic cocci
Erysipelothrix rhusiopathiae Gram-positive aerobic/facultatively anaerobic bacilli
Francisella tularensis Gram-negative aerobic bacilli
Fusobacterium Anaerobes
Haemophilus ducreyi Gram-negative aerobic coccobacilli
Haemophilus influenzae Gram-negative aerobic coccobacilli
Hafnia Gram-negative facultatively anaerobic bacilli
Helicobacter pylori Gram-negative aerobic bacilli
Klebsiella Gram-negative facultatively anaerobic bacilli
Lactobacillus Anaerobes
Legionella pneumophila Gram-negative aerobic bacilli
Leptospira Spirochetes
Listeria monocytogenes Gram-positive aerobic/facultatively anaerobic bacilli
M. avium complex Mycobacteria
M. kansasii Mycobacteria
M. leprae Mycobacteria
M. tuberculosis Mycobacteria
Moraxella catarrhalis Gram-negative aerobic diplococci
Myocoplasma pneumoniae Defective cell wall bacteria
Neisseria gonorrhoeae Gram-negative aerobic diplococci
Neisseria meningitidis Gram-negative aerobic diplococci
Nocardia Gram-positive aerobic/facultatively anaerobic bacilli
Pasteurella multocida Gram-negative facultatively anaerobic bacilli
Peptostreptococcus Anaerobes
Pneumococcus Gram-positive aerobic cocci
Proteus Gram-negative facultatively anaerobic bacilli
Providencia Gram-negative facultatively anaerobic bacilli
Pseudomonas aeruginosa Gram-negative aerobic bacilli
Rickettsia prowazekii Defective cell wall bacteria
Rickettsia rickettsii Defective cell wall bacteria
Rickettsia typhi Defective cell wall bacteria
Salmonella Gram-negative facultatively anaerobic bacilli
Serratia Gram-negative facultatively anaerobic bacilli
Shigella Gram-negative facultatively anaerobic bacilli
Staph aureus (coagulase positive) Gram-positive aerobic cocci
Staph epidermidis (coagulase negative) Gram-positive aerobic cocci
Stenotrophomonas maltophilia Gram-negative aerobic bacilli
Strep agalactiae (Group B) Gram-positive aerobic cocci
Strep pneumoniae (pneumococcus) Gram-positive aerobic cocci
Strep pyogenes (Group A) Gram-positive aerobic cocci
Streptococci Gram-positive aerobic cocci
Treponema pallidum Spirochetes
Ureaplasma urealyticum Defective cell wall bacteria
Vibrio cholerae Gram-negative aerobic bacilli
Yersinia Gram-negative aerobic bacilli

ANTIMICROBIALS

regimen (600 mg PO two times per day) is poorly tolerated. Peds, full-dose regimen: Start with 250 mg/m^2 two times per day and increase q 2 to 3 days by 50 mg/m^2 two times per day to achieve usual dose of 350 to 400 mg/m^2 PO two times per day for age older than 1 mo (up to 600 mg/dose). If 400 mg/m^2 two times per day not tolerated, consider other alternatives. See specific protease inhibitor entries (atazanavir, darunavir, fosamprenavir, tipranavir) for pediatric boosting doses of ritonavir. [Trade only: Caps 100 mg, tabs 100 mg. Oral soln 80 mg/mL (240 mL).] ▶L ♀B ▶– $$$$$

SAQUINAVIR (*Invirase, SQV*) Regimens must contain ritonavir. Saquinavir 1000 mg + ritonavir 100 mg both PO two times per day within 2 h after meals. Saquinavir 1000 mg + Kaletra 400/100 mg PO both two times per day. [Trade only: Invirase (hard gel) Caps 200 mg. Tabs 500 mg.] ▶L ♀B ▶? $$$$$

TIPRANAVIR (*Aptivus, TPV*) 500 mg boosted by ritonavir 200 mg PO two times per day with food. Peds: 14 kg/kg with 6 mg/kg ritonavir PO two times per day; do not exceed adult dose. Hepatotoxicity. [Trade only: Caps 250 mg. Oral soln 100 mg/mL (95 mL in unit-of-use amber glass bottle).] ▶Feces ♀C ▶– $$$$$ ■

Antiviral Agents—Anti-Influenza

AMANTADINE (*Symmetrel,* ✦ *Endantadine*) Parkinsonism: 100 mg PO two times per day. Max 300 to 400 mg/day divided three to four times per day. Prevention/treatment of influenza A: 5 mg/kg/day up to 150 mg/day PO divided two times per day for age 1 to 9 yo and any child wt less than 40 kg. Give 100 mg PO two times per day for adults and children age 10 yo or older; reduce to 100 mg PO daily if age 65 yo or older. The CDC generally recommends against amantadine/rimantadine for treatment/prevention of influenza A in the United States due to high levels of resistance. [Generic only: Caps 100 mg. Tabs 100 mg. Syrup 50 mg/5 mL (480 mL).] ▶K ♀C ▶? $$$$

OSELTAMIVIR (*Tamiflu*) Influenza A/B: For treatment, give each dose two times per day for 5 days starting within 2 days of symptom onset. For prevention, give each dose once daily for 10 days starting within 2 days of exposure. For adults each dose is 75 mg. For peds, age 1 yo or older, each dose is 30 mg for wt 15 kg or less; 45 mg for wt 16 to 23 kg; 60 mg for wt 24 to 40 kg; and 75 mg for wt greater than 40 kg or age 13 yo or older. Influenza treatment in infants age 2 weeks old to 1 yo: 3 mg/kg/dose PO two times per day for 5 days. Influenza prophylaxis in infants 3 to 11 mo: 3 mg/kg/dose PO once daily. Due to limited data, prophylaxis is not recommended for infants younger than 3 mo unless the situation is critical. Can take with food to improve tolerability. [Trade only: Caps 30, 45, 75 mg. Susp 6 mg/mL (60 mL) with 10 mL dosing device. Pharmacist can also compound susp (6 mg/mL).] ▶LK ♀C, but + ▶? $$$$

RIMANTADINE (*Flumadine*) Treatment or prevention of influenza A in adults: 100 mg PO two times per day. Reduce dose to 100 mg PO once daily for age older than 65 yo. Peds influenza A prophylaxis: 5 mg/kg (up to 150 mg/day) PO once daily for age 1 to 9 yo. Use adult dose for age 10 yo or older. The

(cont.)

ANTIVIRAL DRUGS FOR INFLUENZA	Treatment* (Duration of 5 days)	Prevention (Duration of 7 to 10 days post-exposure)[†]
OSELTAMIVIR *(Tamiflu)*		
Adults and adolescents age 13 years and older		
	75 mg PO bid	75 mg PO once daily
Children, 1 year of age and older[‡]		
Body weight ≤15 kg	30 mg PO bid	30 mg PO once daily
Body weight >15 to 23 kg	45 mg PO bid	45 mg PO once daily
Body weight >23 to 40 kg	60 mg PO bid	60 mg PO once daily
Body weight >40 kg	75 mg PO bid	75 mg PO once daily
Infants, newborn to 11 months of age[‡]		
Age 3 to 11 months old	3 mg/kg/dose PO bid	3 mg/kg/dose PO once daily
Age younger than 3 months old[§]	3 mg/kg/dose PO bid	Not for routine prophylaxis in infants <3 mo
ZANAMIVIR *(Relenza)* **		
Adults and children (age 7 years and older for treatment, age 5 years and older for prophylaxis)		
	10 mg (two 5-mg inhalations) bid	10 mg (two 5-mg inhalations) once daily

Adapted from http://www.cdc.gov/mmwr/pdf/rr/rr6001.pdf

*Start treatment as soon as possible; benefit is greatest when started within 2 days of symptom onset. Consider longer treatment for patients who remain severely ill after 5 days of treatment.

[†]Duration is 10 days after household exposure, and 7 days after most recent known exposure in other situations. For long-term care facilities and hospitals, prophylaxis should last a minimum of 14 days and up to 7 days after the most recent known case was identified.

[‡]Tamiflu prescribing information contains instructions for pharmacists to compound a 6 mg/mL suspension when Tamiflu suspension is not available. Tamiflu suspension is provided with a 10 mL oral dispenser measured in mL Capsules can be opened and mixed with sweetened fluids to mask bitter taste. Make sure units of measure on dosing instructions match dosing device provided.

[¶]Oseltamivir is FDA-approved for treatment of influenza in infants 2 weeks of age and older and prevention of influenza in children 1 year of age and older.

[§]This dose is not intended for premature infants. Immature renal function may lead to slow clearance and high concentrations of oseltamivir in this age group.

**Zanamivir should not be used by patients with underlying pulmonary disease. Do not attempt to use *Relenza* in a nebulizer or ventilator; lactose in the formulation may cause the device to malfunction.

bid=two times per day.

CDC generally recommends against amantadine/rimantadine for treatment/prevention of influenza A in the United States due to high levels of resistance. [Generic/Trade: Tabs 100 mg. Pharmacist can compound suspension.] ▶LK ♀C ▶– $$

ZANAMIVIR (*Relenza*) Influenza A/B treatment: 2 puffs two times per day for 5 days for adults and children 7yo or older. Influenza A/B prevention: 2 puffs once daily for 10 days for adults and children 5 yo or older starting within 2 days of exposure. Do not use if chronic airway disease. [Trade only: Rotadisk inhaler 5 mg/puff (20 puffs).] ▶K ♀C ▶? $$$

Antiviral Agents—Other

ADEFOVIR (*Hepsera*) Chronic hepatitis B: 10 mg PO daily. Nephrotoxic; lactic acidosis and hepatic steatosis; discontinuation may exacerbate hepatitis B; may result in HIV resistance in untreated HIV infection. [Trade only: Tabs 10 mg.] ▶K ♀C ▶– $$$$$ ■

BOCEPREVIR (*Victrelis*) Chronic hepatitis C (genotype 1): 800 mg PO three times per day (q 7 to 9 h) in combination with peginterferon and ribavirin. Take with food. Start boceprevir after 4 weeks of peginterferon plus ribavirin. Treatment duration is based on response at weeks 8, 12, and 24. Stop boceprevir if HCV-RNA is 100 International units/mL or greater at week 12 or confirmed detectable at week 24. Neutropenia, anemia. Many drug interactions. [Trade only: Caps 200 mg.] ▶L ♀B ▶– $$$$$

ENTECAVIR (*Baraclude*) Chronic hepatitis B: 0.5 mg PO once daily if treatment-naive; give 1 mg if lamivudine- or telbivudine-resistant, history of viremia despite lamivudine treatment, decompensated liver disease, or HIV coinfected. Give on empty stomach. [Trade only: Tabs 0.5, 1 mg. Oral soln 0.05 mg/mL (210 mL).] ▶K ♀C ▶– $$$$$ ■

INTERFERON ALFA-2B (*Intron A*) Chronic hepatitis B: 5 million units/day or 10 million units 3 times per week SC/IM for 16 weeks if HBeAg+, for 48 weeks if HBeAg–. [Trade only: Powder/soln for injection 10, 18, 50 million units/vial. Soln for injection 18, 25 million units/multidose vial. Multidose injection pens 3, 5, 10 million units/0.2 mL (1.5 mL), 6 doses/pen.] ▶K ♀C ▶?+ $$$$$ ■

PALIVIZUMAB (*Synagis*) Prevention of respiratory syncytial virus pulmonary disease in high-risk infants: 15 mg/kg IM once monthly during RSV season. ▶L ♀C ▶? $$$$$

PEGINTERFERON ALFA-2A (*Pegasys*) Chronic hepatitis C, not previously treated with alfa-interferon: 180 mcg SC in abdomen or thigh once a week. Treat for 24 weeks (genotype 2 or 3 with ribavirin) or 48 weeks (genotype 1 or 4 with ribavirin; any patient receiving peginterferon monotherapy, or HIV-infected patients). Regimen of choice for genotype 1 patients is telaprevir/boceprevir plus peginterferon (FDA-approved indication) and weight-based ribavirin. See telaprevir or boceprevir entries for details. In combination with ribavirin for chronic hepatitis C, peginterferon is preferred over interferon alfa because of substantially higher response rate. Peginterferon monotherapy is only for patients who cannot use combo therapy. Hepatitis B: 180 mcg SC

(cont.)

in abdomen or thigh once a week for 48 weeks. Peds. Chronic hepatitis C, age 5 yo or older: 180 mcg/1.73 m² (max dose of 180 mcg) SC once weekly with PO ribavirin for 24 weeks (genotype 2 or 3) or 48 weeks (genotype 1 or 4). May cause or worsen severe autoimmune, neuropsychiatric, ischemic, and infectious diseases. Frequent clinical and lab monitoring. [Trade only: 180 mcg/1 mL soln in single-use vial; 180 mcg/0.5 mL prefilled syringe; 180 mcg/0.5 mL, 135 mcg/0.5 mL auto-injector.] ▶LK ♀C ▶– $$$$$ ■

PEGINTERFERON ALFA-2B (*PEG-Intron*) Chronic hepatitis C, not previously treated with alfa-interferon: Telaprevir/boceprevir in combination with peginterferon (FDA approved indication) plus weight-based ribavirin is regimen of choice for genotype 1 patients. See telaprevir or boceprevir entries for dosage regimens and duration of therapy. Give peginterferon alfa-2b SC once a week on same day each week. Monotherapy (only for patients who cannot use combo therapy): 1 mcg/kg/week. In combo with oral ribavirin: 1.5 mcg/kg/week with ribavirin 800 to 1400 mg/day PO divided two times per day. Peds, age 3 yo or older: 60 mcg/m² SC once a week with ribavirin 15 mg/kg/day PO divided two times per day. May cause or worsen severe autoimmune, neuropsychiatric, ischemic, and infectious diseases. Frequent clinical and lab monitoring. [Trade only: 50, 80, 120, 150 mcg/0.5 mL single-use vials with diluent, 2 syringes, and alcohol swabs. Disposable single-dose Redipen 50, 80, 120, 150 mcg.] ▶K? ♀C ▶– $$$$$ ■

RIBAVIRIN—ORAL (*Rebetol, Copegus, Ribasphere*) Chronic hepatitis C not previously treated with alfa-interferon: Telaprevir/boceprevir in combination with peginterferon plus weight-based ribavirin is regimen of choice for genotype 1 patients. See telaprevir or boceprevir entries for dosage regimens and duration of therapy. Regimen duration and ribavirin dose in treatment guidelines is based on genotype. Divide daily dose of ribavirin two times per day and give with food. Chronic hepatitis C, genotypes 1 and 4: Treat for 48 weeks, evaluating response after 12 weeks. Ribavirin in combo with peginterferon alfa-2b (PegIntron): 800 mg/day PO for wt 65 kg or less, 1000 mg/day for wt 66 kg to 85 kg, 1200 mg/day for wt 86 kg to 105 kg, 1400 mg/day for wt greater than 105 kg. Ribavirin in combo with peginterferon alfa-2a (Pegasys): 1000 mg/day PO for wt less than 75 kg, 1200 mg/day for wt 75 kg or greater. Chronic hepatitis C, genotypes 2 and 3: Treat for 24 weeks with ribavirin 800 mg/day in combo with peginterferon. Chronic hepatitis C, peds. Rebetol, age 3 yo and older: 15 mg/kg/day PO divided two times per day with peginterferon alfa-2b (PegIntron). Copegus, age 5 yo and older: 15 mg/kg/day PO divided two times per day with peginterferon alfa-2a (Pegasys). Can cause hemolytic anemia; dosage adjustments required based on Hb. [Generic/Trade: Caps 200 mg, Tabs 200 mg. Generic only: Tabs 400, 600 mg. Trade only (Rebetol): Oral soln 40 mg/mL (100 mL).] ▶Cellular, K ♀X ▶– $$$$$ ■

TELAPREVIR (*Incivek*) Chronic hepatitis C (genotype 1): 750 mg PO three times per day (q 7 to 9 h) taken with food (not low-fat). Give with peginterferon and ribavirin for 12 weeks. Give peginterferon and ribavirin for additional 12 to 36 weeks based on HCV RNA levels at weeks 4 and 12, and whether patient was partial/null responder to prior therapy. Stop telaprevir if HCV RNA

(cont.)

ANTIMICROBIALS

is greater than 1000 international units/mL at week 4 or 12, or detectable at week 24. Many drug interactions. Can cause serious skin reactions and anemia. Dosage adjustment for coadministration with efavirenz: 1125 mg PO q 8 h. [Trade only: 375 mg tabs in 28-day blister pack] ▶L ♀B ▶– $$$$$ ■

TELBIVUDINE (*Tyzeka*, ✚ *Sebivo*) Chronic hepatitis B: 600 mg PO once daily. [Trade only: Tabs 600 mg.] ▶K ♀B ▶– $$$$$ ■

Carbapenems

DORIPENEM (*Doribax*) 500 mg IV q 8 h. ▶K ♀B ▶? $$$$$

ERTAPENEM (*Invanz*) 1 g IV/IM q 24 h. Prophylaxis, colorectal surgery: 1 g IV 1 h before incision. Peds, younger than 13 yo: 15 mg/kg IV/IM q 12 h (up to 1 g/day). Infuse IV over 30 min. ▶K ♀B ▶? $$$$$

IMIPENEM-CILASTATIN (*Primaxin*) 250 to 1000 mg IV q 6 to 8 h. Peds, age older than 3 mo: 15 to 25 mg/kg IV q 6 h. Seizures (especially if given with ganciclovir, elderly with renal dysfunction, or cerebrovascular or seizure disorder). ▶K ♀C ▶? $$$$$

MEROPENEM (*Merrem IV*) Complicated skin infections: 10 mg/kg up to 500 mg IV q 8 h. Intra-abdominal infections: 20 mg/kg up to 1 g IV q 8 h. Peds meningitis: 40 mg/kg IV q 8 h for age 3 mo or older; 2 g IV q 8 h for wt greater than 50 kg. ▶K ♀B ▶? $$$$$

Cephalosporins—1st Generation

CEFADROXIL 1 to 2 g/day PO once daily or divided two times per day. Peds: 30 mg/kg/day divided two times per day. [Generic only: Tabs 1 g. Caps 500 mg. Susp 250, 500 mg/5 mL.] ▶K ♀B ▶+ $$$

CEFAZOLIN 0.5 to 1.5 g IM/IV q 6 to 8 h. Peds: 25 to 50 mg/kg/day divided q 6 to 8 h (up to 100 mg/kg/day for severe infections). ▶K ♀B ▶+ $$

CEPHALEXIN (*Keflex*) 250 to 500 mg PO four times per day. Peds: 25 to 50 mg/kg/day. Not for otitis media, sinusitis. [Generic/Trade: Caps 250, 500, 750 mg. Generic only: Tabs 250, 500 mg. Susp 125, 250 mg/5 mL.] ▶K ♀B ▶? $$

Cephalosporins—2nd Generation

CEFACLOR (✚ *Ceclor*) 250 to 500 mg PO three times per day. Peds: 20 to 40 mg/kg/day PO divided three times per day. Group A streptococcal pharyngitis: 20 mg/kg/day PO divided two times per day. Serum sickness-like reactions with repeated use. [Generic only: Caps 250, 500 mg. Susp 125, 187, 250, 375 mg per 5 mL. Tablet Extended Release: 500 mg] ▶K ♀B ▶? $$$$

CEFOXITIN 1 to 2 g IM/IV q 6 to 8 h. Peds: 80 to 160 mg/kg/day IV divided q 4 to 8 h. ▶K ♀B ▶+ $

CEFPROZIL (✚ *Cefzil*) 250 to 500 mg PO two times per day. Peds otitis media: 15 mg/kg/dose PO two times per day. Peds group A streptococcal pharyngitis (2nd line to penicillin): 7.5 mg/kg/dose PO two times per day for 10 days. [Generic only: Tabs 250, 500 mg. Susp 125, 250 mg/5 mL.] ▶K ♀B ▶+ $$$$

CEFUROXIME (*Zinacef*, *Ceftin*) Adult: 750 to 1500 mg IM/IV q 8 h. 250 to 500 mg PO two times per day. Peds: 50 to 100 mg/kg/day IV divided q 6 to 8 h; not

(cont.)

for meningitis; 20 to 30 mg/kg/day susp PO divided two times per day. [Generic/Trade: Tabs 250, 500 mg. Susp 125, 250 mg/5 mL.] ▶K ♀B ▶? $$$$

Cephalosporins—3rd Generation

CEFDINIR 14 mg/kg/day up to 600 mg/day PO once daily or divided two times per day. [Generic only: Caps 300 mg. Susp 125, 250 mg/5 mL.] ▶K ♀B ▶? $$$$

CEFDITOREN (*Spectracef*) 200 to 400 mg PO two times per day with food. [Trade only: Tabs 200, 400 mg.] ▶K ♀B ▶? $$$$$

CEFIXIME (*Suprax*) 400 mg PO once daily. Gonorrhea: 400 mg PO single dose. CDC now considers cefixime 2nd line for treatment of gonorrhea and requires test-of-cure. See STD table. Peds: 8 mg/kg/day once daily or divided two times per day. Use only susp/chew tabs for otitis media (better blood levels). [Trade only: Susp 100, 200, 500 mg/5 mL. Chewable tabs 100, 150, 200 mg. Tabs 400 mg. Caps 400 mg.] ▶K/Bile ♀B ▶? $$$$

CEFOTAXIME (*Claforan*) Usual dose: 1 to 2 g IM/IV q 6 to 8 h. Peds: 50 to 180 mg/kg/day IM/IV divided q 4 to 6 h. AAP dose for pneumococcal meningitis: 225 to 300 mg/kg/day IV divided q 6 to 8 h. ▶KL ♀B ▶+ $$$$

CEFPODOXIME 100 to 400 mg PO two times per day. Peds: 10 mg/kg/day divided two times per day. [Generic: Tabs 100, 200 mg. Susp 50, 100 mg/5 mL.] ▶K ♀B ▶? $$$$

CEFTAZIDIME (*Fortaz, Tazicef*) 1 g IM/IV or 2 g IV q 8 to 12 h. Peds: 30 to 50 mg/kg IV q 8 h. ▶K ♀B ▶+ $$$$

CEFTIBUTEN (*Cedax*) 400 mg PO once daily. Peds: 9 mg/kg (up to 400 mg) PO once daily. [Trade only: Caps 400 mg. Susp 90 mg/5 mL] ▶K ♀B ▶? $$$$$

CEFTIZOXIME 1 to 2 g IV q 8 to 12 h. Peds: 50 mg/kg/dose IV q 6 to 8 h. ▶K ♀B ▶? $$$$$

CEFTRIAXONE (*Rocephin*) 1 to 2 g IM/IV q 24 h. Meningitis: 2 g IV q 12 h. Gonorrhea: 250 mg IM plus azithromycin 1 g PO both single dose. Peds: 50 to 75 mg/kg/day (up to 2 g/day) divided q 12 to 24 h. Peds meningitis: 100 mg/kg/day (up to 4 g/day) IV divided q 12 to 24 h. Otitis media: 50 mg/kg up to 1 g IM single dose. See table for management of acute otitis media in

(cont.)

CEPHALOSPORINS –GENERAL ANTIMICROBIAL SPECTRUM

1st generation	Gram-positive (including *Staphylococcus aureus*); basic Gram-negative coverage
2nd generation	diminished *S. aureus*, improved Gram-negative coverage compared to 1st generation; some with anaerobic coverage
3rd generation	further diminished *S. aureus*, further improved Gram-negative coverage compared to 1st and 2nd generations; some with Pseudomonas coverage and diminished Gram-positive coverage
4th generation	same as 3rd generation plus coverage against *Pseudomonas*
5th generation	Gram-negative coverage similar to 3rd generation; also active against *S. aureus* (including MRSA) and *S. pneumoniae*

ANTIMICROBIALS

children. May dilute in 1% lidocaine for IM. Contraindicated in neonates who require (or are expected to require) IV calcium (including calcium in TPN); fatal lung/kidney precipitation of calcium ceftriaxone has been reported in neonates. In other patients, do not give ceftriaxone and calcium-containing solns simultaneously, but sequential administration is acceptable if lines are flushed with a compatible fluid between infusions. ▶K/Bile ♀B ▶+ $

ACUTE OTITIS MEDIA (AOM) IN CHILDREN: AMERICAN ACADEMY OF PEDIATRICS TREATMENT RECOMMENDATIONS

Initial Treatment [a] (immediate or delayed [b])		Treatment After First Antibiotic Failure [b]	
First-line	Alternative for Penicillin Allergy [c]	First-line	Alternative
Amoxicillin 80–90 mg/kg/day PO divided 2 times per day OR Amoxicillin-clavulanate [c] 90 mg/kg/day PO divided 2 times per day	Cefdinir 14 mg/kg/day PO divided 1 or 2 times per day OR Cefuroxime 30 mg/kg/day PO divided 2 times per day OR Cefpodoxime 10 mg/kg/day PO divided 2 times per day OR Ceftriaxone 50 mg IM/IV once daily for 1 or 3 days	Amoxicillin-clavulanate [c] 90 mg/kg/day PO divided 2 times per day OR Ceftriaxone 50 mg IM/IV once daily for 3 days	Ceftriaxone 50 mg/kg IM/IV once daily for 3 days OR Clindamycin 30-40 mg/kg/day PO divided 3 times per day +/- third-generation cephalosporin
		Treatment After Second Antibiotic Failure	
		Clindamycin 30–40 mg/kg/day PO divided 3 times per day plus third-generation cephalosporin Tympanocentesis [d] Consult specialist [d]	

Adapted from Pediatrics 2013;131:e964-e999. Available online at: http://pediatrics.aappublications.org.

[a] The duration of oral treatment is 10 days for age <2 yo and children of any age with severe symptoms, 7 days for age 2 to 5 yo with mild to moderate symptoms, and 5 to 7 days for age ≥6 yo with mild to moderate symptoms.

[b] This guideline is for uncomplicated AOM in children age 6 mo to 12 yo. Immediate treatment is recommended for children with otorrhea or severe symptoms (moderate to severe pain, pain for ≥48 h, or temperature ≥39°C), and bilateral AOM in children age 6 to 23 mo. Observation for 48 to 72 h before antibiotic therapy is an option for children age 6 to 23mo with unilateral AOM and mild symptoms (mild pain for <48 h and temperature <39°C), or children 2 yo and older with unilateral/bilateral AOM and mild symptoms. Observation must have mechanism for follow-up and initiation of antibiotic if child worsens or does not improve within 48 to 72 h of symptom onset. Do not use observation if follow-up is unsure.

[c] Consider in patients who have received amoxicillin in the past 30 days or who have the otitis-conjunctivitis syndrome. Use the 14:1 formulation of amoxicillin-clavulanate that provides amoxicillin 90 mg/kg/day and clavulanate 6.4 mg/kg/day. In Canada, the 14:1 formulation of amoxicillin-clavulanate is not available, so it is necessary to give the 7:1 ratio formulation with additional amoxicillin. Do not increase the dose of a 4:1 or 7:1 amoxicillin-clavulanate formulation in order to achieve a higher dose of amoxicillin; this strategy gives an excessive dose of clavulanate which increases the risk of diarrhea.

[d] Tympanocentesis/drainage performed by skilled clinician or otolaryngologist. Seek infectious disease spedalist consultation if tympanocentesis reports multidrug-resistant bacteria.

[e] Cefdinir, cefuroxime, cefpodoxime, and ceftriaxone are highly unlikely to cross-react with penicillin. Excluding patients with a history of a severe reaction, the reaction rate in patients who have not undergone penicillin skin testing is estimated at 0.1%. A drug allergy practice parameter (Ann Allergy Asthma Immunol 2010;105:259-73; available at http://www.allergyparameters.org) recommends that a cephalosporin can be given to patients who do not have a history of a severe and/or recent allergic reaction to penicillin. Options for patients with a history of an IgE-mediated reaction to penicillin include substitution of a non-beta-lactam antibiotic, or the performance of penicillin or cephalosporin skin testing to evaluate the risk of cephalosporin administration.

SEXUALLY TRANSMITTED DISEASES & VAGINITIS*

Bacterial vaginosis	(1) metronidazole 5 g of 0.75% gel intravaginally daily for 5 days OR 500 mg PO two times per day for 7 days; (2) clindamycin 5 g of 2% cream intravaginally at bedtime for 7 days. In pregnancy: (1) metronidazole 500 mg PO two times per day for 7 days OR 250 mg PO three times per day for 7 days; (2) clindamycin 300 mg PO two times per day for 7 days.
Candidal vaginitis	(1) intravaginal clotrimazole, miconazole, terconazole, nystatin, tioconazole, or butoconazole; (2) fluconazole 150 mg PO single dose.
Chancroid	(1) azithromycin 1 g PO single dose; (2) ceftriaxone 250 mg IM single dose; (3) ciprofloxacin 500 mg PO two times per day for 3 days.
Chlamydia	First-line: either azithromycin 1 g PO single dose or doxycycline 100 mg PO two times per day for 7 days. Second-line: fluoroquinolones or erythromycin. In pregnancy: (1) azithromycin 1 g PO single dose; (2) amoxicillin 500 mg PO three times per day for 7 days. Repeat NAAT[1] 3 weeks after treatment in pregnant women.
Epididymitis	(1) ceftriaxone 250 mg IM single dose + doxycycline 100 mg PO two times per day for 10 days; (2) ofloxacin 300 mg PO two times per day or levofloxacin 500 mg PO daily for 10 days if enteric organisms suspected, or negative gonococcal culture or NAAT.[4]
Gonorrhea	First-line: Single dose of ceftriaxone 250 mg IM + azithromycin 1 g PO single dose (preferred) or doxycycline 100 mg PO two times per day for 7 days. Second-line: cefixime 400 mg PO (not for pharyngeal) + azithromycin (preferred)/doxycycline if ceftriaxone not available.[2] Test-of-cure (culture and sensitivity preferred over NAAT[1]) required for cefixime. Consult infectious disease expert if severe cephalosporin allergy.
Gonorrhea, disseminated	Initially treat with ceftriaxone 1 g IM/IV q 24 h until 24 to 48 h after improvement. Second-line alternatives: (1) cefotaxime 1 g IV q 8 h; (2) ceftizoxime 1 g IV q 8 h. Complete at least 1 week of treatment with cefixime tabs 400 mg PO two times per day.[1]
Gonorrhea, meningitis	Ceftriaxone 1 to 2 g IV q 12 h for 10 to 14 days.
Gonorrhea, endocarditis	Ceftriaxone 1 to 2 g IV q 12 h for at least 4 weeks.
Granuloma inguinale	Doxycycline 100 mg PO two times per day for at least 3 weeks and until lesions completely healed. Alternative azithromycin 1 g PO once weekly for at least 3 weeks and until lesions completely healed.
Herpes simplex, genital, 1 episode	(1) acyclovir 400 mg PO three times per day for 7 to 10 days; (2) famciclovir 250 mg PO three times per day for 7 to 10 days; (3) valacyclovir 1 g PO two times per day for 7 to 10 days.
Herpes simplex, genital, recurrent	(1) acyclovir 400 mg PO three times per day for 5 days; (2) acyclovir 800 mg PO three times per day for 2 days or two times per day for 5 days; (3) famciclovir 125 mg PO two times per day for 5 days; (4) famciclovir 1 g PO two times per day for 1 day; (5) famciclovir 500 mg PO 1 dose, then 250 mg PO two to three times per day for 2 days; (6) valacyclovir 500 mg PO two times per day for 3 days; (7) valacyclovir 1 g PO daily for 5 days.
Herpes simplex, suppressive therapy	(1) acyclovir 400 mg PO two times per day; (2) famciclovir 250 mg PO two times per day; (3) valacyclovir 500 to 1000 mg PO daily. Valacyclovir 500 mg PO daily may be less effective than other valacyclovir/acyclovir regimens in patients who have 10 or more recurrences per year.

(cont.)

Herpes simplex, genital, recurrent in HIV infection	(1) acyclovir 400 mg PO three times per day for 5 to 10 days; (2) famciclovir 500 mg PO two times per day for 5 to 10 days; (3) valacyclovir 1 g PO two times per day for 5 to 10 days.
Herpes, suppressive therapy in HIV infection	(1) acyclovir 400 to 800 mg PO two to three times per day; (2) famciclovir 500 mg PO two times per day; (3) valacyclovir 500 mg PO two times per day.
Herpes simplex, prevention of transmission	For patients with no more than 9 recurrences per year: Valacyclovir 500 mg PO daily by source partner, in conjunction with safer sex practices.
Lympho-granuloma venereum	doxycycline 100 mg PO two times per day for 21 days. Alternative: erythromycin base 500 mg PO four times per day for 21 days.
Pelvic inflammatory disease (PID), inpatient regimens	(1) cefoxitin 2 g IV q 6 h + doxycycline 100 mg IV/PO q 12 h; (2) clindamycin 900 mg IV q 8 h + gentamicin 2 mg/kg IM/IV loading dose, then 1.5 mg/kg IM/IV q 8 h (can substitute 3 to 5 mg/kg once-daily dosing). Can switch to PO therapy within 24 h of improvement.
Pelvic inflammatory disease (PID), outpatient treatment	Ceftriaxone 250 mg IM single dose + doxycycline 100 mg PO two times per day +/− metronidazole 500 mg PO two times per day for 14 days.
Proctitis, proctocolitis, enteritis	ceftriaxone 250 mg IM single dose + doxycycline 100 mg PO two times per day for 7 days.
Sexual assault prophylaxis	Ceftriaxone 250 mg IM single dose + metronidazole 2 g PO single dose + azithromycin 1 g PO single dose/doxycycline 100 mg PO two times per day for 7 days.
Syphilis, primary and secondary	(1) benzathine penicillin 2.4 million units IM single dose. (2) doxycycline 100 mg PO two times per day for 2 weeks if penicillin-allergic.
Syphilis, early latent, ie, duration less than 1 year	(1) benzathine penicillin 2.4 million units IM single dose; (2) doxycycline 100 mg PO two times per day for 2 weeks if penicillin-allergic.
Syphilis, late latent or unknown duration	(1) benzathine penicillin 2.4 million units IM q week for 3 doses; (2) doxycycline 100 mg PO two times per day for 4 weeks if penicillin-allergic.
Syphilis, tertiary	benzathine penicillin 2.4 million units IM q week for 3 doses. Consult infectious disease specialist for management of penicillin-allergic patients.
Syphilis, neuro	(1) penicillin G 18 to 24 million units/day continuous IV infusion or 3 to 4 million units IV q 4 h for 10 to 14 days; (2) if compliance can be ensured, consider procaine penicillin 2.4 million units IM daily + probenecid 500 mg PO four times per day, both for 10 to 14 days.
Syphilis in pregnancy	Treat only with penicillin regimen for stage of syphilis as noted above. Use penicillin-desensitization protocol if penicillin-allergic.

(cont.)

Trichomoniasis	Metronidazole (can use in pregnancy) or tinidazole, each 2 g PO single dose.
Urethritis, Cervicitis	Test for chlamydia and gonorrhea with NAAT.[1] Treat based on test results or treat presumptively if high risk of infection (chlamydia: age 25 yo or younger, new/multiple sex partners, or unprotected sex; gonorrhea: population prevalence greater than 5%), esp. if NAAT[2] unavailable or patient unlikely to return for follow-up.
Urethritis, persistent/ recurrent	Metronidazole/tinidazole 2 g PO single dose + azithromycin 1 g PO single dose (if not used in 1st episode).

* *MMWR* 2010;59:RR-12 or http://www.cdc.gov/STD/treatment/ and *MMWR* 2012;61(31):590. Treat sexual partners for all except herpes, *Candida*, and bacterial vaginosis.

[1]NAAT = nucleic acid amplification test.

[2]There is a growing threat of multidrug-resistant gonorrhea, with high-level azithromycin resistance and reduced cephalosporin susceptibility reported in the US in 2011. Ceftriaxone is the most effective cephalosporin for treatment of gonorrhea. Cefixime is now 2-line because of increasing risk of resistance. If cefixime treatment failure occurs, retreat with ceftriaxone 250 mg IM plus azithromycin 2 g PO both single dose and obtain infectious disease consultation. If ceftriaxone treatment failure occurs, consult infectious disease expert and CDC. Do not use azithromycin monotherapy for routine treatment of gonorrhea. If azithromycin is used in patients with cephalosporin allergy, use azithromycin 2 g PO single dose and perform culture (preferred) or NAAT in 1 week. Report treatment failure to state/local health department within 24 h. As of April 2007, the CDC no longer recommends fluoroquinolones for gonorrhea or PID because of high resistance rates. Do not consider fluoroquinolone unless antimicrobial susceptibility can be documented by culture. If parenteral cephalosporin not feasible for PID (and NAAT is negative or culture documents fluoroquinolone susceptibility), can consider levofloxacin 500 mg PO once daily or ofloxacin 400 mg PO two times per day +/– metronidazole 500 mg PO two times per day for 14 days.

Cephalosporins—4th Generation

CEFEPIME (*Maxipime*) 0.5 to 2 g IM/IV q 12 h. Peds: 50 mg/kg IV q 8 to 12 h. ▶K ♀B ▶? $$$$

Cephalosporins—5th Generation

CEFTAROLINE (*Teflaro*) Community-acquired bacterial pneumonia, acute bacterial skin and skin structure infections: 600 mg IV q 12 h infused over 1 h. ▶K ♀B ▶? $$$$$

Macrolides

AZITHROMYCIN (*Zithromax, Zmax*) 500 mg IV daily. 10 mg/kg (up to 500 mg) PO on day 1, then 5 mg/kg (up to 250 mg) daily for 4 days. Azithromycin is a poor option for otitis media and sinusitis due to pneumococcal and H influenzae resistance; see otitis media and sinusitis treatment tables for alternatives. Otitis media: 30 mg/kg PO single dose or 10 mg/kg PO daily for 3 days. Peds sinusitis: 10 mg/kg PO daily for 3 days. Group A streptococcal pharyngitis (second-line to penicillin): 12 mg/kg (up to 500 mg) PO daily for 5 days. Adult acute sinusitis or exacerbation of chronic bronchitis: 500 mg PO daily for 3 days. Zmax for community-acquired pneumonia, acute sinusitis: 60 mg/kg (up to 2 g) PO single dose on empty stomach; give adult dose of 2 g for wt 34 kg or greater. Chlamydia (including pregnancy), chancroid: 1 g PO single dose. Prevention of disseminated *Mycobacterium avium* complex disease: 1200 mg PO once a week. Pertussis treatment/post-exposure

(cont.)

prophylaxis: 10 mg/kg PO once daily for 5 days for infants age younger than 6 mo; 10 mg/kg (max 500 mg) PO on day 1, then 5 mg/kg (max 250 mg) PO once daily for 4 days for children 6 mo and older; 500 mg PO on day 1, then 250 mg PO daily for 4 days for adolescents and adults. [Generic/Trade: Tabs 250, 500, 600 mg. Susp 100, 200 mg/5 mL. Packet 1000 mg. Z-Pak: #6, 250 mg tab. Tri-Pak: #3, 500 mg tab. Trade only: Extended-release oral susp: 2 g in 60 mL single-dose bottle.] ▶L ♀B ▶? $$

CLARITHROMYCIN (*Biaxin, Biaxin XL*) 250 to 500 mg PO two times per day. Peds: 7.5 mg/kg PO two times per day. *H. pylori:* See table in GI section. See table for prophylaxis of bacterial endocarditis. *Mycobacterium avium* complex disease prevention: 7.5 mg/kg up to 500 mg PO two times per day. Biaxin XL: 1000 mg PO daily with food. [Generic/Trade: Tabs 250, 500 mg. Extended-release tab 500 mg. Susp 125, 250 mg/ 5 mL. Trade only: Biaxin XL-Pak: #14, 500 mg tabs.] ▶KL ♀C ▶? $$$

ERYTHROMYCIN BASE (*Ery-Tab, P.C.E., ✦ Eryc*) Adult: 250 to 500 mg PO four times per day, 333 mg PO three times per day, or 500 mg PO two times per day. Peds: 30 to 50 mg/kg/day PO divided four times per day. [Generic/Trade: Tabs 250, 500 mg, delayed-release cap 250 mg, delayed-release tab 250, 333, 500 mg.] ▶L ♀B ▶+ $$$$

ERYTHROMYCIN ETHYL SUCCINATE (*EES, EryPed*) 400 mg PO four times per day. Peds: 30 to 50 mg/kg/day PO divided four times per day. [Generic/Trade: Tabs 400. Trade Only: Susp 200, 400 mg/5 mL.] ▶L ♀B ▶+ $

ERYTHROMYCIN LACTOBIONATE (*Erythrocin IV, ✦ Erythrocin IV*) 15 to 20 mg/kg/day (max 4 g) IV divided q 6 h. Peds: 15 to 50 mg/kg/day IV divided q 6 h. ▶L ♀B ▶+ $$$$$

FIDAXOMICIN (*Dificid*) *C. difficile*–associated diarrhea: 200 mg PO two times per day for 10 days. [Trade only: 200 mg tabs.] ▶minimal absorption ♀B ▶? $$$$$

Penicillins—1st generation—Natural

BENZATHINE PENICILLIN (*Bicillin L-A,*) Usual dose: 1.2 million units IM for adults and peds wt greater than 27 kg; 600,000 units IM for peds wt 27 kg or less. Give single dose for group A streptococcal pharyngitis. Give IM q month for secondary prevention of rheumatic fever (every 3 weeks for high-risk patients). See STD table for treatment of syphilis in adults. Dose lasts 2 to 4 weeks. [Trade only: For IM use, 600,000 units/mL; 1, 2, 4 mL syringes.] ▶K ♀B ▶? $$$ ■

BICILLIN C-R (procaine penicillin + benzathine penicillin) For IM use. Not for treatment of syphilis. [Trade only: For IM use 300/300 and 450/150 (Peds) thousand units/mL procaine/benzathine penicillin (600,000 units/mL); 2 mL syringe] ▶K ♀B ▶? $$$$ ■

PENICILLIN G Pneumococcal pneumonia and severe infections: 250,000 to 400,000 units/kg/day (8 to 12 million units/day in adult) IV divided q 4 to 6 h. Pneumococcal meningitis: 250,000 to 400,000 units/kg/day (24 million units/ day in adult) in 4 to 6 divided doses. ▶K ♀B ▶? $$$$

PENICILLIN V Adults: 250 to 500 mg PO four times per day. Peds: 25 to 50 mg/kg/day divided two to four times per day. AHA doses for pharyngitis: 250

(cont.)

PENICILLINS—GENERAL ANTIMICROBIAL SPECTRUM

1st generation	Most streptococci; oral anaerobic coverage
2nd generation	Most streptococci; *S.aureus* (but not MRSA)
3rd generation	Most streptococci; basic Gram-negative coverage
4th generation	*Pseudomonas*

mg (peds 27 kg or less) or 500 mg (adults and peds greater than 27 kg) PO two to three times per day for 10 days. [Generic only: Tabs 250, 500 mg. Oral soln 125, 250 mg/5 mL.] ▶K ♀B ▶? $

PROCAINE PENICILLIN 0.6 to 1 million units IM daily (peak 4 h, lasts 24 h). [Generic: For IM use, 600,000 units/mL; 1, 2 mL syringes.] ▶K ♀B ▶? $$$$$ ■

Penicillins—2nd generation—Penicillinase-Resistant

DICLOXACILLIN 250 to 500 mg PO four times per day. Peds: 12.5 to 25 mg/kg/day PO divided four times per day. [Generic only: Caps 250, 500 mg.] ▶KL ♀B ▶? $$

NAFCILLIN 1 to 2 g IM/IV q 4 h. Peds: 50 to 200 mg/kg/day IM/IV divided q 4 to 6 h. ▶L ♀B ▶? $$$$$

OXACILLIN 1 to 2 g IM/IV q 4 to 6 h. Peds: 150 to 200 mg/kg/day IM/IV divided q 4 to 6 h. ▶KL ♀B ▶? $$$$$

Penicillins—3rd generation—Aminopenicillins

AMOXICILLIN (*Moxatag*) 250 to 500 mg PO three times per day, or 500 to 875 mg PO two times per day. High-dose for community-acquired pneumonia, acute sinusitis: 1 g PO three times per day. See table for management of acute sinusitis in adults and children. Lyme disease: 500 mg PO three times per day for 14 days for early disease, for 28 days for Lyme arthritis. Chlamydia in pregnancy: 500 mg PO three times per day for 7 days. AHA dosing for group A streptococcal pharyngitis: 50 mg/kg (max 1 g) PO once daily for 10 days. Group A streptococcal pharyngitis/ tonsillitis: 775 mg ER tab (Moxatag) PO for 10 days for age 12 yo or older. Peds AAP otitis media: 80 to 90 mg/kg/day divided two times per day. Give 5 to 7 days of therapy for age 6 yo and older with mild to moderate symptoms, 7 days for age 2 to 5 yo with mild to moderate symptoms, and 10 days for age younger than 2 yo and children with severe symptoms. See table for management of acute otitis media in children. Peds infections other than otitis media: 40 mg/kg/day PO divided three times per day or 45 mg/kg/day divided two times per day. [Generic only: Caps 250, 500 mg. Tabs 500, 875 mg. Chewable tabs 125, 200, 250, 400 mg. Susp 125, 250 mg/5 mL. Susp 200, 400 mg/5 mL. Trade only: Moxatag 775 mg extended-release tab.] ▶K ♀B ▶+ $

AMOXICILLIN-CLAVULANATE (*Augmentin, Augmentin ES-600, Augmentin XR, ✦ Clavulin*) Adults, usual dose: 500 or 875 mg PO two times per day or 250 to 500 mg three times per day. Augmentin XR: 2 tabs PO q 12 h with

(cont.)

ACUTE BACTERIAL SINUSITIS IN ADULTS AND CHILDREN[§] IDSA TREATMENT RECOMMENDATIONS

Initial therapy in patients without risk factors for resistance and infection of mild or moderate severity	
Adults: Amoxicillin-clavulanate 500 mg/125 mg PO three times per day or 875 mg/125 mg PO two times per day for 5 to 7 days	Peds: Amoxicillin-clavulanate[§] 45 mg/kg/day PO two times per day for 10 to 14 days
Initial therapy in patients with severe infection, risk factors for resistance,[†] or high endemic rate of invasive penicillin-nonsusceptible *S. pneumonia* (≥10%)	
Adults: Treat for 5 to 7 days with: 1) Amoxicillin-clavulanate* 2000 mg/125 mg PO two times per day 2) Doxycycline 100 mg PO two times per day or 200 mg PO once daily	Peds: Amoxicillin-clavulanate* 90 mg/kg/day PO two times per day for 10 to 14 days
Beta-lactam allergy	
Adults: Treat for 5 to 7 days with: 1) Doxycycline 100 mg PO two times per day or 200 mg PO once daily 2) Levofloxacin 500 mg PO once daily 3) Moxifloxacin 400 mg PO once daily	Peds, type 1 hypersensitivity: Levofloxacin 10 to 20 mg/kg/day PO q 12–24 h for 10 to 14 days Peds, not type 1 hypersensitivity: Clindamycin[‡] 30 to 40 mg/kg/day PO three times per day plus cefixime 8 mg/kg/day PO two times per day or cefpodoxime 10 mg/kg/day PO two times per day for 10 to 14 days
Risk factors for antibiotic resistance[†] or failed first-line therapy	
Adults: Treat for 5 to 7 days with: 1) Amoxicillin-clavulanate* 2000 mg/125 mg PO two times per day 2) Levofloxacin 500 mg PO once daily 3) Moxifloxacin 400 mg PO once daily	Peds: Treat for 10 to 14 days with: 1) Amoxicillin-clavulanate* 90 mg/kg/day PO two times per day 2) Clindamycin[‡] 30 to 40 mg/kg/day PO three times per day plus cefixime 8 mg/kg/day PO two times per day or cefpodoxime 10 mg/kg/day PO two times per day 3) Levofloxacin 10 to 20 mg/kg/day PO q 12 to 24 h
Severe infection requiring hospitalization	
Adults: 1) Ampicillin-sulbactam 1.5 to 3 g N q 6 h 2) Levofloxacin 500 mg PO or IV once daily 3) Moxifloxacin 400 mg PO or IV once daily 4) Ceftriaxone 1 to 2 g IV q 12 to 24 h 5) Cefotaxime 2 g IV q 4 to 6 h	Peds: 1) Ampicillin-sulbactam 200 to 400 mg/kg/day IV q 6 h 2) Ceftriaxone 50 mg/kg/day IV q 12 h 3) Cefotaxime 100 to 200 mg/kg/day IV q 6 h 4) Levofloxacin 10 to 20 mg/kg/day IV q 12 to 24 h

Adapted from *Clin Infect Dis* 2012;54(8):e72-e112. Available online at: http://www.idsociety.org.

*High-dose amoxicillin-clavulanate recommended for geographic regions with high endemic rates (at least 10%) of invasive penicillin-nonsusceptible *S. pneumoniae*, those with severe infection (eg, evidence of systemic toxicity with fever of 39° C or higher, and threat of suppurative complications), or risk factors for antibiotic resistance. (Use the 14:1 formulation of amoxicillin-clavulanate that provides amoxicillin 90 mg/kg/day and clavulanate 6.4 mg/kg/day. In Canada, the 14:1 formulation of amoxicillin-clavulanate is not available, so it is necessary to give the 7:1 formulation with additional amoxicillin. Do not increase the dose of the 4:1 or 7:1 amoxicillin-clavulanate formulation in order to achieve a higher dose of amoxicillin; this strategy gives an excessive dose of clavulanate which increases the risk of diarrhea.)

†Risk factors for antibiotic resistance include attendance at daycare, age younger than 2 yo or older than 65 yo, recent hospitalization, antibiotic use within the past month, or patients who are immunocompromised.

‡ Clindamycin resistance in *S. pneumoniae* is common in some areas of US the United states.

§ American Academy of Pediatrics guideline for management of sinusitis in children (Pediatrics 2013;132:e262-e280; available online at: http://pediatrics.aappublications.org) recommends amoxicillin as first-line treatment of uncomplicated acute sinusitis when antimicrobial resistance is not suspected. Amoxicillin 45 mg/kg/day dosed two times per day is recommended for mild-moderate sinusitis in children 2 years old or older who do not attend daycare and have not been treated with an antibiotic in the last 4 weeks. Amoxicillin 80 to 90 mg/kg/day divided two times daily (max 2 g/dose) is recommended in communities with a high prevalence of nonsusceptible *S. pneumoniae* (at least 10%). Amoxicillin-clavulanate 80 to 90 mg/kg/day divided two times per day (max 2 g/dose) is an option for moderate-severe sinusitis, and sinusitis in children less than 2 years old, attending daycare, or who have received an antibiotic in the last 4 weeks.

PROPHYLAXIS FOR BACTERIAL ENDOCARDITIS*

Limited to dental or respiratory tract procedures in patients at highest risk. All regimens are single doses administered 30–60 minutes prior to procedure.	
Standard regimen	Amoxicillin 2 g PO
Unable to take oral meds	Ampicillin 2 g IM/IV; or cefazolin† or ceftriaxone† 1 g IM/IV
Allergic to penicillin	Clindamycin 600 mg PO; or cephalexin† 2 g PO; or azithromycin or clarithromycin 500 mg PO
Allergic to penicillin and unable to take oral meds	Clindamycin 600 mg IM/IV; or cefazolin† or ceftriaxone† 1 g IM/IV
Pediatric drug doses	Pediatric dose should not exceed adult dose. Amoxicillin 50 mg/kg, ampicillin 50 mg/kg, azithromycin 15 mg/kg, cephalexin† 50 mg/kg, cefazolin† 50 mg/kg, ceftriaxone† 50 mg/kg, clarithromycin 15 mg/kg, clindamycin 20 mg/kg.

*For additional details of the 2007 AHA guidelines, see http://www.americanheart.org.
†Avoid cephalosporins if prior penicillin-associated anaphylaxis, angioedema, or urticaria.

meals. See table for management of acute sinusitis in adults and children. Peds, usual dose: 45 mg/kg/day PO divided two times per day or 40 mg/kg/day divided three times per day. High-dose for community-acquired pneumonia, otitis media, sinusitis: 90 mg/kg/day PO divided two times per day (max dose of 2 g PO two times per day for age 5 yo and older). Treat pneumonia for up to 10 days; sinusitis for 10 to 14 days. For oral therapy of acute otitis media, AAP recommends 5 to 7 days of therapy for children 6 yo and older with mild to moderate symptoms, 7 days for children 2 to 5 yo with mild to moderate symptoms, and 10 days for children younger than 2 yo and those with severe symptoms. See table for management of acute otitis media in children. [Generic/Trade: (amoxicillin-clavulanate) Tabs 250/125, 500/125, 875/125 mg. Chewables, Susp 200/28.5, 400/57 mg per tab or 5 mL, 250/62.5 mg per 5 mL. (ES) Susp 600/42.9 mg per 5 mL. Extended-release tabs 1000/62.5 mg. Trade only: Susp 125/31.25 per 5 mL, 250/62.5 mg per 5mL.] ▶K ♀B ▶? $$$

AMPICILLIN Usual dose: 1 to 2 g IV q 4 to 6 h. Sepsis, meningitis: 150 to 200 mg/kg/day IV divided q 3 to 4 h. Peds: 100 to 400 mg/kg/day IM/IV divided q 4 to 6 h. [Generic only: Caps 250, 500 mg. Susp 125, 250 mg/5 mL.] ▶K ♀B ▶? $ PO $$$$$ IV

AMPICILLIN-SULBACTAM (*Unasyn*) 1.5 to 3 g IM/IV q 6 h. Peds: 100 to 400 mg/kg/day of ampicillin divided q 6 h. ▶K ♀B ▶? $$$

Penicillins—4th generation—Extended Spectrum

PIPERACILLIN-TAZOBACTAM (*Zosyn*, ✦*Tazocin*) 3.375 to 4.5 g IV q 6 h. Peds appendicitis or peritonitis: 80 mg/kg IV q 8 h for age 2 to 9 mo, 100 mg/kg piperacillin IV q 8 h for age older than 9 mo, use adult dose for wt greater than 40 kg. ▶K ♀B ▶? $$$$$

TICARCILLIN-CLAVULANATE (*Timentin*) 3.1 g IV q 4 to 6 h. Peds: 50 mg/kg up to 3.1 g IV q 4 to 6 h. ▶K ♀B ▶? $$$$$

QUINOLONES—GENERAL ANTIMICROBIAL SPECTRUM

1st generation	1st-generation quinolones are no longer available
2nd generation	Gram-negative (including *Pseudomonas*); *S. aureus* (but not MRSA or *Pneumococcus*); some atypicals
3rd generation	Gram-negative (including *Pseudomonas*); Gram-positive, including *Pneumococcus* and *S. aureus* (but not MRSA); expanded atypical coverage
4th generation	same as 3rd generation plus enhanced coverage of *Pneumococcus*, decreased *Pseudomonas* activity

Quinolones—2nd Generation

CIPROFLOXACIN (*Cipro, Cipro XR*) 200 to 400 mg IV q 8 to 12 h. 250 to 750 mg PO two times per day. Simple UTI: 250 mg two times per day for 3 days or Cipro XR 500 mg PO daily for 3 days. Cipro XR for pyelonephritis or complicated UTI: 1000 mg PO daily for 7 to 14 days. [Generic/Trade: Tabs 100, 250, 500, 750 mg. Extended-release tabs 500, 1000 mg.] ▶LK ♀C but teratogenicity unlikely ▶?+ $ ■
NORFLOXACIN (*Noroxin*) Simple UTI: 400 mg PO two times per day for 3 days. [Trade only: Tabs 400 mg.] ▶LK ♀C ▶? $$ ■
OFLOXACIN 200 to 400 mg PO two times per day. [Generic only: Tabs 200, 300, 400 mg.] ▶LK ♀C ▶?+ $$$ ■

Quinolones—3rd Generation

LEVOFLOXACIN (*Levaquin*) IV and PO doses are the same. Usual adult dose: 250 to 750 mg PO/IV daily. Simple UTI: 250 mg once daily for 3 days. Complicated UTI or pyelonephritis: 250 mg once daily for 10 days or 750 mg once daily for 5 days. Community-acquired pneumonia: 750 mg once daily for 5 days or 500 mg once daily for 7 to 14 days. See table for management of acute sinusitis in adults and children. Peds. Community-acquired pneumonia: 8 to 10 mg/kg two times per day for age 6 mo to 5 yo; 8 to 10 mg/kg once daily (max 750 mg once daily) for age 5 to 16 yo. [Generic/Trade: Tabs 250, 500, 750 mg. Oral soln 25 mg/mL] ▶KL ♀C ▶? $$$

Quinolones—4th Generation

GEMIFLOXACIN (*Factive*) 320 mg PO daily for 5 to 7 days. [Trade only: Tabs 320 mg.] ▶Feces, K ♀C ▶− $$$$$ ■
MOXIFLOXACIN (*Avelox*) 400 mg PO/IV daily for 5 days (chronic bronchitis exacerbation), 5 to 14 days (complicated intra-abdominal infection), 7 days (uncomplicated skin infections), 10 days (acute sinusitis), 7 to 14 days (community-acquired pneumonia), 7 to 21 days (complicated skin infections). See table for management of acute sinusitis. [Trade only: Tabs 400 mg.] ▶LK ♀C ▶− $$$$ ■

Sulfonamides

TRIMETHOPRIM-SULFAMETHOXAZOLE (*Bactrim, Septra, Sulfatrim, cotrimoxazole*) Usual adult dose: 1 tab PO two times per day, double-strength

(cont.)

C difficile Infection (CDI) in Adults: IDSA/SHEA and ACG Treatment Recommendations		
Severity Initial episode	**Clinical signs**	**Treatment**
Mild to moderate	IDSA: WBC ≤15,000 AND serum creatinine<1.5 times premorbid level ACG: Diarrhea with signs or symptoms not meeting severe or complicated criteria	Metronidazole 500 mg PO q8h for 10 to 14 days[a] ACG: If unable to take metronidazole, use vancomycin 125 mg PO q6h for 10 days. If no response to metronidazole in 5 to 7 days, consider vancomycin.
Severe[b]	IDSA: WBC ≥15,000 OR serum creatinine ≥1.5 times premorbid level ACG: Serum albumin<3 g/dL plus ONE of the following: WBC ≥15,000 Abdominal tenderness	Vancomycin 125 mg PO q 6 h for 10 to 14 days[a]
Severe and complicated[c]	IDSA: Hypotension or shock, ileus, megacolon ACG: Any of the following attributable to CDI: ICU admission for CDI Hypotension +/- required use of vasopressors Fever ≥38.5° C Ileus or significant abdominal distention Mental status changes WBC ≥35,000 or <2000 Serum lactate >2.2mmol/L End organ failure (mechanical ventilation, renal failure, etc)	Vancomycin 500 mg PO/NGq6hplus metronidazole 500 mg IV q8h IDSA: Consider adding vancomycin 500 mg/100 mL[c] normal saline retention enema q 6 h id complete ileus. ACG: Add vancomycin 500 mg/500 mL[c] normal saline enema q6h if complicated CDI with ileus or toxic colon and/or significant abdominal distention.
Recurrent episodes		
First recurrence	--	Same as initial episode, stratified by severity. IDSA: Use vancomycin if WBC ≥15,000 or serum creatinine is increasing.
Second recurrence	--	Vancomycin taper and/or pulsed regimen[d]

Adapted from: *Infect Control HospEpidemiol*2010; 31:431. Available online at:http://www.idsociety.org. *Am J Gastroenterol*2013;108:478-98. Available online at: http://gi.org.

[a] ACG recommends 10 days of therapy on the basis that clinical trials only evaluated 10 days of treatment.

[b] IDSA: Consider colectomy in patients with severe CDI.ACG: Get surgical consultation for patients with complicated CDI.Consider surgery for patients with any of the following attributed to CDI: hypotension requiring vasopressors, clinical signs of sepsis and organ dysfunction (renal and pulmonary), mental status changes, WBC ≥50,000, lactate ≥5 mmol/L, or failure to improve on medical therapy after 5 days.

[c] IDSA recommends diluting vancomycin in 100 mL for administration as enema. ACG recommends diluting vancomycin in a larger volume (500 mL) in order to ensure delivery to ascending and transverse colon.

[d] IDSA taper example: Vancomycin 125 mg PO QID for 10 to 14 days, then 125 mg two times per day for 7 days, then 125 mg once daily for 7 days, then 125 mg every 2 or 3 days for 2 to 8 weeks. ACG proposed pulse regimen: Vancomycin 125 mg PO q6h for 10 days, then 125 mg once every 3 days for 10 doses. Note: If there is a third recurrence after a pulsed vancomycin regimen, ACG recommends considering fecal microbiota transplant.

(DS, 160 mg/800 mg) or single-strength (SS, 80 mg/400 mg). TMP-SMX is a poor option for otitis media and sinusitis due to pneumococcal and H influenzae resistance; see otitis media and sinusitis treatment tables for alternatives. Community-acquired MRSA skin infections, adults: 1 to 2 DS tabs PO two times per day for 7 to 10 days. Peds: 1 to 1.5 mL/kg/day PO divided two times per day. Pneumocystis pneumonia treatment: 15 to 20 mg/kg/day (based on TMP) IV divided q 6 to 8 h or PO divided three times per day for 21 days total. Pneumocystis pneumonia prophylaxis, adults: 1 DS tab PO daily. Peds usual dose: 1 mL/kg/day susp PO divided two times per day (up to 20 mL DS PO two times per day). Use adult dose for wt greater than 40 kg. [Generic/Trade: Tabs 80 mg TMP/400 mg SMX (SS), 160 mg TMP/800 mg SMX (DS). Susp 40 mg TMP/200 mg SMX per 5 mL. 20 mL susp = 2 SS tabs = 1 DS tab.] ▶K ♀C ▶+ $

(cont.)

Tetracyclines

DEMECLOCYCLINE   Usual dose: 150 mg PO four times per day or 300 mg PO two times per day on empty stomach. SIADH: 600 to 1200 mg/day PO given in 3 to 4 divided doses. [Generic only: Tabs 150, 300 mg.] ▶K, feces ♀D ▶?+ $$$$

DOXYCYCLINE   (*Doryx, Monodox, Oracea, Vibramycin, Vibra-Tabs, Adoxa, ✦Doxycin, Periostat, Apprilon*) 100 mg PO two times per day on 1st day, then 50 mg two times per day or 100 mg daily. Severe infections: 100 mg PO/IV two times per day. See table for management of acute sinusitis. Community-acquired MRSA skin infections: 100 mg PO two times per day. Lyme disease: 100 mg PO two times per day for 14 days for early disease, for 28 days for Lyme arthritis. Chlamydia, nongonococcal urethritis: 100 mg PO two times per day for 7 days. Doryx for chlamydia urethritis/cervicitis: 200 mg PO once daily for 7 days. Acne: Up to 100 mg PO two times per day. Oracea ($$$$$) for inflammatory rosacea: 40 mg PO once q am on empty stomach. Periostat for periodontitis: 20 mg PO two times per day. Malaria prophylaxis: 2 mg/kg/day up to 100 mg PO daily starting 1 to 2 days before exposure until 4 weeks after. Avoid in children younger than 8 yo due to teeth staining. [Monohydrate Salt: Generic/Trade: Caps 50, 75, 100, 150 mg. Tabs 50, 75, 100, 150 mg. Trade only: Delayed-release caps 40 mg (Oracea $$$$$). Susp 25 mg/5 mL (Vibramycin) Hyclate Salt. Tabs Generic/Trade: 20 mg. Generic only: 100 mg. Capsules: Generic only: 50 mg. Generic/Trade: 100 mg. Delayed-release tabs. Generic only: 75, 100 mg. Generic/Trade: 150 mg. Trade only: 200 mg (Doryx $$$$$). Delayed-release caps: Generic only: 75, 100 mg. Calcium Salt. Trade only: 50 mg/5 ml] ▶LK ♀D ▶?+ $

MINOCYCLINE   (*Minocin, Dynacin, Solodyn,   ✦Enca*) 200 mg IV/PO initially, then 100 mg q 12 h. Community-acquired MRSA skin infections: 200 mg PO first dose, then 100 mg PO two times per day for 5 to 10 days. Acne (traditional dosing, not Solodyn): 50 mg PO two times per day. Solodyn ($$$$$) for inflammatory acne in adults and children 12 yo and older: 1 mg/kg PO once daily. [Generic/Trade: Caps, Tabs ($) 50, 75, 100 mg. Tabs, extended-release ($$$$$) 45, 90, 135 mg. Trade only: Tabs, extended-release (Solodyn-$$$$$) 55, 65, 80, 105, 115 mg.] ▶LK ♀D ▶?+ $

Other Antimicrobials

AZTREONAM   (*Azactam, Cayston*) 0.5 to 2 g IM/IV q 6 to 12 h. Peds: 30 mg/kg IV q 6 to 8 h. [Trade only (Cayston): 75 mg/vial with diluent for inhalation.] ▶K ♀B ▶+ $$$$$

CHLORAMPHENICOL   50 to 100 mg/kg/day IV divided q 6 h. Aplastic anemia. ▶LK ♀C ▶– $$$$$ ■

CLINDAMYCIN   (*Cleocin,   ✦Dalacin C*) 150 to 450 mg PO four times per day. 600 to 900 mg IV q 8 h. Community-acquired MRSA skin infections: 300 to 450 mg PO three times per day for 5 to 10 days for adults; 10 to 13 mg/kg/dose PO q 6 to 8 h (max 40 mg/kg/day) for peds. Peds usual dose: 20 to 40 mg/kg/day IV divided q 6 to 8 h or give 8 to 25 mg/kg/day susp PO divided q 6 to 8 h. See table for management of acute otitis media in children. [Generic/Trade: Caps 75, 150, 300 mg. Oral soln 75 mg/5 mL (100 mL).] ▶L ♀B ▶?+ $$$ ■

DAPTOMYCIN (*Cubicin*) Complicated skin infections (including MRSA): 4 mg/kg IV daily for 7 to 14 days. *S. aureus* bacteremia (including MRSA): 6 mg/kg IV daily for at least 2 to 6 weeks. Infuse over 30 min. Not for pneumonia (inactivated by surfactant). Not approved in children. ▶K ♀B ▶? $$$$$

FOSFOMYCIN (*Monurol*) Simple UTI: One 3 g packet PO single dose. [Trade only: 3 g packet of granules.] ▶K ♀B ▶? $$

LINEZOLID (*Zyvox*, ✦*Zyvoxam*) Pneumonia, complicated skin infections (including MRSA), vancomycin-resistant *E. faecium* infections: 10 mg/kg (up to 600 mg) IV/PO q 8 h for age younger than 12 yo, 600 mg IV/PO q 12 h for adults and age 12 yo or older. Myelosuppression, drug interactions due to MAO inhibition. Limit tyramine foods to less than 100 mg/meal. [Trade only: Tabs 600 mg. Susp 100 mg/ 5 mL.] ▶Oxidation/K ♀C ▶? $$$$$

METRONIDAZOLE (*Flagyl*, *Flagyl ER*, ✦*Florazole ER*, *Trikacide*, *Nidazol*) Bacterial vaginosis: 500 mg PO two times per day or Flagyl ER 750 mg PO daily for 7 days. *H. pylori*: See table in GI section. Anaerobic bacterial infections: Load 1 g or 15 mg/kg IV, then 500 mg or 7.5 mg/kg (up to 4 g/day) IV/PO q 6 to 8 h, each IV dose over 1 h. Peds: 7.5 mg/kg IV q 6 h. *C. difficile*–associated diarrhea: Adults: 500 mg PO three times per day for 10 to 14 days. Peds: 30 mg/kg/day PO divided four times per day for 10 to 14 days. See table for management of *C. difficile* infection in adults. Trichomoniasis: 2 g PO single dose for patient and sex partners (may be used in pregnancy per CDC). Giardia: 250 mg (5 mg/kg/dose for peds) PO three times per day for 5 to 7 days. [Generic/Trade: Tabs 250, 500 mg. Caps 375 mg. Trade only: Tabs, extended-release 750 mg.] ▶KL ♀B ▶?– $$$$$

NITROFURANTOIN (*Furadantin*, *Macrodantin*, *Macrobid*) Uncomplicated UTI: 50 to 100 mg PO four times per day for 7 days. Peds: 5 to 7 mg/kg/day divided four times per day. Macrobid for uncomplicated UTI: 100 mg PO two times per day for 7 days. Take nitrofurantoin with food. [Generic/Trade (Macrodantin): Caps 25, 50, 100 mg. Generic/Trade (Macrobid): Caps 100 mg. Generic/Trade (Furadantin): Susp 25 mg/5 mL.] ▶KL ♀B ▶+? $

RIFAXIMIN (*Xifaxan*) Traveler's diarrhea: 200 mg PO three times per day for 3 days. Prevention of recurrent hepatic encephalopathy ($$$$$): 550 mg PO two times per day. [Trade only: Tabs 200, 550 mg.] ▶Feces, no GI absorption ♀C ▶? $$$

SYNERCID (quinupristin + dalfopristin) 7.5 mg/kg IV q 12 h, each dose over 1 h. MRSA bacteremia (2nd line): 7.5 mg/kg IV q 8 h. Not active against *E. faecalis*. ▶Bile ♀B ▶? $$$$$

TELAVANCIN (*Vibativ*) Complicated skin infections including MRSA: 10 mg/kg IV once daily for 7 to 14 days. Hospital-acquired/ventilator-associated *S. aureus* pneumonia (not first-line): 10 mg/kg IV once daily for 7 to 21 days. Infuse over 1 h. Teratogenic; get serum pregnancy test before use in women of childbearing potential. Nephrotoxic; monitor renal function. Do not use if CrCl is 50 mL/min or lower unless potential benefit exceeds risk. Not approved in children. ▶K ♀C ▶? $$$$$ ■

TELITHROMYCIN (*Ketek*) 800 mg PO daily for 7 to 10 days for community-acquired pneumonia. No longer indicated for acute sinusitis or acute exacerbation of chronic bronchitis (risks exceed potential benefit).

(cont.)

Contraindicated in myasthenia gravis. [Trade only: Tabs 300, 400 mg. Ketek Pak: #10, 400 mg tabs.] ▶LK ♀C ▶? $$$ ∎

TIGECYCLINE (*Tygacil*) Complicated skin infections, complicated intra-abdominal infections, community-acquired pneumonia: 100 mg IV first dose, then 50 mg IV q 12 h. Infuse over 30 to 60 min. Consider other antibiotics for severe infection because mortality is higher with tigecycline, especially in ventilator-associated pneumonia. ▶Bile, K ♀D ▶+ $$$$$

TRIMETHOPRIM (*Primsol*) 100 mg PO two times per day or 200 mg PO daily. [Generic only: Tabs 100 mg. Trade only (Primsol): Oral soln 50 mg/5 mL.] ▶K ♀C ▶– $

VANCOMYCIN (*Vancocin*) Usual dose: 15 to 20 mg/kg IV q 8 to 12 h; consider loading dose of 25 to 30 mg/kg for severe infection. Infuse over 1 h; infuse over 1.5 to 2 h if dose greater than 1 g. Peds: 10 to 15 mg/kg IV q 6 h. *C. difficile* diarrhea: 40 mg/kg/day PO up to 2 g/day divided four times per day for at least 10 days. IV administration ineffective for this indication. Dose depends on severity and complications, see table for management of *C. difficile* infection in adults. [Generic/Trade: Caps 125, 250 mg.] ▶K ♀C ▶? $$$$$

CARDIOVASCULAR

HTN Therapy[1]

Area of Concern	BP Target	Preferred Therapy[2]	Comments
General CAD prevention	<140/90 mm Hg	ACEI, ARB, CCB, thiazide, or combination	Start 2 drugs if systolic BP ≥ 160 or diastolic BP ≥ 100
High CAD risk[3]	<130/80 mm Hg		
Stable angina, unstable angina, MI	<130/80 mm Hg	Beta-blocker[4] + (ACEI or ARB)[5]	May add dihydropyridine CCB or thiazide
Left heart failure[6,7]	<120/80 mm Hg	Beta-blocker + (ACEI or ARB) + diuretic[8] + aldosterone antagonist[9]	

[1]ACEI = angiotensin-converting enzyme inhibitor; ARB = angiotensin-receptor blocker; CCB = calcium-channel blocker; MI = myocardial infarction. Adapted from *Circulation* 2007;115:2761–2788.
[2]All patients should attempt lifestyle modifications: optimize wt, healthy diet, sodium restriction, exercise, smoking cessation, alcohol moderation.
[3]DM, chronic kidney disease, known CAD or risk equivalent (eg, peripheral artery disease, abdominal aortic aneurysm, carotid artery disease, and prior ischemic CVA/TIA), 10-year Framingham risk score ≥ 10%.
[4]Use only if hemodynamically stable. If beta-blocker contraindications or intolerable side effects (and no bradycardia or heart failure), may substitute verapamil or diltiazem.
[5]Preferred if anterior wall MI, persistent HTN, heart failure, or DM.
[6]Avoid verapamil, diltiazem, clonidine, alpha-blockers.
[7]For blacks with NYHA class III or IV HF, consider adding hydralazine/isosorbide dinitrate.
[8]Loop or thiazide.
[9]Use if NYHA class III or IV, or if clinical heart failure + LVEF < 40%.

ACE Inhibitors

NOTE: *See also Antihypertensive Combinations. Contraindicated in pregnancy or with history of angioedema. Do not use with aliskiren in patients with DM or CrCl < 60 mL/min. Dual inhibition of renin-angiotensin system increases risk of renal impairment, hypotension, and hyperkalemia. Hyperkalemia possible,*

(cont.)

especially if used concomitantly with other drugs that increase K+ (including K+ containing salt substitutes) and in patients with heart failure, DM, or renal impairment. Concomitant NSAIDs, including selective COX-2 inhibitors, may further deteriorate renal function and decrease antihypertensive effects.

BENAZEPRIL (*Lotensin*) HTN: Start 10 mg PO daily, usual maintenance dose 20 to 40 mg PO daily or divided two times per day, max 80 mg/day. [Generic/ Trade: Tabs unscored 5, 10, 20, 40 mg.] ▶LK ♀D ▶? $$ ■

CAPTOPRIL (*Capoten*) HTN: Start 25 mg PO two to three times per day, usual maintenance dose 25 to 150 mg two to three times per day, max 450 mg/day. Heart failure: Start 6.25 to 12.5 mg PO three times per day, usual dose 50 to 100 mg PO three times per day, max 450 mg/day. Diabetic nephropathy: 25 mg PO three times per day. [Generic/Trade: Tabs, scored 12.5, 25, 50, 100 mg.] ▶LK ♀D ▶+ $ ■

CILAZAPRIL (❧*Inhibace*) Canada only. HTN: 1.25 to 10 mg PO daily. [Generic/Trade: Tabs, scored 1, 2.5, 5 mg.] ▶LK ♀D ▶? $ ■

ENALAPRIL (enalaprilat, *Vasotec*) HTN: Start 5 mg PO daily, usual maintenance dose 10 to 40 mg PO daily or divided two times per day, max 40 mg/day. If oral therapy not possible, can use enalaprilat 1.25 mg IV q 6 h over 5 min, and increase up to 5 mg IV q 6 h if needed. Renal impairment or concomitant diuretic therapy: Start 2.5 mg PO daily. Heart failure: Start 2.5 mg PO two times per day, usual dose 10 to 20 mg PO two times per day, max 40 mg/day. [Generic/Trade: Tabs, scored 2.5, 5 mg, unscored 10, 20 mg.] ▶LK ♀D ▶+ $$ ■

FOSINOPRIL (*Monopril*) HTN: Start 10 mg PO daily, usual maintenance dose 20 to 40 mg PO daily or divided two times per day, max 80 mg/day. Heart failure:

(cont.)

ACE INHIBITOR DOSING	HTN		Heart Failure	
	Initial	Max/day	Initial	Max/day
benazepril (*Lotensin*)	10 mg daily*	80 mg	-	-
captopril (*Capoten*)	25 mg bid to tid	450 mg	6.25 mg tid	450 mg
enalapril (*Vasotec*)	5 mg daily*	40 mg	2.5 mg bid	40 mg
fosinopril (*Monopril*)	10 mg daily*	80 mg	5–10 mg daily	40 mg
lisinopril (*Zestril/ Prinivil*)	10 mg daily	80 mg	2.5–5 mg daily	40 mg
moexipril (*Univasc*)	7.5 mg daily*	30 mg	-	-
perindopril (*Aceon*)	4 mg daily*	16 mg	2 mg daily	16 mg
quinapril (*Accupril*)	10–20 mg daily*	80 mg	5 mg bid	40 mg
ramipril (*Altace*)	2.5 mg daily*	20 mg	1.25–2.5 mg bid	10 mg
trandolapril (*Mavik*)	1–2 mg daily*	8 mg	1 mg daily	4 mg

bid = two times per day; tid = three times per day.
Data taken from prescribing information and
http://circ.ahajournals.org/content/early/2013/06/03/CIR.0b013e31829e8776.citation.
* May require twice daily dosing for 24-h BP control.

Start 5 to 10 mg PO daily, usual dose 20 to 40 mg PO daily, max 40 mg/day. [Generic/Trade: Tabs, scored 10, unscored 20, 40 mg.] ▶LK ♀D ▶? $ ■

LISINOPRIL (*Prinivil, Zestril*) HTN: Start 10 mg PO daily, usual maintenance dose 20 to 40 mg PO daily, max 80 mg/day. Heart failure, acute MI: Start 2.5 to 5 mg PO daily, usual dose 5 to 20 mg PO daily, max dose 40 mg. [Generic/Trade: Tabs, unscored (Zestril) 2.5, 5, 10, 20, 30, 40 mg. Tabs, scored (Prinivil) 10, 20, 40 mg.] ▶K ♀D ▶? $ ■

MOEXIPRIL (*Univasc*) HTN: Start 7.5 mg PO daily, usual maintenance dose 7.5 to 30 mg PO daily or divided two times per day, max 30 mg/day. [Generic/Trade: Tabs, scored 7.5, 15 mg.] ▶LK ♀D ▶? $$ ■

PERINDOPRIL (*Aceon*, ◆*Coversyl*) HTN: Start 4 mg PO daily, usual maintenance dose 4 to 8 mg PO daily or divided two times per day, max 16 mg/day. Reduction of cardiovascular events in stable CAD: Start 4 mg PO daily for 2 weeks, max 8 mg/day. Elderly (age older than 65 yo): 4 mg PO daily, max 8 mg/day. [Generic/Trade: Tabs scored 2, 4, 8 mg.] ▶K ♀D ▶? $ ■

QUINAPRIL (*Accupril*) HTN: (Start 10 to 20 mg PO daily (start 10 mg/day if elderly), usual maintenance dose 20 to 80 mg PO daily or divided two times per day, max 80 mg/day. Heart failure: Start 5 mg PO two times per day, usual maintenance dose 10 to 20 mg PO two times per day. [Generic/Trade: Tabs, scored 5, unscored 10, 20, 40 mg.] ▶LK ♀D ▶? $$ ■

RAMIPRIL (*Altace*) HTN: 2.5 mg PO daily, usual maintenance dose 2.5 to 20 mg PO daily or divided two times per day, max 20 mg/day. Heart failure post-MI: Start 2.5 mg PO two times per day, usual maintenance dose 5 mg PO two times per day. Reduce risk of MI, CVA, death from cardiovascular causes: 2.5 mg PO daily for 1 week, then 5 mg daily for 3 weeks, increase as tolerated to max 10 mg/day. [Generic/Trade: Caps 1.25, 2.5, 5, 10 mg.] ▶LK ♀D ▶? $$$ ■

TRANDOLAPRIL (*Mavik*) HTN: Start 1 mg PO daily, usual maintenance dose 2 to 4 mg PO daily or divided two times per day, max 8 mg/day. Heart failure/post-MI: Start 1 mg PO daily, usual maintenance dose 4 mg PO daily. Renal impairment or concomitant diuretic therapy: Start 0.5 mg PO daily. [Generic/Trade: Tabs, scored 1, unscored 2, 4 mg.] ▶LK ♀D ▶? $$ ■

Aldosterone Antagonists

NOTE: *Hyperkalemia possible, especially if used concomitantly with other drugs that increase K+ (including K+ containing salt substitutes) and in patients with heart failure, DM, or renal impairment.*

EPLERENONE (*Inspra*) HTN: Start 50 mg PO daily; max 50 mg two times per day. Improve survival of stable patients with LV systolic dysfunction (LVEF 40% or less) and heart failure post MI: Start 25 mg PO daily; titrate to target dose 50 mg daily within 4 weeks, if tolerated. [Generic/trade: Tabs unscored 25, 50 mg.] ▶L ♀B ▶? $$$

SPIRONOLACTONE (*Aldactone*) HTN: 50 to 100 mg PO daily or divided two times per day. Edema: 25 to 200 mg/day. Hypokalemia: 25 to 100 mg PO daily. Primary hyperaldosteronism, maintenance: 100 to 400 mg/day PO. Heart failure, NYHA III or IV: 25 to 50 mg PO daily. [Generic/Trade: Tabs, unscored 25 mg scored 50, 100 mg.] ▶LK ♀D ▶+ $ ■

Angiotensin Receptor Blockers (ARBs)

NOTE: *See also antihypertensive combinations. Avoid concomitant ACE inhibitor use. Contraindicated in pregnancy. Do not use with aliskerin in patients with DM or CrCl < 60 mL/min. Dual inhibition of renin-angiotensin system increases risk of renal impairment, hypotension, and hyperkalemia. Hyperkalemia possible, especially if used concomitantly with other drugs that increase K+ (including K+ containing salt substitutes) and in patients with heart failure, DM, or renal impairment. Concomitant NSAID, including selective COX-2 inhibitors, may further deteriorate renal function and decrease antihypertensive effects.*

AZILSARTAN (*Edarbi*) HTN: 80 mg daily. [Trade only: Tabs, unscored 40, 80 mg.] ▶L – ♀D ▶? $$$ ■

CANDESARTAN (*Atacand*) HTN: Start 16 mg PO daily, maximum 32 mg/day. Heart failure (NYHA II–IV and LVEF 40% or less): Start 4 mg PO daily, maximum 32 mg/day. [Trade only: Tabs, unscored 4, 8, 16, 32 mg.] ▶K ♀D ▶? $$$ ■

EPROSARTAN (*Teveten*, ✦*Teveten*) HTN: Start 600 mg PO daily, maximum 800 mg/day given daily or divided two times per day. [Generic/Trade: Tabs, unscored 400, 600 mg.] ▶Fecal excretion ♀D ▶? $$$$ ■

IRBESARTAN (*Avapro*) HTN: Start 150 mg PO daily, maximum 300 mg/day. Type 2 diabetic nephropathy: Start 150 mg PO daily, target dose 300 mg daily. [Generic/Trade: Tabs, unscored 75, 150, 300 mg.] ▶L ♀D ▶? $ ■

LOSARTAN (*Cozaar*) HTN: Start 50 mg PO daily, max 100 mg/day given daily or divided two times per day. Volume-depleted patients or history of hepatic impairment: Start 25 mg PO daily. CVA risk reduction in patients with HTN and LV hypertrophy (may not be effective in black patients): Start 50 mg PO daily. If need more BP reduction add HCTZ 12.5 mg PO daily, then increase losartan to 100 mg/day, then increase HCTZ to 25 mg/day. Type 2 diabetic nephropathy: Start 50 mg PO daily, target dose 100 mg daily. [Generic/Trade: Tabs, unscored 25, 50, 100 mg.] ▶L ♀D ▶? $$$ ■

OLMESARTAN (*Benicar*, ✦*Olmetec*) HTN: Start 20 mg PO daily, max 40 mg/day. [Trade only: Tabs, unscored 5, 20, 40 mg.] ▶K ♀D ▶? $$$ ■

TELMISARTAN (*Micardis*) HTN: Start 40 mg PO daily, max 80 mg/day. Cardiovascular risk reduction: Start 80 mg PO daily, max 80 mg/day. [Trade only: Tabs, unscored 20, 40, 80 mg.] ▶L ♀D ▶? $$$ ■

VALSARTAN (*Diovan*) HTN: Start 80 to 160 mg PO daily, max 320 mg/day. Heart failure: Start 40 mg PO two times per day, target dose 160 mg two times per day. Reduce mortality/morbidity post-MI with LV systolic dysfunction/failure: Start 20 mg PO two times per day, target dose 160 mg two times per day. [Trade only: Tabs, scored 40, unscored 80, 160, 320 mg.] ▶L ♀D ▶? $$$ ■

Anti-Dysrhythmics/Cardiac Arrest

ADENOSINE (*Adenocard*) PSVT conversion (not A-fib): Adult and peds wt 50 kg or greater: 6 mg rapid IV and flush, preferably through a central line. If no response after 1 to 2 min, then 12 mg. A 3rd dose of 12 mg may be given prn.

(cont.)

SELECTED DRUGS THAT MAY PROLONG THE QT INTERVAL

alfuzosin	erythromycin*†	lithium	quinidine*†
amantadine	escitalopram	methadone*†	ranolazine
amiodarone*†	famotidine	mirtazapine	risperidone
arsenic trioxide*	felbamate	moexipril/HCTZ	saquinavir
atazanavir	fingolimod	moxifloxacin*	sevoflurane
azithromycin*	flecainide*	nicardipine	sotalol*†
bedaquiline	foscarnet	nilotinib	sunitinib
chloroquine*	fosphenytoin	ofloxacin	tacrolimus
chlorpromazine*	gatifloxacin	olanzapine	tamoxifen
cisapride*	gemifloxacin	ondansetron	telithromycin
citalopram*	granisetron	oxytocin	thioridazine*†
clarithromycin*	halofantrine*†	paliperidone	tizanidine
clozapine	haloperidol*	pentamidine*†	tolterodine
disopyramide*†	ibutilide*†	perflutren lipid microspheres	vandetanib*
dofetilide*†	iloperidone	phenothiazines‡	vardenafil
dolasetron	indapamide	pimozide*†	venlafaxi‑ne
dronedarone	isradipine	procainamide*	voriconazole
droperidol*	lapatinib	quetiapine	ziprasidone
eribulin	levofloxacin		

NOTE: This table may not include all drugs that prolong the QT interval or cause torsades. Risk of drug-induced QT prolongation may be increased in women, elderly, hypokalemia, hypomagnesemia, bradycardia, starvation, CHF, and CNS injuries. Hepatorenal dysfunction and drug interactions can increase the concentration of QT interval-prolonging drugs. Coadministration of QT interval prolonging drugs can have additive effects. Avoid these (and other) drugs in congenital prolonged QT syndrome (www.qtdrugs.org).
*Torsades reported in product labeling/case reports.
†Increased in women.

Peds wt less than 50 kg: Initial dose 50 to 100 mcg/kg, subsequent doses 100 to 200 mcg/kg q 1 to 2 min prn up to a max single dose of 300 mcg/kg or 12 mg, whichever is less. Half-life is less than 10 sec. Give doses by rapid IV push followed by NS flush. Need higher dose if on theophylline or caffeine, lower dose if on dipyridamole or carbamazepine ▶Plasma ♀C ▶? $$$
AMIODARONE (Cordarone, Pacerone) Proarrhythmic. Life-threatening ventricular arrhythmia without cardiac arrest: Load 150 mg IV over 10 min, then 1 mg/min for 6 h, then 0.5 mg/min for 18 h. Mix in D5W. Oral loading dose 800 to 1600 mg PO daily for 1 to 3 weeks, reduce to 400 to 800 mg PO daily for 1 month when arrhythmia is controlled, reduce to lowest effective dose thereafter, usually 200 to 400 mg PO daily. Photosensitivity with oral therapy. Pulmonary and hepatic toxicity. Hypo- or hyperthyroidism possible. Coadministration of fluoroquinolones, macrolides, loratadine, trazodone,

(cont.)

azoles, or Class IA and III antiarrhythmic drugs may prolong QTc. May increase digoxin levels; discontinue digoxin or decrease dose by 50%. May increase INR with warfarin; decrease warfarin dose by 33 to 50%. Do not use with grapefruit juice. Do not use with simvastatin dose greater than 20 mg/day, lovastatin dose greater than 40 mg/day; may increase atorvastatin level; increases risk of myopathy and rhabdomyolysis. Caution with beta-blockers and calcium channel blockers. IV therapy may cause hypotension. Contraindicated with marked sinus bradycardia and 2nd or 3rd degree heart block in the absence of a functioning pacemaker. [Trade only (Pacerone): tabs, unscored 100 mg. Generic/Trade: Tabs, scored 200, 400 mg.] ▶L ♀D ▶– $$$$ ■

ATROPINE (*AtroPen*) Bradyarrhythmia/CPR: 0.5 to 1 mg IV q 3 to 5 min to max 0.04 mg/kg (3 mg). Peds: 0.02 mg/kg/dose; minimum single dose, 0.1 mg; max cumulative dose, 1 mg. [Trade only: Prefilled auto-injector pen: 0.25 mg (yellow), 0.5 mg (blue), 1 mg (dark red), 2 mg (green).] ▶K ♀C ▶– $

DIGOXIN (*Lanoxin, Lanoxicaps, Digitek, ✚ Toloxin*) Proarrhythmic. Systolic heart failure/rate control of chronic A-fib: Younger than 70 yo: 0.25 mg PO daily; age 70 yo or older: 0.125 mg PO daily; impaired renal function: 0.0625 to 0.125 mg PO daily. Rapid A-fib: Total loading dose (TLD), 10 to 15 mcg/kg IV/PO, give in 3 divided doses q 6 to 8 h; give ~50% TLD for 1 dose, then ~25% TLD for 2 doses (eg, 70 kg with normal renal function: 0.5 mg, then 0.25 mg q 6 to 8 h for 2 doses). Impaired renal function, 6 to 10 mcg/kg IV/PO TLD, given in 3 divided 0.125 to 0.375 mg IV/PO daily. [Generic/Trade: Tabs, scored (Lanoxin, Digitek) 0.125, 0.25 mg; elixir 0.05 mg/mL. Trade only: Caps (Lanoxicaps), 0.1, 0.2 mg.] ▶K ♀C ▶+ $

DIGOXIN IMMUNE FAB (*Digibind, DigiFab*) Digoxin toxicity: Acute ingestion of known amount: 1 vial binds approximately 0.5 mg digoxin. Acute ingestion of unknown amount: 10 vials IV, may repeat once. Toxicity during chronic therapy: 6 vials usually adequate; one formula is: Number vials = (serum dig level in ng/mL) × (kg)/100. ▶K ♀C ▶? $$$$$

DISOPYRAMIDE (*Norpace, Norpace CR, ✚ Rythmodan, Rythmodan-LA*) Proarrhythmic. Rarely indicated, consult cardiologist. Ventricular arrhythmia: 400 to 800 mg PO daily in divided doses (immediate-release is divided q 6 h; extended-release is divided q 12 h). [Generic/Trade: Caps, immediate-release 100, 150 mg; extended-release 150 mg. Trade only: Caps, extended-release 100 mg.] ▶KL ♀C ▶+ $$$$ ■

DOFETILIDE (*Tikosyn*) Proarrhythmic. Conversion of A-fib/flutter: Specialized dosing based on CrCl and QTc interval. Available only to hospitals and prescribers who have received appropriate dosing and treatment-initiation education. [Trade only: Caps, 0.125, 0.25, 0.5 mg.] ▶KL ♀C ▶– $$$$ ■

DRONEDARONE (*Multaq*) Proarrhythmic. Reduce hospitalization risk for patients with atrial fib who are in sinus rhythm and have a history of paroxysmal or persistent atrial fib: 400 mg PO two times per day with morning and evening meals. Do not use with permanent atrial fibrillation. NYHA Class IV heart failure or NYHA Class II to III heart failure with recent decompensation requiring hospitalization or referral to heart failure clinic; 2nd or 3rd degree AV block or sick sinus syndrome without functioning pacemaker; bradycardia less than 50 bpm;

(cont.)

QTc Bazett interval longer than 500 ms; liver or lung toxicity related to previous amiodarone use; severe hepatic impairment; pregnancy; lactation; grapefruit juice; drugs or herbals that increase QT interval; Class I or III antiarrhythmic agents; potent inhibitors of CYP3A4 enzyme system (clarithromycin, itraconazole, ketoconazole, nefazodone, ritonavir, voriconazole); or inducers of CYP3A4 enzyme system (carbamazepine, phenytoin, phenobarbital, rifampin, St. John's wort). Correct hypo/hyperkalemia and hypomagnesemia before giving. Monitor EKG q 3 months; if in atrial fib, then either discontinue dronedarone or cardiovert. May initiate or worsen heart failure symptoms. May be associated with hepatic injury; discontinue if hepatic injury is suspected. Serum creatinine and/or BUN may increase during 1st weeks, but does not reflect change in renal function; reversible when discontinued. Give with appropriate antithrombotic therapy. May increase INR when used with warfarin. May increase dabigatran level. May increase digoxin level; discontinue digoxin or decrease dose by 50%. Use cautiously with beta-blockers (BB) and calcium channel blockers (CCB); initiate lower doses of BB or CCB; initiate at low dose and monitor EKG. Do not use with more than 10 mg of simvastatin. May increase level of sirolimus, tacrolimus, or CYP3A4 substrates with narrow therapeutic index. [Trade: Tabs, unscored 400 mg.] ▶L ♀X $$$$ ■

FLECAINIDE (*Tambocor*) Proarrhythmic. Prevention of paroxysmal atrial fib/flutter or PSVT, with symptoms and no structural heart disease: Start 50 mg PO q 12 h, may increase by 50 mg two times per day q 4 days, max 300 mg/day. Use with AV nodal slowing agent (beta-blocker, verapamil, diltiazem) to minimize risk of 1:1 atrial flutter. Life-threatening ventricular arrhythmias without structural heart disease: Start 100 mg PO q 12 h, may increase by 50 mg two times per day q 4 days, max 400 mg/day. With CrCl less than 35 mL/min: Start 50 mg PO two times per day. [Generic/Trade: Tabs, unscored 50 mg, scored 100, 150 mg.] ▶K ♀C ▶– $$$$ ■

IBUTILIDE (*Corvert*) Proarrhythmic. Recent onset A-fib/flutter: 0.01 mg/kg up to 1 mg IV over 10 min, may repeat once if no response after 10 min. Keep on cardiac monitor at least 4 h. ▶K ♀C ▶? $$$$$ ■

ISOPROTERENOL (*Isuprel*) Refractory bradycardia or 3rd degree AV block: Bolus method: 0.02 to 0.06 mg IV; infusion method, dilute 2 mg in 250 mL D5W (8 mcg/mL); a rate of 37.5 mL/h delivers 5 mcg/min. Peds infusion method: 0.05 to 2 mcg/kg/min. Using the same concentration as adult for a 10 kg child; a rate of 8 mL/h delivers 0.1 mcg/kg/min. ▶LK ♀C ▶? $$$

LIDOCAINE (*Xylocaine, Xylocard*) Ventricular arrhythmia: Load 1 mg/kg IV, then 0.5 mg/kg q 8 to 10 min prn to max 3 mg/kg. IV infusion: 4 g in 500 mL D5W (8 mg/mL) run at rate of 7.5 to 30 mL/h to deliver 1 to 4 mg/min. Peds: 20 to 50 mcg/kg/min. ▶LK ♀B ▶? $

MEXILETINE (*Mexitil*) Proarrhythmic. Rarely indicated, consult cardiologist. Ventricular arrhythmia: Start 200 mg PO q 8 h with food or antacid, max dose 1200 mg/day. [Generic only: Caps 150, 200, 250 mg.] ▶L ♀C ▶– $$$ ■

PROCAINAMIDE (*Pronestyl, ✦Procan SR*) Proarrhythmic. Ventricular arrhythmia: Loading dose: 100 mg IV q 10 min or 20 mg/min (150 mL/h) until QRS widens more than 50%, dysrhythmia suppressed, hypotension, or total of

(cont.)

17 mg/kg or 1000 mg delivered. Infusion: dilute 2 g in 250 mL D5W (8 mg/mL) rate of 15 to 45 mL/h to deliver 2 to 6 mg/min. ▶LK ♀C ▶? $ ■

PROPAFENONE (*Rythmol, Rythmol SR*) Proarrhythmic. Prevention of paroxysmal atrial fib/flutter or PSVT, with symptoms and no structural heart disease; or life-threatening ventricular arrhythmias: Start (immediate-release) 150 mg PO q 8 h; may increase after 3 to 4 days to 225 mg PO q 8 h; max 900 mg/day. Prolong time to recurrence of symptomatic atrial fib without structural heart disease: 225 mg SR PO q 12 h, may increase after 5 days to 325 mg SR PO q 12 h, max 425 mg SR PO q 12 h. Consider using with AV nodal blocking agent (beta-blocker, verapamil, diltiazem) to minimize risk of 1:1 atrial flutter. [Generic/Trade: Tabs, immediate-release scored 150, 225, 300 mg. Trade only: Tabs, SR, Caps 225, 325, 425 mg.] ▶L ♀C ▶? $$$$ ■

QUINIDINE Proarrhythmic. Arrhythmia: Gluconate, extended-release: 324 to 648 mg PO q 8 to 12 h; sulfate, immediate-release: 200 to 400 mg PO q 6 to 8 h; sulfate, extended-release: 300 to 600 mg PO q 8 to 12 h. [Generic gluconate: Tabs, extended-release unscored 324 mg. Generic sulfate: Tabs, scored immediate-release 200, 300 mg, Tabs, extended-release 300 mg.] ▶LK ♀C ▶+ $$$-gluconate, $-sulfate ■

SODIUM BICARBONATE Severe acidosis: 1 mEq/kg IV up to 50 to 100 mEq/ dose. ▶K ♀C ▶? $

SOTALOL (*Betapace, Betapace AF, ✦ Rylosol*) Proarrhythmic. Ventricular arrhythmia (Betapace), A-fib/A-flutter (Betapace AF): Start 80 mg PO two times per day, max 640 mg/day. Initiate or re-initiate this product in a facility with cardiac resuscitation capacity, continuous EKG and CrCl monitoring. Do not substitute Betapace for Betapace AF. [Generic/Trade: Tabs, scored 80, 120, 160, 240 mg, Tabs, scored (Betapace AF) 80, 120, 160 mg.] ▶K ♀B ▶− $$$$ ■

Anti-Hyperlipidemic Agents—Bile Acid Sequestrants

CHOLESTYRAMINE (*Questran, Questran Light, Prevalite, LoCHOLEST, LoCHOLEST Light, ✦ Olestyr*) Elevated LDL-C: Powder: Start 4 g PO daily to two times per day before meals, increase up to max 24 g/day. [Generic/ Trade: Powder for oral susp, 4 g cholestyramine resin/9 g powder (Questran, LoCHOLEST), 4 g cholestyramine resin/5 g powder (Questran Light), 4 g cholestyramine resin/5.5 g powder (Prevalite, LoCHOLEST Light). Each available in bulk powder and single-dose packets.] ▶Not absorbed ♀C ▶+ $$$

COLESEVELAM (*Welchol, ✦ Lodalis*) LDL-C reduction or glycemic control of type 2 diabetes: 3.75 g once daily or 1.875 g PO two times per day, max 3.75 g/day. Give with meal and 4 to 8 ounces of water, fruit juice, or diet soft drink. 3.75 g is equivalent to 6 tabs; 1.875 g is equivalent to 3 tabs. Powder packets contain phenylalanine. [Trade only: Tabs, unscored 625 mg. Powder, single-dose packets 1.875, 3.75 g] ▶Not absorbed ♀B ▶+ $$$$$

COLESTIPOL (*Colestid, Colestid Flavored*) Elevated LDL-C: Tabs: Start 2 g PO daily to two times per day with full glass of liquid, max 16 g/day. Granules: Start 5 g PO daily to two times per day, max 30 g/day. Mix granules in at least

(cont.)

90 mL of non-carbonated liquid. Administer other drugs at least 1 h before or 4 to 6 h after colestipol. [Generic/Trade: Tabs 1 g. Granules for oral susp, 5 g/7.5 g powder.] ▶Not absorbed ♀B ▶+ $$$$

LIPID REDUCTION BY CLASS/AGENT[1]

Drug class/agent	LDL-C	HDL-C	TG
Bile acid sequestrants[2]	↓ 15–30%	↑ 3–5%	No change or ↑
Cholesterol absorption inhibitor[3]	↓ 18%	↑ 1%	↓ 8%
Fibrates[4]	↓ 5–20%	↑ 10–20%	↓ 20–50%
Lovastatin+ER niacin[5]*	↓ 30–42%	↑ 20–30%	↓ 32–44%
Niacin[5]*	↓ 5–25%	↑ 15–35%	↓ 20–50%
Omega 3 fatty acids[7]	↓ 5% or ↑ 44%	↓ 4% or ↑ 9%	↓ 27–45 %
Statins[8]	↓ 18–63%	↑ 5–15%	↓ 7–35%
Simvastatin+ezetimibe[9]	↓ 45–59%	↑ 6–10%	↓ 23–31%

[1]LDL = low density lipoprotein. HDL = high density lipoprotein. TG = triglycerides. ER = extended-release. Adapted from NCEP: JAMA 2001; 285:2486 and prescribing information.
[2]Cholestyramine (4–16 g), colestipol (5–20 g), colesevelam (2.6–3.8 g).
[3]Ezetimibe (10 mg). When added to statin therapy, will ↓ LDL 25%, ↑ HDL 3%, ↓ TG 14% in addition to statin effects.
[4]Fenofibrate (145–200 mg), gemfibrozil (600 mg two times per day).
[5]Advicor® (20/1000–40/2000 mg).
[6]Extended-release nicotinic acid (Niaspan® 1–2 g), immediate-release (crystalline) nicotinic acid (1.5–3 g), sustained-release nicotinic acid (Slo-Niacin® 1–2 g).
[7]Lovaza (4 g), Vascepa (4 g)
[8]Atorvastatin (10–80 mg), fluvastatin (20–80 mg), lovastatin (20–80 mg), pravastatin (20–80 mg), rosuvastatin (5–40 mg), simvastatin (20–40 mg).
[9]Vytorin® (10/10–10/40 mg).
*Lowers lipoprotein a.

Anti-Hyperlipidemic Agents—Fibrates

NOTE: *Contraindicated with active liver disease, gall bladder disease, and/or CrCl less than 30 mL/min. Monitor LFTs periodically. Increased risk of myopathy and rhabdomyolysis when used with a statin or colchicine. May increase cholesterol excretion into bile, leading to cholelithiasis. May increase the effect of warfarin; monitor INR. Take either at least 2 h before or 4 h after bile acid sequestrants.*

BEZAFIBRATE (◆ *Bezalip SR*) Canada only. Hyperlipidemia/hypertriglyceridemia: 400 mg of sustained-release PO daily. [Canada Trade only: Sustained-release tab 400 mg.] ▶K ♀D ▶– $$$
FENOFIBRATE (*TriCor, Antara, Fenoglide, Lipofen, Triglide,* ◆ *Lipidil Micro, Lipidil Supra, Lipidil EZ*) Hypertriglyceridemia: TriCor tabs: 48 to 145 mg PO daily, max 145 mg daily. Antara: 43 to 130 mg PO daily; max 130 mg daily. Fenoglide: 40 to 120 mg PO daily; max 120 mg daily. Lipofen: 50 to 150 mg PO daily, max 150 mg daily. Triglide: 50 to 160 mg PO daily, max 160 mg daily. Generic tabs: 54 to 160 mg, max 160 mg daily. Generic caps: 67 to 200 mg PO

(cont.)

daily; max 200 mg daily. Hypercholesterolemia/mixed dyslipidemia: TriCor tabs: 145 mg PO daily. Antara: 130 mg PO daily. Fenoglide: 120 mg daily. Lipofen: 150 mg daily. Triglide: 160 mg daily. Generic tabs: 160 mg daily. Generic caps 200 mg PO daily. All formulations, except Antara, TriCor, and Triglide, should be taken with food. [Generic only: Tabs, unscored 54, 160 mg. Generic caps 67, 134, 200 mg. Generic/Trade: Tabs (TriCor), unscored 48, 145 mg. Caps (Antara) 43, 130 mg. Trade only: Tabs (Fenoglide), unscored 40, 120 mg. Tabs (Lipofen), unscored 50, 150 mg. Tabs (Triglide), unscored 50, 160 mg.]   ▶LK ♀C ▶– $$$

LDL CHOLESTEROL GOALS[1]

Risk Category	Patient characteristics	LDL-C goal	Treatment[a]
Very high risk	Atherosclerosis[b] (CAD or PAD)	< 70	drug[c] if above goal
High risk	DM; CKD; or ≥ 2 RF + 10-year CHD risk > 20%	< 100 (optional < 70 if baseline < 100)	drug[c] if above goal
Moderately high risk	≥ 2 RF + 10-year CHD risk 10–20%[e]	<130 (optional < 100 if baseline 100–129)[f]	drug[c] if above goal
Moderate risk	≥ 2 RF + 10-year CHD risk <10%[e]	<130	drug[c] if LDL-C ≥ 160
Lower risk	≤ 1 RF (almost all have 10-year CHD risk < 10%[e]	< 160	drug[c] if LDL-C ≥ 190

Adapted from: NCEP: *JAMA* 2001;285:2486–97. NCEP Report: *Circulation* 2004;110:227-39. *Circulation* 2011;123:1243-1262. *Stroke* 2011;42:227-276. *Am J Kidney* Dis 2003;41(4 suppl 3):I-IV, S1-S91. *Circulation* 2011;124:2458-2473. *Circulation*. 2006;113:e463-e654. *Stroke*. 2011;42:517-584. *JAMA* 2007;297(6):611-619. *Circulation* 2008;118:2243-2251.

CAD = coronary artery disease (includes prior myocardial infarction, percutaneous coronary intervention, or bypass surgery; angina pectoris; silent ischemia). CHD = coronary heart disease. CKD = chronic kidney disease. DM = diabetes mellitus. LDL-C = low-density lipoprotein cholesterol. PAD = peripheral artery disease (includes carotid artery disease, history of ischemic stroke or transient ischemic attack, abdominal aortic aneurysm, renal artery stenosis). RF = risk factors [age (men ≥45 yo, women ≥55 yo); current cigarette smoking; hypertension (SBP ≥ 140, DBP ≥ 90, or on medication to lower blood pressure); HDL-C (men < 40 mg/dL, women < 50 mg/dL. If HDL-C ≥ 60 mg/dL, this is desirable and counts as a negative risk factor; subtract 1 point.); family history of premature coronary heart disease (men, 1st-degree relative < 55 yo; women, 1st -degree relative < 65 yo)].

[a] When lifestyle-related risk factors (obesity, physical inactivity, ☒ triglycerides, ☒ HDL, metabolic syndrome, tobacco use) are present, recommend dietary modification, weight reduction, exercise, tobacco cessation regardless of LDL-C.

[b] LDL-C goal of less than 70 mg/dL is reasonable for any patient with evidence of atherosclerotic disease.

[c] Statins preferred; achieve at least a 30–40% LDL-C reduction.

[d] If baseline LDL-C is below 100 mg/dL, LDL-C–lowering therapy is an option based on clinical trials.

[e] 10-year risks for patients without CAD, PAD, diabetes, and/or CKD are based on either Framingham stratification (electronic calculators are available at www.nhlbi.nih.gov/guidelines/cholesterol) or Reynolds Risk Score (electronic calculator is available at www.reynoldsriskscore.org/).

[f] At baseline or after lifestyle changes, initiating therapy to achieve LDL-C less than 100 mg/dL is an option based on clinical trials.

CARDIOVASCULAR

FENOFIBRIC ACID   (*Fibricor, TriLipix*) In combination with statin for mixed dyslipidemia and CHD or CHD risk equivalent: TriLipix: 135 mg PO daily. Hypertriglyceridemia: Fibricor: 35 to 105 mg PO daily, max 105 mg daily. TriLipix: 45 to 135 mg PO daily, max 135 mg daily. Hypercholesterolemia/mixed dyslipidemia: Fibricor: 105 mg PO daily. TriLipix: 135 mg PO daily. [Trade only: Caps (TriLipix) delayed-release 45, 135 mg. Tabs (Fibricor) 35, 105 mg. Generic only: Tabs 35, 105 mg.] ▶LK ♀C ▶– $$$

GEMFIBROZIL   (*Lopid*) Hypertriglyceridemia/primary prevention of CAD: 600 mg PO two times per day 30 min before meals. Not as safe as fenofibrate or fenofibric acid when used in combination with a statin. [Generic/Trade: Tabs, scored 600 mg.] ▶LK ♀C ▶? $$$

Anti-Hyperlipidemic Agents—HMG-CoA Reductase Inhibitors ("Statins") and Combinations

NOTE: *Each statin has restricted maximum doses that are lower than typical maximum doses when used with certain interacting medications; see prescribing information for complete information. Muscle issues: Measure creatine kinase before starting therapy. Evaluate muscle symptoms before starting therapy, 6 to 12 weeks after starting/increasing therapy and at each follow-up visit. Risk of muscle issues increase with advanced age (65 yo or older), female gender, uncontrolled hypothyroidism, renal impairment, higher statin doses, and concomitant use of certain medicines (eg, fibrates, niacin 1 g or more, colchicine, or ranolazine). Teach patients to report promptly unexplained muscle pain, tenderness, or weakness; rule out common causes; discontinue if myopathy diagnosed or suspected. Obtain creatine kinase, TSH, vitamin D level when patient complains of muscle soreness, tenderness, weakness, or pain. Hepatotoxicity: Rare. Monitor LFTs before initiating statin therapy and as clinically indicated thereafter. Statins may increase the risk of hyperglycemia (and type 2 diabetes) or transient memory problems; benefits usually outweigh risks.*

ADVICOR   (*lovastatin + niacin*) Hyperlipidemia: 1 tab PO at bedtime, max 40/2000 mg/day. [Trade only: Tabs, unscored extended-release lovastatin/niacin 20/500, 20/750, 20/1000, 40/1000 mg.] ▶LK ♀X ▶– $$$$

ATORVASTATIN   (*Lipitor*) Hyperlipidemia/prevention of cardiovascular events, including type 2 DM: Start 10 to 40 mg PO daily, max 80 mg/day. Do not give with cyclosporine, tipranavir + ritonavir, or telaprevir. Use with caution and lowest dose necessary with lopinavir + ritonavir. Do not exceed 20 mg/day when given with clarithromycin, itraconazole, other protease inhibitors (saquinavir + ritonavir, darunavir + ritonavir, fosamprenavir, or fosamprenavir + ritonavir). Do not exceed 40 mg/day when given with boceprevir or nelfinavir. [Generic/Trade Tabs, unscored 10, 20, 40, 80 mg.] ▶L ♀X ▶– $

CADUET   (*amlodipine + atorvastatin*) Simultaneous treatment of HTN and hypercholesterolemia: Establish dose using component drugs first. Dosing

(cont.)

interval: Daily. [Trade only: Tabs, 2.5/10, 2.5/20, 2.5/40, 5/10, 5/20, 5/40, 5/80, 10/10, 10/20, 10/40, 10/80 mg.] ▶L ♀X ▶– $$$$

FLUVASTATIN (*Lescol, Lescol XL*) Hyperlipidemia: Start 20 to 80 mg PO at bedtime, max 80 mg daily (XL) or divided two times per day. Post-percutaneous coronary intervention: 80 mg of extended-release PO daily, max 80 mg daily. Do not exceed 20 mg/day when given with cylosporine or fluconazole. [Generic/Trade: Caps 20, 40 mg. Trade only: Tabs, extended-release unscored 80 mg.] ▶L ♀X ▶– $$$$

LIPTRUZET (**ezetimibe + atorvastatin**) Start 10/10 or 10/20 mg PO daily, max 10/80 mg/day. See component drugs for other dose restrictions. [Trade only: Tabs, unscored ezetimibe/atorvastatin 10/10, 10/20, 10/40, 10/80 mg.] ▶L – ♀X ▶– $$$$

LOVASTATIN (*Mevacor, Altoprev*) Hyperlipidemia/prevention of cardiovascular events: Start 20 mg PO q pm, max 80 mg/day daily or divided two times per day. Do not use with boceprevir, clarithromycin, cyclosporine, erythromycin, gemfibrozil, grapefruit juice, HIV protease inhibitors, itraconazole, ketoconazole, nefazodone, posaconazole, telaprevir, telithromycin, or voriconazole; increases risk of myopathy. Do not exceed 20 mg/day when used with danazol, diltiazem, dronedarone, verapamil, or CrCl less than 30 mL/min. Do not exceed 40 mg/day when used with amiodarone. [Generic/Trade: Tabs, unscored 20, 40 mg. Trade only: Tabs, extended-release (Altoprev) 20, 40, 60 mg.] ▶L ♀X ▶– $

PITAVASTATIN (*Livalo*) Hyperlipidemia: Start 2 mg PO at bedtime, max 4 mg daily. CrCl 15 to 59 mL/min or on dialysis: Max start 1 mg PO daily, max 2 mg daily. Do not use with cyclosporine. Do not exceed 1 mg/day when given with erythromycin. Do not exceed 2 mg/day when given with rifampin. [Trade only: Tabs 1, 2, 4 mg.] ▶L – ♀X ▶– $$$$

PRAVASTATIN (*Pravachol*) Hyperlipidemia/prevention of cardiovascular events: Start 40 mg PO daily, max 80 mg/day. Do not exceed 20 mg/day when given with cyclosporine. Do not exceed 40 mg/day when given with clarithromycin. [Generic/Trade: Tabs, unscored 10, 20, 40, 80 mg.] ▶L ♀X ▶– $

(cont.)

LDL-C reduction by statin dose

Statin	Dose to get at least 30-40% LDL-C reduction(LDL-C reduction)*	Dose to get at least 50% LDL-C reduction(LDL-C reduction)
atorvastatin	10 mg (−39%)	40 mg (-50%)
fluvastatin	40 mg twice daily (−36%)	n/a
fluvastatin XL	80 mg (−35%)	n/a
lovastatin	40 mg (−31%)	n/a
pitavastatin	2 mg (−36%)	n/a
pravastatin	40 mg (−34%)	n/a
rosuvastatin	5 mg (−45%)	10 mg (-52%)
simvastatin	20 mg (−38%)	n/a

LDL = low-density lipoprotein. Will get ~6% decrease in LDL with every doubling of dose.
*Adapted from *Circulation* 2004;110:227-239 and prescribing information.

CARDIOVASCULAR

ROSUVASTATIN (*Crestor*) Hyperlipidemia/slow progression of atherosclerosis/primary prevention of cardiovascular disease: Start 10 to 20 mg PO daily, max 40 mg/day. Renal impairment (CrCl less than 30 mL/min and not on hemodialysis): Start 5 mg PO daily, max 10 mg/day. Asians: Start 5 mg PO daily. When given with atazanavir with or without ritonavir or lopinavir with ritonavir, do not exceed 10 mg/day. When given with cyclosporine, do not exceed 5 mg/day. Avoid using with gemfibrozil; if used concomitantly, do not exceed 10 mg/day. [Trade only: Tabs, unscored 5, 10, 20, 40 mg.] ▶L ♀X ▶– $$$$

SIMCOR (simvastatin + niacin) Hyperlipidemia: 1 tab PO at bedtime with a low-fat snack, max 40/2000 mg/day. If niacin-naive or switching from immediate-release niacin, start: 20/500 mg PO q pm. If receiving extended-release niacin, do not start with more than 40/2000 mg PO q pm. Do not use with boceprevir, clarithromycin, cyclosporine, danazol, diltiazem, erythromycin, fenofibrate, gemfibrozil, grapefruit juice, HIV protease inhibitors, itraconazole, ketoconazole, nefazodone, posaconazole, strong CYP3A4 inhibitors, telaprevir, telithromycin, verapamil; increases risk of myopathy. Do not exceed 20/1000 mg/day when used in Chinese patients or with amiodarone, amlodipine, or ranolazine; increases risk of myopathy. Immediate-release aspirin or NSAID 30 min prior may decrease niacin-flushing reaction. Niacin may worsen glucose control, peptic ulcer disease, gout, headaches, and menopausal flushing. Swallow whole; do not break, chew, or crush. [Trade only: Tabs, unscored extended-release simvastatin/niacin 20/500, 20/750, 20/1000 mg.] ▶LK ♀X ▶– $$$

SIMVASTATIN (*Zocor*) Do not initiate therapy with or titrate to 80 mg/day; only use 80 mg/day in patients who have taken this dose for more than 12 months without evidence of muscle toxicity. Hyperlipidemia: Start 10 to 20 mg PO q pm, max 40 mg/day. Reduce cardiovascular mortality/events in high risk for coronary heart disease event: Start 40 mg PO q pm, max 40 mg/day. Severe renal impairment: Start 5 mg/day, closely monitor. Chinese patients: Do not exceed 20 mg/day with niacin 1 g or more daily. Do not use with boceprevir, clarithromycin, cyclosporine, danazol, erythromycin, gemfibrozil, grapefruit juice, HIV protease inhibitors, itraconazole, ketoconazole, nefazodone, posaconazole, strong CYP3A4 inhibitors, telaprevir, telithromycin, voriconazole; increases risk of myopathy. Do not exceed 10 mg/day when used with diltiazem, dronedarone, or verapamil. Do not exceed 20 mg/day when used with amiodarone, amlodipine, or ranolazine. [Generic/Trade: Tabs, unscored 5, 10, 20, 40, 80 mg.] ▶L ♀X ▶– $$$$

VYTORIN (ezetimibe + simvastatin) Hyperlipidemia: Start 10/10 or 10/20 mg PO q pm, max 10/40 mg/day. Restrict the use of the 10/80 mg dose to patients who have taken it at least 12 months without muscle toxicity. See simvastatin monograph for other dose restrictions. [Trade only: Tabs, unscored ezetimibe/simvastatin 10/10, 10/20, 10/40, 10/80 mg.] ▶L ♀X ▶– $$$$

Anti-Hyperlipidemic Agents—Other

EZETIMIBE (*Zetia*, ✦*Ezetrol*) Hyperlipidemia: 10 mg PO daily. [Trade only: Tabs, unscored 10 mg.] ▶L ♀C ▶? $$$$

ICOSAPENT ETHYL (*Vascepa*) Hypertriglyceridemia (500 mg/dL or above): 2 caps PO twice daily. Swallow whole. [Trade only: Caps 1 g.] ▶L – ♀C ▶? $$$$$

OMEGA-3-ACID ETHYL ESTERS (*Lovaza, fish oil, omega 3 fatty acids*) Hypertriglyceridemia (500 mg/dL or above): 4 caps PO daily or divided two times per day. [Trade only: (Lovaza) 1 g cap (total 840 mg EPA + DHA).] ▶L ♀C ▶? $

Antiadrenergic Agents

CLONIDINE (*Catapres, Catapres-TTS, Kapvay, ✦Dixarit*) Immediate-release, HTN: Start 0.1 mg PO two times per day, usual maintenance dose 0.2 to 0.6 mg/day in 2 to 3 divided doses, max 2.4 mg daily. Transdermal (Catapres-TTS), HTN: Start 0.1 mg/24 h patch once a week, titrate to desired effect, max effective dose 0.6 mg/24 h (two 0.3 mg/24 h patches). Transdermal Therapeutic System (TTS) is designed for 7-day use so that a TTS-1 delivers 0.1 mg/day for 7 days. May supplement 1st dose of TTS with oral for 2 to 3 days while therapeutic level is achieved. Extended-release (Kapvay), ADHD (6 to 17 yo): Start 0.1 mg PO at bedtime; may increase by 0.1 mg/day each week; give two times per day with equal or higher dose at bedtime, max 0.4 mg daily. Immediate-release, ADHD (unapproved peds): Start 0.05 mg PO at bedtime, titrate based on response over 8 weeks to max 0.2 mg/day (for wt less than 45 kg) or to max 0.4 mg/day (for wt 45 kg or greater) in 2 to 4 divided doses. Tourette syndrome (unapproved peds and adult): 3 to 5 mcg/kg/day PO divided two to four times per day. Opioid withdrawal, adjunct: 0.1 to 0.3 mg PO three to four times per day or 0.1 to 0.2 mg PO q 4 h for 3 days tapering off over 4 to 10 days. Alcohol withdrawal, adjunct: 0.1 to 0.2 mg PO q 4 h prn. Smoking cessation: Start 0.1 mg PO two times per day, increase 0.1 mg/day at weekly intervals to 0.75 mg/day as tolerated; transdermal (Catapres TTS): 0.1 to 0.2 mg/24 h patch once a week for 2 to 3 weeks after cessation. Menopausal flushing: 0.1 to 0.4 mg PO divided two to three times per day. Transdermal system applied weekly: 0.1 mg/day. May cause dizziness, drowsiness, or lightheadedness. Monitor for bradycardia when taking concomitant digitalis, nondihydropyridine calcium channel blockers, or beta blockers. [Generic/Trade: Tabs, immediate-release unscored (Catapres) 0.1, 0.2, 0.3 mg. Transdermal weekly patch 0.1 mg/day (TTS-1), 0.2 mg/day (TTS-2), 0.3 mg/day (TTS-3). Trade only: Tabs, extended-release unscored (Kapvay) 0.1, 0.2 mg.] ▶LK ♀C ▶? $$

DOXAZOSIN (*Cardura, Cardura XL*) BPH: Immediate-release: Start 1 mg PO at bedtime, max 8 mg/day. Extended-release (not approved for HTN): 4 mg PO q am with breakfast, max 8 mg/day. HTN: Start 1 mg PO at bedtime, max 16 mg/day. Take 1st dose at bedtime to minimize orthostatic hypotension. [Generic/Trade: Tabs scored 1, 2, 4, 8 mg. Trade only (Cardura XL): Tabs, extended-release 4, 8 mg.] ▶L ♀C ▶? $$ ■

METHYLDOPA (*Aldomet*) HTN: Start 250 mg PO two to three times per day, max 3000 mg/day. May be used to manage BP during pregnancy. [Generic only: Tabs, unscored 125, 250, 500 mg.] ▶LK ♀B ▶+ $

PRAZOSIN (*Minipress*) HTN: Start 1 mg PO two to three times per day, max 40 mg/day. Take 1st dose at bedtime to minimize orthostatic hypotension. [Generic/Trade: Caps 1, 2, 5 mg.] ▶L ♀C ▶? $$ ■

TERAZOSIN (*Hytrin*) HTN: Start 1 mg PO at bedtime, usual effective dose 1 to 5 mg PO daily or divided two times per day, max 20 mg/day. Take first dose at bedtime to minimize orthostatic hypotension. BPH: Start 1 mg PO at bedtime, usual effective dose 10 mg/day, max 20 mg/day. [Generic/Trade: Tabs/Caps 1, 2, 5, 10 mg.] ▶LK ♀C ▶? $$ ■

Antihypertensive Combinations

NOTE: *Dosage should first be adjusted by using each drug separately. See component drugs for further details.*

BY TYPE: ACE Inhibitor/Diuretic: *Accuretic, Capozide, Inhibace Plus, Lotensin HCT, Monopril HCT, Prinzide, Uniretic, Vaseretic, Zestoretic.* **ACE Inhibitor/Calcium Channel Blocker:** *Lexxel, Lotrel, Tarka.* **Angiotensin Receptor Blocker/Diuretic:** *Atacand HCT, Avalide, Benicar HCT, Diovan HCT, Edarbyclor, Hyzaar Micardis HCT, Teveten HCT.* **Angiotensin Receptor Blocker/Calcium Channel Blocker:** *Azor, Exforge, Twynsta.* **Angiotensin Receptor Blocker/Calcium Channel Blocker/Diuretic:** *Exforge HCT, Tribenzor.* **Beta-blocker/Diuretic:** *Corzide, Dutoprol, Inderide, Lopressor HCT, Tenoretic, Ziac.* **Calcium Channel Blocker/Statin:** *Caduet.* **Direct renin inhibitor/Calcium Channel Blocker:** *Tekamlo.* **Direct renin inhibitor/Calcium Channel Blocker/Diuretic:** *Amturnide.* **Direct renin inhibitor/Diuretic:** *Rasilez HCT, Tekturna HCT.* **Diuretic combinations:** *Aldactazide, Dyazide, Maxzide, Moduretic.* **Diuretic/miscellaneous antihypertensive:** *Aldoril, Apresazide, Clorpres, Minizide.*

BY NAME: Accuretic (quinapril + HCTZ): Generic/Trade: Tabs, scored 10/12.5, 20/12.5, unscored 20/25 mg. *Aldactazide* (spironolactone + HCTZ): Generic/Trade: Tabs, unscored 25/25, scored 50/50 mg. *Aldoril* (methyldopa + HCTZ): Generic: Tabs, unscored 250/15, 250/25 mg. *Amturnide* (aliskiren + amlodipine + HCTZ): Trade only: Tabs, unscored 150/5/12.5, 300/5/12.5, 300/5/25, 300/10/12.5, 300/10/25 mg. *Apresazide* (hydralazine + HCTZ): Generic only: Caps 25/25, 50/50 mg. *Atacand HCT* (candesartan + HCTZ, ◆*Atacand Plus*): Trade only: Tab, unscored 16/12.5, 32/12.5, 32/25 mg. *Avalide* (irbesartan + HCTZ): Generic/Trade: Tabs, unscored 150/12.5, 300/12.5, 300/25 mg. *Azor* (amlodipine + olmesartan): Trade only: Tabs, unscored 5/20, 5/40, 10/20, 10/40 mg. *Benicar HCT* (olmesartan + HCTZ): Trade only: Tabs, unscored 20/12.5, 40/12.5, 40/25 mg. *Caduet* (amlodipine + atorvastatin): Trade only: 2.5/10, 2.5/20, 2.5/40, 5/10, 5/20, 5/40, 5/80, 10/10, 10/20, 10/40, 10/80 mg. *Capozide* (captopril + HCTZ): Generic/Trade: Tabs, scored 25/15, 25/25, 50/15, 50/25 mg. *Clorpres* (clonidine + chlorthalidone): Trade only: Tabs, scored 0.1/15, 0.2/15, 0.3/15 mg. *Corzide* (nadolol + bendroflumethiazide): Generic/Trade: Tabs 40/5, 80/5 mg. *Diovan HCT* (valsartan + HCTZ): Generic/Trade: Tabs, unscored 80/12.5, 160/12.5, 160/25, 320/12.5, 320/25 mg. *Dutoprol* (metoprolol succinate + HCTZ): Trade: Tabs, 25/12.5, 50/12.5, 100/12.5 mg. *Dyazide* (triamterene + HCTZ): Generic/Trade: Caps, (Dyazide) 37.5/25, (generic only) 50/25 mg. *Edarbyclor* (azilsartan + chlorthalidone): Trade: Tabs, unscored 40/12.5, 40/25 mg. *Exforge* (amlodipine + valsartan): Trade only: Tabs, unscored 5/160, 5/320, 10/160, 10/320 mg. *Exforge HCT* (amlodipine + valsartan + HCTZ): Trade
(cont.)

only: Tabs, unscored 5/160/12.5, 5/160/25, 10/160/12.5, 10/160/25, 10/320/25 mg. *Hyzaar* (losartan + HCTZ): Generic/Trade: Tabs, unscored 50/12.5, 100/12.5, 100/25 mg. *Inderide* (propranolol + HCTZ): Generic/Trade: Tabs, scored 40/25, 80/25 mg. ✚*Inhibace Plus* (cilazapril + HCTZ): Trade only: Tabs, scored 5/12.5 mg. **Lexxel** (enalapril + felodipine): Trade only: Tabs, unscored 5/2.5, 5/5 mg. **Lopressor HCT** (metoprolol + HCTZ): Generic/Trade: Tabs, scored 50/25, 100/25, 100/50 mg. *Lotensin HCT* (benazepril + HCTZ): Generic/ Trade: Tabs, scored 5/6.25, 10/12.5, 20/12.5, 20/25 mg. *Lotrel* (amlodipine + benazepril): Generic/Trade: Cap, 2.5/10, 5/10, 5/20, 10/20 mg. Trade only: Cap, 5/40, 10/40 mg. **Maxzide** (triamterene + HCTZ, ✚*Triazide*): Generic/ Trade: Tabs, scored (Maxzide-25) 37.5/25 (Maxzide) 75/50 mg. *Micardis HCT* (telmisartan + HCTZ, ✚*Micardis Plus*): Trade only: Tabs, unscored 40/12.5, 80/12.5, 80/25 mg. **Minizide** (prazosin + polythiazide): Trade only: cap, 1/0.5, 2/0.5, 5/0.5 mg. *Moduretic* (amiloride + HCTZ, ✚*Moduret*): Generic/Trade: Tabs, scored 5/50 mg. *Monopril HCT* (fosinopril + HCTZ): Generic/Trade: Tabs, unscored 10/12.5, scored 20/12.5 mg. **Prinzide** (lisinopril + HCTZ): Generic/Trade: Tabs, unscored 10/12.5, 20/12.5, 20/25 mg. *Tarka* (trandolapril + verapamil): Trade only: Tabs, unscored 2/180, 1/240, 2/240, 4/240 mg. *Tekamlo* (aliskiren + amlodipine): Trade only: Tabs, unscored 150/5, 150/10, 300/5, 300/10 mg. *Tekturna HCT* (aliskiren + HCTZ, ✚*Rasilez HCT*): Trade only: Tabs, unscored 150/12.5, 150/25, 300/12.5, 300/25 mg. *Tenoretic* (atenolol + chlorthalidone): Generic/Trade: Tabs, scored 50/25, unscored 100/25 mg. *Teveten HCT* (eprosartan + HCTZ): Trade only: Tabs, unscored 600/12.5, 600/25 mg. *Tribenzor* (amlodipine + olmesartan + HCTZ): Trade only: Tabs, unscored 5/20/12.5, 5/40/12.5, 5/40/25,10/40/12.5,10/40/25 mg. *Twynsta* (amlodipine + telmisartan): Trade only: Tabs, unscored 5/40, 5/80, 10/40, 10/80 mg. *Uniretic* (moexipril + HCTZ): Generic/ Trade: Tabs, scored 7.5/12.5, 15/12.5, 15/25 mg. *Vaseretic* (enalapril + HCTZ): Generic/Trade: Tabs, scored 5/12.5, 10/25 mg. *Zestoretic* (lisinopril HCTZ): Generic/Trade: Tabs, unscored 10/12.5, 20/12.5, 20/25 mg. *Ziac* (bisoprolol + HCTZ): Generic/Trade: Tabs, unscored 2.5/6.25, 5/6.25, 10/6.25 mg.

Antihypertensives—Other

ALISKIREN (*Tekturna*, ✚*Rasilez*) HTN: 150 mg PO daily, max 300 mg/ day. Contraindicated in pregnancy. Do not use with ACE inhibitors or angiotensin receptor blockers in patients with DM or CrCl less than 60 mL/ min. Do not use with cyclosporine or itraconazole. Concomitant NSAIDs, including selective COX-2 inhibitors, may further deteriorate renal function and decrease antihypertensive effects. Dual inhibition of renin-angiotensin system increases risk of renal impairment, hypotension, and hyperkalemia. Hyperkalemia possible, especially if used concomitantly with other drugs that increase K+ (including K+ containing salt substitutes) and in patients with heart failure, DM, or renal impairment. Monitor potassium and renal function periodically. [Trade only: Tabs, unscored 150, 300 mg.] ▶LK ♀D ▶–? $$$ ■
FENOLDOPAM (*Corlopam*) Severe HTN: 10 mg in 250 mL D5W (40 mcg/mL), start at 0.1 mcg/kg/min titrate q 15 min, usual effective dose 0.1 to 1.6 mcg/ kg/min. ▶LK ♀B ▶? $$$

HYDRALAZINE   (*Apresoline*) Hypertensive emergency: 10 to 20 mg IV or 10 to 50 mg IM, repeat prn. HTN: Start 10 mg PO two to four times per day, max 300 mg/day. Headaches, peripheral edema, systemic lupus erythematosus-like syndrome. [Generic only: Tabs, unscored 10, 25, 50, 100 mg.] ▶LK ♀C ▶+ $

NITROPRUSSIDE   (*Nitropress*) Hypertensive emergency: Dilute 50 mg in 250 mL D5W (200 mcg/mL); rate of 6 mL/h for 70 kg adult delivers starting dose of 0.3 mcg/kg/min. Max 10 mcg/kg/min. Protect from light. Cyanide toxicity with high doses (10 mcg/kg/min), hepatic/renal impairment, and prolonged infusions (longer than 3 to 7 days); check thiocyanate levels. ▶RBCs ♀C ▶– $ ■

PHENTOLAMINE   (*Regitine, Rogitine*) Extravasation: 5 to 10 mg in 10 mL NS, inject 1 to 5 mL SC (in divided doses) around extravasation site. ▶Plasma ♀C ▶? $$$

Antiplatelet Drugs

ABCIXIMAB   (*ReoPro*) Platelet aggregation inhibition, percutaneous coronary intervention: 0.25 mg/kg IV bolus via separate infusion line before procedure, then 0.125 mcg/kg/min (max 10 mcg/min) IV infusion for 12 h. ▶Plasma ♀C ▶? $$$$$

AGGRENOX   (acetylsalicylic acid + dipyridamole) Prevention of CVA after TIA/CVA: 1 cap PO two times per day. Headaches are common adverse effect. [Trade only: Caps, 25 mg aspirin/200 mg extended-release dipyridamole.] ▶LK ♀D ▶? $$$$

CLOPIDOGREL   (*Plavix*) Reduction of thrombotic events, recent acute MI/CVA, established peripheral arterial disease: 75 mg PO daily. Non-ST segment elevation acute coronary syndrome: 300 to 600 mg loading dose, then 75 mg PO daily in combination with aspirin. ST segment elevation MI: Start with/without 300 mg loading dose, then 75 mg PO daily in combination with aspirin, with/without thrombolytic. Avoid drugs that are strong or moderate CYP2C19 inhibitors (eg, omeprazole, esomeprazole, cimetidine, etravirine, felbamate, fluconazole, fluoxetine, fluvoxamine, ketoconazole, voriconazole). [Generic/Trade: Tabs, unscored 75, 300 mg.] ▶LK ♀B ▶? $ ■

DIPYRIDAMOLE   (*Persantine*) Antithrombotic: 75 to 100 mg PO four times per day. [Generic/Trade: Tabs unscored 25, 50, 75 mg.] ▶L ♀B ▶? $$$

EPTIFIBATIDE   (*Integrilin*) Acute coronary syndrome: Load 180 mcg/kg IV bolus, then infusion 2 mcg/kg/min for up to 72 h. Discontinue infusion prior to CABG. Percutaneous coronary intervention: Load 180 mcg/kg IV bolus just before procedure, followed by infusion 2 mcg/kg/min and a 2nd 180 mcg/kg IV bolus 10 min after the 1st bolus. Continue infusion for up to 18 to 24 h (minimum 12 h) after procedure. CrCl less than 50 mL/min not on dialysis: Reduce infusion rate to 1 mcg/kg/min. Dialysis: contraindicated. Thrombocytopenia possible; monitor platelets. ▶K ♀B ▶? $$$$$

PRASUGREL   (*Effient*) Reduction of thrombotic events after acute coronary syndrome managed with percutaneous coronary intervention (PCI): 60 mg loading dose, then 10 mg PO daily in combination with aspirin. Wt less than 60 kg: Consider lower maintenance dose, 5 mg PO daily. May cause significant, fatal bleeding. Do not use with active bleeding or history of TIA or CVA. Generally

(cont.)

not recommend for patients 75 yo and older. Risk factors for bleeding: Body wt less than 60 kg, propensity to bleed, concomitant medications that increase bleeding risk. [Trade: Tabs, unscored 5, 10 mg.] ▶LK ♀B ▶? \$\$\$\$ ■

TICAGRELOR (*Brilinta*) Reduction of thrombotic events in patients with acute coronary syndrome (MI or unstable angina): 180 mg loading dose, then 90 mg PO two times daily in combination with aspirin. After any initial dose, use with aspirin 75 to 100 mg max per day. Do not use with history of intracranial hemorrhage, active bleeding, severe hepatic impairment, strong CYP3A inhibitors, or CYP3A inducers. Monitor digoxin levels when initiating or changing ticagrelor therapy. Do not use with strong CYP3A inhibitors (eg, clarithromycin, HIV protease inhibitors, itraconazole, ketoconazole, nefazodone, telithromycin, voriconazole), CYP3A inducers (eg, carbamazepine, dexamethasone, phenobarbital, phenytoin, rifampin), or severe hepatic impairment. [Trade only: Tabs, unscored 90 mg.] ▶L – ♀C ▶? \$\$\$\$\$ ■

TICLOPIDINE (*Ticlid*) Due to high incidence of neutropenia and thrombotic thrombocytopenia purpura, other antiplatelet agents preferred. Platelet aggregation inhibition/reduction of thrombotic CVA: 250 mg PO twice daily with food. [Generic/Trade: Tabs, unscored 250 mg.] ▶L ♀B ▶? \$\$\$\$ ■

TIROFIBAN (*Aggrastat*) Acute coronary syndromes: Start 0.4 mcg/kg/min IV infusion for 30 min, then decrease to 0.1 mcg/kg/min for 48 to 108 h or until 12 to 24 h after coronary intervention. Half dose with CrCl less than 30 mL/min. Use concurrent heparin to keep PTT 2 × normal. ▶K ♀B ▶? \$\$\$\$\$ ■

Beta-Blockers

NOTE: *See also Antihypertensive Combinations. Not 1st line for HTN (unless to treat angina, post MI, LV dysfunction, or heart failure). Abrupt discontinuation may precipitate angina, MI, arrhythmias, or rebound HTN; discontinue by tapering over 1 to 2 weeks. Avoid use of nonselective beta-blockers in patients with asthma/COPD. For patients with asthma/COPD, use agents with beta-1 selectivity and monitor cautiously. Beta-1 selectivity diminishes at high doses. Avoid initiating beta-blocker therapy in acute decompensated heart failure, sick sinus syndrome without pacer, and severe peripheral artery disease.*

ACEBUTOLOL (*Sectral*) HTN: Start 400 mg PO daily or 200 mg PO two times per day, maximum 1200 mg/day. Beta-1 receptor selective; has mild intrinsic sympathomimetic activity. [Generic/Trade: Caps 200, 400 mg.] ▶LK ♀B ▶– \$\$ ■

ATENOLOL (*Tenormin*) Acute MI: 50 to 100 mg PO daily or in divided doses. HTN: Start 25 to 50 mg PO daily or divided two times per day, max 100 mg/day. Beta-1 receptor selective. May be less effective for HTN and lowering CV event risk than other beta-blockers. [Generic/Trade: Tabs, unscored 25, 100 mg; scored, 50 mg.] ▶K ♀D ▶– \$ ■

BISOPROLOL (*Zebeta*, ✦*Monocor*) HTN: Start 2.5 to 5 mg PO daily, max 20 mg/day. Highly beta-1 receptor selective. [Generic/Trade: Tabs, scored 5 mg, unscored 10 mg.] ▶LK ♀C ▶? \$\$ ■

CARVEDILOL (*Coreg, Coreg CR*) Heart failure, immediate-release: Start 3.125 mg PO two times per day, double dose q 2 weeks as tolerated up to max of 25 mg two times per day (for wt 85 kg or less) or 50 mg two times per day (for wt greater than 85 kg). Heart failure, sustained-release: Start 10 mg PO daily, double dose q 2 weeks as tolerated to max of 80 mg/day. LV dysfunction following acute MI, immediate-release: Start 3.125 to 6.25 mg PO two times per day, double dose q 3 to 10 days as tolerated to max of 25 mg two times per day. LV dysfunction following acute MI, sustained-release: Start 10 to 20 mg PO daily, double dose q 3 to 10 days as tolerated to max of 80 mg/day. HTN, immediate-release: Start 6.25 mg PO two times per day, double dose q 7 to 14 days as tolerated to max 50 mg/day. HTN, sustained-release: Start 20 mg PO daily, double dose q 7 to 14 days as tolerated to max 80 mg/day. Take with food to decrease orthostatic hypotension. Give Coreg CR in the morning. Alpha-1, beta-1, and beta-2 receptor blocker. [Generic/ Trade: Tabs, immediate-release unscored 3.125, 6.25, 12.5, 25 mg. Trade only: Caps, extended-release 10, 20, 40, 80 mg.] ▶L ♀C ▶? $$$$ ■

ESMOLOL (*Brevibloc*) SVT/HTN emergency: Load 500 mcg/kg over 1 min (dilute 5 g in 500 mL to make a soln of 10 mg/mL) and give 3.5 mL to deliver 35 mg bolus for 70 kg patient) then start infusion 50 to 200 mcg/kg/min (40 mL/h delivers 100 mcg/kg/min for 70 kg patient). Half-life is 9 min. Beta-1 receptor selective. ▶K ♀C ▶? $ ■

LABETALOL (*Trandate*) HTN: Start 100 mg PO two times per day, max 2400 mg/day. HTN emergency: Start 20 mg IV slow injection, then 40 to 80 mg IV q 10 min prn up to 300 mg or IV infusion 0.5 to 2 mg/min. Peds: Start 0.3 to 1 mg/kg/dose (max 20 mg). May be used to manage BP during pregnancy. Alpha-1, beta-1, and beta-2 receptor blocker. [Generic/Trade: Tabs, scored 100, 200, 300 mg.] ▶LK ♀C ▶+ $$$ ■

METOPROLOL (*Lopressor, Toprol-XL, ✦Betaloc*) Acute MI: 50 to 100 mg PO q 12 h; or 5-mg increments IV q 5 to 15 min up to 15 mg followed by oral therapy. HTN (immediate-release): Start 100 mg PO daily or in divided doses, increase prn up to 450 mg/day; may require multiple daily doses to maintain 24 h BP control. HTN (extended-release): Start 25 to 100 mg PO daily, increase prn up to 400 mg/ day. Heart failure: Start 12.5 to 25 mg (extended-release) PO daily, double dose q 2 weeks as tolerated up to max 200 mg/day. Angina: Start 50 mg PO two times per day (immediate-release) or 100 mg PO daily (extended-release), increase prn up to 400 mg/day. IV to PO conversion: 1 mg IV is equivalent to 2.5 mg PO (divided four times per day). The immediate-(metoprolol tartrate) and extended-release (metoprolol succinate) products may not give same clinical response on mg:mg basis; monitor response and side effects when interchanging between metoprolol products. Extended-release tabs may be broken in half, but do not chew or crush. Beta-1 receptor selective. Take with food. [Generic/Trade: Tabs, scored 50, 100 mg, extended-release 25, 50, 100, 200 mg. Generic only: Tabs, scored 25 mg.] ▶L ♀C ▶? $$$ ■

NADOLOL (*Corgard*) HTN: Start 20 to 40 mg PO daily, max 320 mg/day. Prevent rebleeding esophageal varices: 40 to 160 mg PO daily; titrate dose to reduce heart rate to 25% below baseline. Beta-1 receptor blocker. [Generic/Trade: Tabs, scored 20, 40, 80, 120, 160 mg.] ▶K ♀C ▶– $$ ■

NEBIVOLOL (*Bystolic*) HTN: Start 5 mg PO daily, maximum 40 mg/day. At doses of 10 mg or less or for extensive metabolizers: beta-1 receptor selective. At doses greater than 10 mg or poor metabolizers: beta-1 and beta-2 receptor blocker. [Trade only: Tabs unscored 2.5, 5, 10, 20 mg.] ▶L ♀C ▶– $$$ ■

PROPRANOLOL (*Inderal, Inderal LA, InnoPran XL*) HTN: Start 20 to 40 mg PO two times per day or 60 to 80 mg PO daily, max 640 mg/day; extended-release (Inderal LA) max 640 mg/day; extended-release (InnoPran XL) 80 mg at bedtime (10 pm), max 120 mg at bedtime (chronotherapy). Supraventricular tachycardia or rapid atrial fibrillation/flutter: 1 mg IV q 2 min. Max of 2 doses in 4 h. Migraine prophylaxis: Start 40 mg PO two times per day or 80 mg PO daily (extended-release), max 240 mg/day. Prevent rebleeding esophageal varices: 20 to 180 mg PO two times per day; titrate dose to reduce heart rate to 25% below baseline. Beta-1 and beta-2 receptor blocker. [Generic/Trade: Tabs, scored 40, 60, 80. Caps, extended-release 60, 80, 120, 160 mg. Generic only: Soln 20, 40 mg/5 mL. Tabs, 10, 20 mg. Trade only: (InnoPran XL at bedtime) 80, 120 mg.] ▶L ♀C ▶+ $$ ■

Calcium Channel Blockers (CCBs)—Dihydropyridines

NOTE: *See also Antihypertensive Combinations. Avoid in decompensated heart failure. May increase proteinuria, edema. Extended/controlled/sustained-release forms: swallow whole; do not chew/crush.*

AMLODIPINE (*Norvasc*) HTN: Start 5 mg PO daily, max 10 mg/day. Elderly, small, frail, or with hepatic insufficiency: Start 2.5 PO daily. [Generic/Trade: Tabs, unscored 2.5, 5, 10 mg.] ▶L ♀C ▶? $

CLEVIDIPINE (*Cleviprex*) HTN: Start 1 to 2 mg/h IV, titrate q 1.5 to 10 min to BP response, usual maintenance dose 4 to 6 mg/h, max 32 mg/h IV. An increase of 1 to 2 mg/h will decrease SBP approximately 2 to 4 mmHg. ▶KL ♀C ▶? $$$

FELODIPINE (*Plendil, ✦ Renedil*) HTN: Start 2.5 to 5 mg PO daily, maximum 10 mg/day. [Generic/Trade: Tabs, extended-release, unscored 2.5, 5, 10 mg.] ▶L ♀C ▶? $$

ISRADIPINE (*DynaCirc, DynaCirc CR*) HTN: Start 2.5 mg PO two times per day, max 20 mg/day (max 10 mg/day in elderly). Controlled-release: 5 to 20 mg PO daily. Immediate-release: Tabs, controlled-release 5, 10 mg. Generic only: Immediate-release caps 2.5, 5 mg.] ▶L ♀C ▶? $$$$

NICARDIPINE (*Cardene, Cardene SR*) HTN emergency: Begin IV infusion at 5 mg/h, titrate to effect, max 15 mg/h. HTN: Start 20 mg PO three times per day, max 120 mg/day. Sustained-release: Start 30 mg PO two times per day, max 120 mg/day. Short-term management of HTN, patient receiving PO nicardipine: If using 20 mg PO q 8 h, give 0.5 mg/h IV; if using 30 mg PO q 8 h, give 1.2 mg/h IV; if using 40 mg PO q 8 h, give 2.2 mg/h. [Generic/Trade: Caps, immediate-release 20, 30 mg. Trade only: Caps, sustained-release 30, 45, 60 mg.] ▶L ♀C ▶? $$

NIFEDIPINE (*Procardia, Adalat, Procardia XL, Adalat CC, Afeditab CR, ✦ Adalat XL, Adalat PA*) HTN/angina: Extended-release: 30 to 60 mg PO daily, max 120 mg/day. Angina: Immediate-release: Start 10 mg PO three times per day, max

(cont.)

120 mg/day. Avoid sublingual administration, may cause excessive hypotension, acute MI, CVA. Do not use immediate-release caps for treating HTN, hypertensive emergencies, or ST-elevation MI. Preterm labor: Loading dose: 10 mg PO q 20 to 30 min if contractions persist, up to 40 mg within the first h. Maintenance dose: 10 to 20 mg PO q 4 to 6 h or 60 to 160 mg extended-release PO daily. [Generic/Trade: Caps 10, 20 mg. Tabs, extended-release (Adalat CC, Afeditab CR, Procardia XL) 30, 60 mg, (Adalat CC, Procardia XL) 90 mg.] ▶L ♀C ▶– $$

NISOLDIPINE (*Sular*) HTN: Start 17 mg PO daily, max 34 mg/day. Take on an empty stomach. [Trade only: Tabs, extended-release 8.5, 17, 25.5, 34 mg. These replace the former 10, 20, 30, 40 mg tabs. Generic only: Tabs, extended-release 20, 30, 40 mg.] ▶L ♀C ▶? $$$

Calcium Channel Blockers (CCBs)—Non-Dihydropyridines

NOTE: *See also Antihypertensive Combinations. Avoid in decompensated heart failure, sick sinus syndrome or 2nd/3rd degree heart block without pacemaker, acute MI and pulmonary congestion, or systolic blood pressure less than 90 mm Hg.*

DILTIAZEM (*Cardizem, Cardizem LA, Cardizem CD, Cartia XT, Dilacor XR, Diltiazem CD, Diltzac, Diltia XT, Tiazac, Taztia XT*) Atrial fibrillation/flutter, PSVT: Bolus 20 mg (0.25 mg/kg) IV over 2 min. Rebolus 15 min later (if needed) 25 mg (0.35 mg/kg). Infusion 5 to 15 mg/h. HTN, once daily, extended-release: Start 120 to 240 mg PO daily, max 540 mg/day. HTN, once daily, graded extended-release (Cardizem LA): Start 180 to 240 mg PO daily, max 540 mg/day. HTN, twice daily, sustained-release: Start 60 to 120 mg PO two times per day, max 360 mg/day. Angina, immediate-release: Start 30 mg PO four times per day, max 360 mg/day divided three to four times per day; Angina, extended-release: Start 120 to 240 mg PO daily, max 540 mg/day. Angina, once daily, graded extended-release (Cardizem LA): Start 180 mg PO daily; doses more than 360 mg may provide no additional benefit. [Generic/Trade: Tabs, immediate-release, unscored (Cardizem) 30, scored 60, 90, 120 mg; Caps extended-release (Cardizem CD, Cartia XT daily) 120, 180, 240, 300, 360 mg, (Diltzac, Taztia XT, Tiazac daily) 120, 180, 240, 300, 360, 420 mg, (Dilacor XR, Diltia XT) 120, 180, 240 mg. Trade only: Tabs, extended-release graded (Cardizem LA daily) 120, 180, 240, 300, 360, 420 mg.] ▶L ♀C ▶+ $$

VERAPAMIL (*Isoptin SR, Calan, Covera-HS, Verelan, Verelan PM*) SVT adults: 5 to 10 mg IV over 2 min; SVT peds (age 1 to 15 yr): 2 to 5 mg (0.1 to 0.3 mg/kg) IV, max dose 5 mg. Angina: Immediate-release, start 40 to 80 mg PO three to four times per day, max 480 mg/day. Angina, sustained-release, start 120 to 240 mg PO daily, max 480 mg/day (use twice daily dosing for doses greater than 240 mg/day with Isoptin SR and Calan SR); (Covera-HS) 180 mg PO at bedtime, max 480 mg/day. HTN: Same as angina, except (Verelan PM) 100 to 200 mg PO at bedtime, max 400 mg/day; immediate-release tabs should be avoided in treating HTN. Use cautiously in impaired renal/hepatic function. [Generic/Trade: Tabs, immediate-release,

(cont.)

scored (Calan) 40, 80, 120 mg; Tabs, sustained-release, unscored (Isoptin SR) 120, scored 180, 240 mg; Caps, sustained-release (Verelan) 120, 180, 240, 360 mg; Caps, extended-release (Verelan PM) 100, 200, 300 mg. Trade only: Tabs, extended-release (Covera-HS) 180, 240 mg.] ▶L ♀C ▶- $$

Diuretics—Carbonic Anhydrase Inhibitors

ACETAZOLAMIDE (*Diamox, Diamox Sequels*) Glaucoma: 250 mg PO up to four times per day (immediate-release) or 500 mg PO up to two times per day (sustained-release). Max 1 g/day. Acute glaucoma: 250 mg IV q 4 h or 500 mg IV initially with 125 to 250 mg q 4 h, followed by oral therapy. Mountain sickness prophylaxis: 125 to 250 mg PO two to three times per day, beginning 1 to 2 days prior to ascent and continuing at least 5 days at higher altitude. Edema: Rarely used, start 250 to 375 mg IV/PO q am given intermittently (every other day or 2 consecutive days followed by none for 1 to 2 days) to avoid loss of diuretic effect. Urinary alkalinization: 5 mg/kg IV, may repeat two or three times daily prn to maintain an alkaline diuresis. [Generic only: Tabs 125, 250 mg. Generic/Trade: Caps, extended-release 500 mg.] ▶LK ♀C ▶+ $

Diuretics—Loop

NOTE: *Thiazides are preferred diuretics for HTN. With decreased renal function (CrCl less than 30 mL/min), loop diuretics may be more effective than thiazides for HTN. Rare hypersensitivity in patients allergic to sulfa-containing drugs, except ethacrynic acid.*

BUMETANIDE (*Bumex, ✦ Burinex*) Edema: 0.5 to 1 mg IV/IM; 0.5 to 2 mg PO daily. 1 mg bumetanide is roughly equivalent to 40 mg furosemide. [Generic/ Trade: Tabs, scored 0.5, 1, 2 mg.] ▶K ♀C ▶? $

ETHACRYNIC ACID (*Edecrin*) Can be safely used in patients with true sulfa allergy. Edema: 0.5 to 1 mg/kg IV, max 100 mg/dose; 25 to 100 mg PO daily to two times per day. [Trade only: Tabs, scored 25 mg.] ▶K ♀B ▶? $$$

FUROSEMIDE (*Lasix*) HTN: Start 10 to 40 mg PO twice daily, max 600 mg daily. Edema: Start 20 to 80 mg IV/IM/PO, increase dose by 20 to 40 mg in 6 to 8 h until desired response is achieved, max 600 mg/day. Ascites: 40 mg PO daily in combination with spironolactone; may increase dose after 2 to 3 days if no response. [Generic/Trade: Tabs, unscored 20, scored 40, 80 mg. Generic only: Oral soln 10 mg/mL, 40 mg/5 mL.] ▶K ♀C ▶? $

TORSEMIDE (*Demadex*) HTN: Start 5 mg PO daily, increase prn q 4 to 6 weeks, max 10 mg daily. Edema: 10 to 20 mg IV/PO daily, max 200 mg IV/PO daily. [Generic/Trade: Tabs, scored 5, 10, 20, 100 mg.] ▶LK ♀B ▶? $

Diuretics—Thiazide Type

NOTE: *See also Antihypertensive Combinations. Possible hypersensitivity in sulfa allergy. Should be used for most patients with HTN, alone or combined with other antihypertensive agents. Thiazides are not recommended for gestational HTN.*

(cont.)

Coadministration with NSAIDs, including selective COX-2 inhibitors, may reduce the antihypertensive, diuretic, and natriuretic effects of thiazides. Thiazide-induced hypokalemia is associated with increased fasting blood glucose and new onset diabetes; keep potassium 4.0 mg/dL or greater to minimize risk; may use thiazide in combination with oral potassium supplementation, ACE inhibitor, ARB, or potassium-sparing diuretic to maintain K+ level.

CHLORTHALIDONE (**Thalitone**) HTN: 12.5 to 25 mg PO daily, max 50 mg/day. Edema: 50 to 100 mg PO daily, max 200 mg/day. Nephrolithiasis (unapproved use): 25 to 50 mg PO daily. [Trade only: Tabs unscored (Thalitone) 15 mg. Generic only: Tabs unscored 25, 50 mg.] ▶L ♀B, D if used in pregnancy-induced HTN ▶+ $

HYDROCHLOROTHIAZIDE (**HCTZ, Oretic, Microzide**) HTN: 12.5 to 25 mg PO daily, max 50 mg/day. Edema: 25 to 100 mg PO daily, max 200 mg/day. [Generic/Trade: Tabs scored 25, 50 mg; Caps 12.5 mg.] ▶L ♀B, D if used in pregnancy-induced HTN ▶+ $

INDAPAMIDE (**Lozol**, ✦ **Lozide**) HTN: 1.25 to 5 mg PO daily, max 5 mg/day. Edema: 2.5 to 5 mg PO q am. [Generic only: Tabs unscored 1.25, 2.5 mg.] ▶L ♀B, D if used in pregnancy-induced HTN ▶? $

METOLAZONE (**Zaroxolyn**) Edema: 5 to 10 mg PO daily, max 10 mg/day in heart failure, 20 mg/day in renal disease. If used with loop diuretic, start with 2.5 mg PO daily. [Generic/Trade: Tabs 2.5, 5, 10 mg.] ▶L ♀B, D if used in pregnancy-induced HTN ▶? $$$

Nitrates

ISOSORBIDE DINITRATE (**Isordil, Dilatrate-SR**) Angina prophylaxis: 5 to 40 mg PO three times per day (7 am, noon, 5 pm), sustained-release: 40 to 80 mg PO two times per day (8 am, 2 pm). Acute angina, SL Tabs: 2.5 to 10 mg SL q 5 to 10 min prn, up to 3 doses in 30 min. [Generic/Trade: Tabs, scored 5, 10, 20, 30 mg. Trade only: Tabs, (Isordil) 40 mg, Caps, extended-release (Dilatrate-SR) 40 mg. Generic only: Tabs, sustained-release 40 mg, Tabs, sublingual 2.5, 5 mg.] ▶L ♀C ▶? $

ISOSORBIDE MONONITRATE (**ISMO, Monoket, Imdur**) Angina: 20 mg PO two times per day (8 am and 3 pm). Extended-release: Start 30 to 60 mg PO daily, maximum 240 mg/day. Do not use for acute angina. [Generic/Trade: Tabs, unscored (ISMO, two times per day dosing) 20 mg, scored (Monoket, two times per day dosing) 20 mg, 20 mg extended-release, scored (Imdur, daily dosing) 30, 60, unscored 120 mg.] ▶L ♀C ▶? $$

NITROGLYCERIN INTRAVENOUS INFUSION Perioperative HTN, acute MI/Heart failure, acute angina: Mix 50 mg in 250 mL D5W (200 mcg/mL), start at 10 to 20 mcg/min (3 to 6 mL/h), then titrate upward by 10 to 20 mcg/min prn. ▶L ♀C ▶? $

NITROGLYCERIN OINTMENT (**Nitro-BID**) Angina prophylaxis: Start 0.5 inch q 8 h, maintenance 1 to 2 inch q 8 h, maximum 4 inch q 4 to 6 h; 15 mg/inch. Allow for a nitrate-free period of 10 to 14 h to avoid nitrate tolerance. 1 inch of ointment contains about 15 mg. Do not use for acute angina attack. [Trade only: Ointment, 2%, tubes 1, 30, 60 g (Nitro-BID).] ▶L ♀C ▶? $

NITROGLYCERIN SPRAY *(Nitrolingual, NitroMist)* Acute angina: 1 to 2 sprays under the tongue prn, max 3 sprays in 15 min. [Trade only: Nitrolingual soln, 4.9, 12 mL. 0.4 mg/spray (60 or 200 sprays/canister); NitroMist aerosol 0.4 mg/spray (230 sprays/canister).] ▶L ♀C ▶? $$$$

NITROGLYCERIN SUBLINGUAL *(Nitrostat, NitroQuick)* Acute angina: 0.4 mg SL under tongue, repeat dose q 5 min prn up to 3 doses in 15 min. [Generic/ Trade: Sublingual tabs, unscored 0.3, 0.4, 0.6 mg; in bottles of 100 or package of 4 bottles with 25 tabs each.] ▶L ♀C ▶? $

NITROGLYCERIN TRANSDERMAL *(Minitran, Nitro-Dur, ✦ Trinipatch, Transderm-Nitro)* Angina prophylaxis: 1 patch 12 to 14 h each day. Allow for a nitrate-free period of 10 to 14 h each day to avoid nitrate tolerance. Do not use for acute angina attack. [Generic/Trade: Transdermal system 0.1, 0.2, 0.4, 0.6 mg/h. Trade only: (Nitro-Dur) 0.3, 0.8 mg/h.] ▶L ♀C ▶? $$

Pressors/Inotropes

DOBUTAMINE Inotropic support: 2 to 20 mcg/kg/min. Dilute 250 mg in 250 mL D5W (1 mg/mL); a rate of 21 mL/h delivers 5 mcg/kg/min for a 70 kg patient. ▶Plasma ♀D ▶– $

DOPAMINE Pressor: Start at 5 mcg/kg/min, increase prn by 5 to 10 mcg/kg/min increments at 10-min intervals, max 50 mcg/kg/min. Mix 400 mg in 250 mL D5W (1600 mcg/mL); a rate of 13 mL/h delivers 5 mcg/kg/min in a 70 kg patient. Doses in mcg/kg/min: 2 to 4 (traditional renal dose, apparently ineffective) dopaminergic receptors; 5 to 10 (cardiac dose) dopaminergic and beta-1 receptors; more than 10 dopaminergic, beta-1, and alpha-1 receptors. ▶Plasma ♀C ▶– $ ■

EPINEPHRINE *(EpiPen, EpiPen Jr, Auvi-Q, adrenalin)* Cardiac arrest: 1 mg IV q 3 to 5 min. Anaphylaxis: 0.1 to 0.5 mg SC/IM, may repeat SC dose q 10 to 15 min. Acute asthma and hypersensitivity reactions: Adults: 0.1 to 0.3 mg of 1:1000 soln SC or IM; Peds: 0.01 mg/kg (up to 0.3 mg) of 1:1000 soln SC or IM. [Soln for injection: 1:1000 (1 mg/mL in 1 mL amps or 10 mL vial). Trade only: EpiPen Auto-injector delivers one 0.3 mg (1:1000, 0.3 mL) IM/SQ dose. EpiPen Jr. Autoinjector delivers one 0.15 mg (1:2000, 0.3 mL) IM/SQ dose. Auvi-Q Autoinjector delivers one 0.15 mg (1:1000, 0.15 mL) or 0.3 mg (1:1000, 0.3 mL) IM/ SQ dose. Epipen and Auvi-Q only available in a 2-pack] ▶Plasma ♀C ▶– $

CARDIAC PARAMETERS AND FORMULAS

Cardiac output (CO) = heart rate × CVA volume [normal 4 to 8 L/min]

Cardiac index (CI) = CO/BSA [normal 2.8 to 4.2 L/min/m²]

MAP (mean arterial press) = [(SBP − DBP)/3] + DBP [normal 80 to 100 mmHg]

SVR (systemic vasc resis) = (MAP − CVP) × (80)/CO [normal 800 to 1200 dyne × sec/cm⁵]

PVR (pulm vasc resis) = (PAM − PCWP) × (80)/CO [normal 45 to 120 dyne × sec/cm⁵]

QTc = QT/square root of RR [normal 0.38 to 0.42]

Right atrial pressure (central venous pressure) [normal 0 to 8 mmHg]

Pulmonary artery systolic pressure (PAS) [normal 20 to 30 mmHg]

Pulmonary artery diastolic pressure (PAD) [normal 10 to 15 mmHg]

Pulmonary capillary wedge pressure (PCWP) [normal 8 to 12 mmHg (post-MI ~16 mmHg)]

CARDIOVASCULAR

MIDODRINE (✦ *Amatine*) Orthostatic hypotension: 10 mg PO three times per day. The last daily dose should be no later than 6 pm to avoid supine HTN during sleep. [Generic: Tabs, scored 2.5, 5, 10 mg.] ▶LK ♀C ▶? $$$$$ ■

MILRINONE (*Primacor*) Systolic heart failure (NYHA class III, IV): Load 50 mcg/kg IV over 10 min, then begin IV infusion of 0.375 to 0.75 mcg/kg/min. ▶K ♀C ▶? $$

NOREPINEPHRINE (*Levophed*) Acute hypotension: Start 8 to 12 mcg/min, adjust to maintain BP, average maintenance rate 2 to 4 mcg/min. Mix 4 mg in 500 mL D5W (8 mcg/mL), a rate of 22.5 mL/h delivers 3 mcg/min. Ideally through central line. ▶Plasma ♀C ▶? ■

PHENYLEPHRINE—INTRAVENOUS Severe hypotension: Infusion: 20 mg in 250 mL D5W (80 mcg/mL), start 100 to 180 mcg/min (75 to 135 mL/h), usual dose once BP is stabilized 40 to 60 mcg/min. ▶Plasma ♀C ▶–$ ■

Pulmonary Arterial Hypertension

SILDENAFIL (*Revatio*) Pulmonary arterial hypertension: 20 mg PO three times per day; or 10 mg IV three times per day. Contraindicated with nitrates. Coadministration is not recommended with ritonavir, potent CYP3A inhibitors, or other phosphodiesterase-5 inhibitors. Teach patients to seek medical attention for vision loss, hearing loss, or in men if erections last longer than 4 h. [Generic/Trade: Tabs 20 mg. Trade only: Susp 10 mg/mL.] ▶LK ♀B ▶– $$$$

TADALAFIL (*Adcirca*) Pulmonary arterial hypertension: 40 mg PO daily. Contraindicated with nitrates. Coadministration is not recommended with potent CYP3A inhibitors (itraconazole, ketoconazole), potent CYP3A inducers (rifampin), other phosphodiesterase-5 inhibitors. Caution with ritonavir, see prescribing info for specific dose adjustments. Teach patients to seek medical attention for vision loss, hearing loss, or in men if erections last longer than 4 h. [Trade only (Adcirca): Tabs 20 mg.] ▶L ♀B ▶– $$$$

Thrombolytics

ALTEPLASE (*tpa, t-PA, Activase, Cathflo,* ✦ *Activase rt-PA*) Acute MI: wt 67 kg or less, give 15 mg IV bolus, then 0.75 mg/kg (max 50 mg) over 30 min, then 0.5 mg/kg (max 35 mg) over the next 60 min; wt greater than 67 kg, give 15 mg IV bolus, then 50 mg over 30 min, then 35 mg over the next 60 min. Acute ischemic stroke with symptoms 3 h or less: 0.9 mg/kg (max 90 mg); give 10% of total dose as an IV bolus, and the remainder IV over 60 min. Multiple exclusion criteria. Acute pulmonary embolism: 100 mg IV over 2 h, then restart heparin when PTT twice normal or less. Occluded central venous access device: 2 mg/mL in catheter for 2 h. May use second dose if needed. ▶L ♀C ▶? $$$$$

RETEPLASE (*Retavase*) Acute MI: 10 units IV over 2 min; repeat once in 30 min. ▶L ♀C ▶? $$$$$

STREPTOKINASE (*Streptase, Kabikinase*) Acute MI: 1.5 million units IV over 60 min. ▶L ♀C ▶? $$$$$

THROMBOLYTIC THERAPY FOR ACUTE MI

Indications (if high-volume cath lab unavailable)	Clinical history and presentation strongly suggestive of MI within 12 h plus at least 1 of the following: 1 mm ST elevation in at least 2 contiguous leads; new left BBB; or 2 mm ST depression in V1–4 suggestive of true posterior MI.
Absolute contraindications	Previous cerebral hemorrhage, known cerebral aneurysm or arteriovenous malformation, known intracranial neoplasm, recent (<3 months) ischemic CVA (except acute ischemic CVA <3 h), aortic dissection, active bleeding or bleeding diathesis (excluding menstruation), significant closed head or facial trauma (<3 months).
Relative contraindications	Severe uncontrolled HTN (>180/110 mm Hg) on presentation or chronic severe HTN; prior ischemic CVA (>3 months), dementia, other intracranial pathology; traumatic/prolonged (>10 min) cardiopulmonary resuscitation; major surgery (<3 weeks); recent (within 2–4 weeks) internal bleeding; puncture of noncompressible vessel; pregnancy; active peptic ulcer disease; current use of anticoagulants. For streptokinase/anistreplase: prior exposure (>5 days ago) or prior allergic reaction.

Reference: *Circulation* 2004;110:588-636.

TENECTEPLASE (*TNKase*) Acute MI: Single IV bolus dose over 5 sec based on body wt: wt less than 60 kg: 30 mg; wt 60 kg to 69 kg: 35 mg; wt 70 to 79 kg: 40 mg; wt 80 to 89 kg: 45 mg; wt 90 kg or more: 50 mg. ▶L ♀C ▶? $$$$$
UROKINASE (*Kinlytic*) PE: 4400 units/kg IV loading dose over 10 min, followed by IV infusion 4400 units/kg/h for 12 h. Occluded IV catheter: 5000 units in catheter, for 1 to 4 h. ▶L ♀B ▶? $$$$$

Volume Expanders

ALBUMIN (*Albuminar, Buminate, Albumarc,* ✚ *Plasbumin*) Shock, burns: 500 mL of 5% soln IV infusion as rapidly as tolerated, repeat in 30 min if needed. ▶L ♀C ▶? $$$$$
DEXTRAN (*Rheomacrodex, Gentran, Macrodex*) Shock/hypovolemia: up to 20 mL/kg in first 24 h, then up to 10 mL/kg for 4 days. ▶K ♀C ▶? $$
HETASTARCH (*Hespan, Hextend*) Shock/hypovolemia: 500 to 1000 mL IV infusion, usually should not exceed 20 mL/kg/day (1500 mL) ▶K ♀C ▶? $$ ■
PLASMA PROTEIN FRACTION (*Plasmanate, Protenate, Plasmatein*) Shock/hypovolemia: 5% soln 250 to 500 mL IV prn. ▶L ♀C ▶? $$$

Other

BIDIL (hydralazine + isosorbide dinitrate) Heart failure (adjunct to standard therapy in black patients): Start 1 tab PO three times per day, increase as tolerated to max 2 tabs three times per day. May decrease to ½ tab three times per day with intolerable side effects. [Trade only: Tabs, scored 37.5/20 mg.] ▶LK ♀C ▶? $$$$$

CILOSTAZOL (*Pletal*) Intermittent claudication: 100 mg PO two times per day on empty stomach. 50 mg PO two times per day with CYP3A4 inhibitors (eg, ketoconazole, itraconazole, erythromycin, diltiazem) or CYP2C19 inhibitors (eg, omeprazole). Contraindicated in heart failure of any severity due to decreased survival. [Generic/Trade: Tabs 50, 100 mg.] ▶L ♀C ▶? $$$$ ■

NESIRITIDE (*Natrecor*) Hospitalized patients with decompensated heart failure with dyspnea at rest: 2 mcg/kg IV bolus over 1 min, then 0.01 mcg/kg/min IV infusion for up to 48 h. Do not initiate at higher doses. Limited experience with increased doses. Mix 1.5 mg vial in 250 mL D5W (6 mcg/mL) a bolus of 23.3 mL is 2 mcg/kg for a 70 kg patient, infusion set at rate 7 mL/h delivers a 0.01 mcg/kg/min for a 70 kg patient. Symptomatic hypotension. May increase mortality. Not indicated for outpatient infusion, for scheduled repetitive use, to improve renal function, or to enhance diuresis. May worsen renal impairment. ▶K, plasma ♀C ▶? $$$$$

PENTOXIFYLLINE (*Trental*) Intermittent claudication: 400 mg PO three times per day with meals. Contraindicated with recent cerebral/retinal bleed. [Generic/Trade: Tabs, extended-release 400 mg.] ▶L ♀C ▶? $$$

RANOLAZINE (*Ranexa*) Chronic angina: 500 mg PO two times per day, max 1000 mg two times per day. Max 500 mg two times per day, if used with diltiazem, verapamil, or moderate CYP3A inhibitors. Baseline and follow-up ECGs; may prolong QT interval. Contraindicated with hepatic cirrhosis, potent CYP3A4 inhibitors, CYP3A inducers. Increases level of cyclosporine, lovastatin, simvastatin, sirolimus, tacrolimus, antipsychotics, TCA(s). Swallow whole; do not crush, break, or chew. Teach patients to report palpitations or fainting spells. [Trade only: Tabs, extended-release 500, 1000 mg.] ▶LK ♀C ▶? $$$$$

CONTRAST MEDIA

MRI Contrast—Gadolinium-based

NOTE: *Avoid gadolinium-based contrast agents if severe renal insufficiency (GFR less than 30 mL/min/1.73 m²) due to risk of nephrogenic systemic fibrosis/nephrogenic fibrosing dermopathy. Similarly avoid in acute renal insufficiency of any severity due to hepatorenal syndrome or during the perioperative phase of liver transplant.*

GADOBENATE (*MultiHance*) ▶K ♀C ▶? $$$$ ■
GADOBUTROL (*Gadavist*) 0.1 mL/kg for age 2 yo or older ▶K – ♀C ▶?©V $$$$ ■
GADODIAMIDE (*Omniscan*) ▶K ♀C ▶? $$$$ ■
GADOPENTETATE (*Magnevist*) ▶K ♀C ▶? $$$ ■
GADOTERIDOL (*Prohance*) ▶K ♀C ▶? $$$$ ■
GADOVERSETAMIDE (*OptiMARK*) ▶K ♀C ▶– $$$$ ■

MRI Contrast—Other

FERUMOXIDES (*Feridex*) Non-iodinated, nonionic, iron-based IV contrast for hepatic MRI. ▶L ♀C ▶? $$$$

FERUMOXSIL (*GastroMARK*) Non-iodinated, nonionic, iron-based, oral GI contrast for MRI. ▶L ♀B ▶? $$$$
MANGAFODIPIR (*Teslascan*) Non-iodinated manganese-based IV contrast for MRI. ▶L ♀– ▶– $$$$

Radiography Contrast

NOTE: *Beware of allergic or anaphylactoid reactions. Avoid IV contrast in renal insufficiency or dehydration. Hold metformin (Glucophage) prior to or at the time of iodinated contrast dye use and for 48 h after procedure. Restart after procedure only if renal function is normal.*

BARIUM SULFATE Non iodinated GI (eg, oral, rectal) contrast. ▶Not absorbed ♀? ▶+ $
DIATRIZOATE (*Cystografin, Gastrografin, Hypaque, MD-Gastroview, RenoCal, Reno-DIP, Reno-60, Renografin*) Iodinated, ionic, high osmolality IV, or GI contrast. ▶K ♀C ▶? $
IODIXANOL (*Visipaque*) Iodinated, nonionic, iso-osmolar IV contrast. ▶K ♀B ▶? $$$
IOHEXOL (*Omnipaque*) Iodinated, nonionic, low osmolality IV, and oral/body cavity contrast. ▶K ♀B ▶? $$$
IOPAMIDOL (*Isovue*) Iodinated, nonionic, low osmolality IV contrast. ▶K ♀? ▶? $$
IOPROMIDE (*Ultravist*) Iodinated, nonionic, low osmolality IV contrast. ▶K ♀B ▶? $$$
IOTHALAMATE (*Conray*) Iodinated, ionic, high osmolality IV contrast. ▶K ♀B ▶– $
IOVERSOL (*Optiray*) Iodinated, nonionic, low osmolality IV contrast. ▶K ♀B ▶? $$
IOXAGLATE (*Hexabrix*) Iodinated, ionic, low osmolality IV contrast. ▶K ♀B ▶– $$$
IOXILAN (*Oxilan*) Iodinated, nonionic, low osmolality IV contrast. ▶K ♀B ▶– $$$

DERMATOLOGY

Acne Preparations

ACANYA (clindamycin + benzoyl peroxide, ✦ *Clindoxyl*) Apply daily. [Trade only: Gel (clindamycin 1.2% + benzoyl peroxide 2.5%) 50 g.] ▶K ♀C ▶+ $$$$
ADAPALENE (*Differin*) Apply at bedtime. [Generic/Trade: Gel 0.1%. Cream 0.1% (45 g). Trade only: Gel 0.3% (45 g). Soln 0.1%(59mL).] ▶Bile ♀C ▶? $$$$
AZELAIC ACID (*Azelex, Finacea, Finevin*) Apply two times per day. [Trade only: Cream 20%, 30, 50 g (Azelex). Gel 15% 50 g (Finacea).] ▶K ♀B ▶? $$$$

BENZACLIN (clindamycin + benzoyl peroxide) Apply two times per day. [Generic/Trade: Gel (clindamycin 1% + benzoyl peroxide 5%) 50 g (jar). Trade only: 25, 35 g (jar) and 50 g (pump).] ▶K ♀C ▶+ $$$$

BENZAMYCIN (erythromycin base + benzoyl peroxide) Apply two times per day. [Generic/Trade: Gel (erythromycin 3% + benzoyl peroxide 5%) 23.3, 46.6 g. Trade only: Benzamycin Pak, #60 gel pouches.] ▶LK ♀C ▶? $$$

BENZOYL PEROXIDE (Benzac, Benzagel 10%, Desquam, Clearasil, ✦ Solugel) Apply once daily; increase to two to three times per day if needed. [OTC and Rx generic: Liquid 2.5, 5, 10%. Bar 5, 10%. Mask 5%. Lotion 4, 5, 8, 10%. Cream 5, 10%. Gel 2.5, 4, 5, 6, 10, 20%. Pad 3, 4, 6, 8, 9%. Other strengths available.] ▶LK ♀C ▶? $

CLENIA (sulfacetamide + sulfur, ✦ Sulfacet-R) Apply daily to three times per day. [Generic only: Lotion (sodium sulfacetamide 10%/sulfur 5%) 25, 30, 45, 60 g. Trade only: Cream (sodium sulfacetamide 10%/sulfur 5%) 28 g. Generic/Trade: Foaming Wash 170, 340 g.] ▶K ♀C ▶? $$$

CLINDAMYCIN—TOPICAL (Cleocin T, Clindagel, ClindaMax, Evoclin, ✦ Dalacin T) Apply daily (Evoclin, Clindagel, Clindamax) or two times per day (Cleocin T). [Generic/Trade: Gel 1% 30, 60 g. Lotion 1% 60 mL. Soln 1% 30, 60 mL. Trade only: Foam 1% 50, 100 g (Evoclin). Gel 1% 40, 75 mL (Clindagel).] ▶L ♀B ▶– $

DIANE-35 (cyproterone + ethinyl estradiol, ✦ Cyestra-35) Canada only. 1 tab PO daily for 21 consecutive days, stop for 7 days, repeat cycle. [Canada Generic/Trade: Blister pack of 21 tabs 2 mg cyproterone acetate/0.035 mg ethinyl estradiol.] ▶L ♀X ▶– $$

DUAC (clindamycin + benzoyl peroxide, ✦ Clindoxyl) Apply at bedtime. [Trade only: Gel (clindamycin 1% + benzoyl peroxide 5%) 45 g.] ▶K ♀C ▶+ $$$$

EPIDUO (adapalene + benzoyl peroxide, ✦ Tactuo) Apply daily. [Trade only: Gel (0.1% adapalene + benzoyl peroxide 2.5%) 45 g.] ▶Bile, K ♀C ▶? $$$$$

ERYTHROMYCIN—TOPICAL (Eryderm, Erycette, Erygel, A/T/S, ✦ Erysol) Apply two times per day. [Generic/Trade: Soln 2% 60 mL. Pads 2%. Gel 2% 30, 60 g. Ointment 2% 25 g. Generic only: Soln 1.5% 60 mL.] ▶L ♀B ▶? $

ISOTRETINOIN (Amnesteem, Claravis, Sotret, Absorica, Myorisan, Zenatane, ✦ Accutane Roche, Clarus) 0.5 to 2 mg/kg/day PO divided two times per day for 15 to 20 weeks. Typical target dose is 1 mg/kg/day. Potent teratogen; use extreme caution. Can only be prescribed by healthcare professionals who are registered with the iPLEDGE program. May cause depression. Not for long-term use. [Generic: Caps 10, 20, 40 mg. Generic only (Sotret, Absorica, and Claravis): Caps 30 mg.] ▶LK ♀X ▶– $$$$$

ROSULA (sulfacetamide + sulfur) Apply daily to three times per day. [Trade only: Gel (sodium sulfacetamide 10%/sulfur 5%) 45 g. Aqueous cleanser (sodium sulfacetamide 10%/sulfur 5%) 355 mL. Soap (sodium sulfacetamide 10%/sulfur 4%) 473 mL.] ▶K ♀C ▶? $$$$

SALICYLIC ACID (Akurza, Clearasil Cleanser, Stridex Pads) Apply/wash area up to three times per day. [OTC Generic/Trade: Pads, Gel, Lotion, Liquid, Mask scrub, 0.5%, 1%, 2%. Rx Trade only (Akurza): Cream 6% 340 g. Lotion 6%, 355 mL.] ▶Not absorbed ♀? ▶? $

SULFACET-R (sulfacetamide + sulfur) Canada only: Apply one to three times per day. [Generic/Trade: Lotion (sodium sulfacetamide 10%/sulfur 5%) 25 g.] ▶K ♀C ▶? $$$

SULFACETAMIDE—TOPICAL (*Klaron*) Apply two times per day. [Generic/Trade: Lotion 10% 118 mL.] ▶K ♀C ▶? $$$$

TAZAROTENE (*Tazorac, Avage*) Acne (Tazorac): Apply 0.1% cream at bedtime. Psoriasis: Apply 0.05% cream at bedtime, increase to 0.1% prn. [Trade only (Tazorac): Cream 0.05% and 0.1% 30, 60 g. Gel 0.05% and 0.1% 30, 100 g. Trade only (Avage): Cream 0.1% 15, 30 g.] ▶L ♀X ▶? $$$$

TRETINOIN—TOPICAL (*Retin-A, Retin-A Micro, Renova, Retisol-A, ✦ Stieva-A, Rejuva-A, Vitamin A Acid Cream*) Acne, wrinkles: Apply at bedtime. [Generic/Trade: Cream 0.025% 20, 45 g, 0.05% 20, 45 g, 0.1% 20, 45 g. Gel 0.025% 15, 45 g, 0.01% 15, 45 g. Micro gel 0.04%, 0.1% 20, 45g, and 50 g pump. Trade only: Renova cream 0.02% 40, 60 g.] ▶LK ♀C ▶? $$$

VELTIN (clindamycin + tretinoin) Acne: Apply at bedtime. [Trade: Gel clindamycin 1.2% + tretinoin 0/025%, 30 g.] ▶LK – ♀C ▶? $$$$

ZIANA (clindamycin + tretinoin) Acne: Apply at bedtime. [Trade only: Gel clindamycin 1.2% + tretinoin 0.025% 30, 60 g.] ▶LK ♀C ▶? $$$$

Actinic Keratosis Preparations

DICLOFENAC—TOPICAL (*Solaraze, Voltaren, Pennsaid*) Solaraze: Actinic/solar keratoses: Apply two times per day to lesions for 60 to 90 days. Voltaren: Osteoarthritis of areas amenable to topical therapy: 2 g (upper extremities) to 4 g (lower extremities) four times per day. Pennsaid: 40 gtts to knee(s) four times daily. [Trade only: Gel 3% 50 g (Solaraze), 100 g (Solaraze, Voltaren). 1.5% soln 150 mL (Pennsaid).] ▶L ♀B ▶? $$$$$

FLUOROURACIL—TOPICAL (*5-FU, Carac, Efudex, Fluoroplex*) Actinic keratoses: Apply two times per day for 2 to 6 weeks. Superficial basal cell carcinomas: Apply 5% cream/soln two times per day. [Trade only: Cream 0.5% 30 g (Carac), 5% 25 g (Efudex), 1% 30 g (Fluoroplex). Generic/Trade: Soln 2%, 5% 10 mL (Efudex). Cream 5% 40 g.] ▶L ♀X ▶– $$$

INGENOL (*Picato*) Apply 0.015% gel to affected area on face and scalp once daily for 3 days or 0.05% gel on affected areas of trunk and extremities once daily for 2 days. [Trade: Gel 0.015% 0.25 g, 0.05% 0.25g.] ▶not absorbed – ♀C ▶? $$$

METHYLAMINOLEVULINATE (*Metvix, Metvixia*) Actinic keratosis: Apply cream to non-hyperkeratotic actinic keratoses lesion and surrounding area on face or scalp; cover with dressing for 3 h; remove dressing and cream and perform illumination therapy. Repeat in 7 days. [Trade only: Cream 16.8%, 2 g tube.] ▶Not absorbed ♀C ▶?

Antibacterials (Topical)

BACITRACIN Apply daily to three times per day. [OTC Generic/Trade: Ointment 500 units/g 1, 15, 30 g.] ▶Not absorbed ♀C ▶? $

+ FUSIDIC ACID—TOPICAL (*Fucidin*) Canada only. Apply three to four times per day. [Canada trade only: Cream 2% fusidic acid 5, 15, 30 g. Ointment 2% sodium fusidate 5, 15, 30 g.] ▶L ♀? ▶? $

GENTAMICIN—TOPICAL (*Garamycin*) Apply three to four times per day. [Generic only: Ointment 0.1% 15, 30 g. Cream 0.1% 15, 30 g.] ▶K ♀D ▶? $

MAFENIDE (*Sulfamylon*) Apply one to two times per day. [Generic/Trade: Topical Soln 50 g packets. Trade only: Cream 5% 57, 114, 454 g.] ▶LK ♀C ▶? $$$

METRONIDAZOLE—TOPICAL (*Noritate, MetroCream, MetroGel, MetroLotion, + Rosasol*) Rosacea: Apply daily (1%) or two times per day (0.75%). [Trade only: Gel (MetroGel) 1% 45, 60 g. Cream (Noritate) 1% 60 g. Generic/Trade: Gel 0.75% 45 g. Cream 0.75% 45 g. Lotion (MetroLotion) 0.75% 59 mL.] ▶KL ♀B (− in 1st trimester) ▶− $$$

MUPIROCIN (*Bactroban, Centany*) Impetigo/infected wounds: Apply three times per day. Nasal MRSA eradication: 0.5 g in each nostril two times per day for 5 days. [Generic/Trade: Ointment 2% 22 g. Nasal ointment 2% 1 g single-use tubes (for MRSA eradication). Trade only: Cream 2% 15, 30 g.] ▶Not absorbed ♀B ▶? $$

NEOSPORIN CREAM (neomycin + polymyxin + bacitracin) Apply one to three times per day. [OTC Trade only: neomycin 3.5 mg/g + polymyxin 10,000 units/g 15 g and unit dose 0.94 g.] ▶K ♀C ▶? $

NEOSPORIN OINTMENT (bacitracin + neomycin + polymyxin) Apply one to three times per day. [OTC Generic/Trade: bacitracin 400 units/g + neomycin 3.5 mg/g + polymyxin 5000 units/g 15, 30 g and "to go" 0.9 g packets.] ▶K ♀C ▶? $

POLYSPORIN (bacitracin + polymyxin, + *Polytopic*) Apply one to three times per day. [OTC Trade only: Ointment 15, 30 g and unit dose 0.9 g. Powder 10 g.] ▶K ♀C ▶? $

RETAPAMULIN (*Altabax*) Impetigo: Apply thin layer two times per day for 5 days. [Trade only: Ointment 1% 5, 10, 15 g.] ▶Not absorbed ♀B ▶? $$$

SILVER SULFADIAZINE (*Silvadene, + Flamazine*) Apply one to two times per day. [Generic/Trade: Cream 1% 20, 50, 85, 400, 1000 g.] ▶LK ♀B ▶− $$

Antifungals (Topical)

BUTENAFINE (*Lotrimin Ultra, Mentax*) Treatment of tinea pedis: Apply daily for 4 weeks or two times per day for 7 days. Tinea corporis, tinea versicolor, or tinea cruris: Apply daily for 2 weeks. Apply one to two times per day. [Rx Trade only: Cream 1% 15, 30 g (Mentax). OTC Trade only: Cream 1% 12, 24 g (Lotrimin Ultra).] ▶L ♀B ▶? $

CICLOPIROX (*Loprox, Loprox TS, Penlac, + Stieprox shampoo*) Tinea pedis, cruris, corporis, and versicolor; candidiasis (cream, lotion): Apply two times per day. Fungal nail infection (Penlac): Apply daily to affected nails; apply over previous coat; remove with alcohol q 7 days. Seborrheic dermatitis (Loprox shampoo): Shampoo two times per week for 4 weeks. [Trade only: Shampoo (Loprox) 1% 120 mL. Generic/Trade: Gel 0.77% 30, 45, 100 g. Nail soln (Penlac) 8% 6.6 mL. Cream (Loprox) 0.77% 15, 30, 90 g. Lotion (Loprox TS) 0.77% 30, 60 mL.] ▶K ♀B ▶? $$$$

CLOTRIMAZOLE—TOPICAL (*Lotrimin AF, Mycelex,* **← *Canesten, Clotrimaderm*)** Treatment of tinea pedis, cruris, corporis, and versicolor; cutaneous candidiasis: Apply two times per day. [Note that Lotrimin brand cream, lotion, soln are clotrimazole, while Lotrimin powders and liquid spray are miconazole. Rx Generic only: Cream 1% 15, 30, 45 g. Soln 1% 10, 30 mL. OTC Generic only: Cream 1% 12, 24 g. Soln 1% 10 mL.] ▶L ♀B ▶? $

ECONAZOLE Tinea pedis, tinea cruris, tinea corporis, tinea versicolor: Apply daily. Cutaneous candidiasis: Apply two times per day. [Generic only: Cream 1% 15, 30, 85 g.] ▶Not absorbed ♀C ▶? $$

KETOCONAZOLE—TOPICAL (*Extina, Nizoral, Nizoral AD, Xolegel,* **← *Ketoderm*)** Tinea/candidal infections: Apply daily. Seborrheic dermatitis: Apply cream one to two times per day for 4 weeks or gel daily for 2 weeks or foam two times per day for 4 weeks. Dandruff (Nizoral AD): Apply shampoo twice a week. Tinea versicolor: Apply shampoo to affected area, leave on for 5 min, rinse. [Generic/Trade: Cream 2% 15, 30, 60 g. Shampoo 2% 120 mL. Trade only: Shampoo 1% 120, 210 mL (OTC Nizoral AD). Gel 2% 15 g (Xolegel). Foam 2% 50, 100 g (Extina).] ▶L ♀C ▶? $$$

MICONAZOLE—TOPICAL (*Micatin, Lotrimin AF, ZeaSorb AF*) Tinea, candida: Apply two times per day. [Note that Lotrimin brand cream, lotion, soln are clotrimazole, while Lotrimin powders and liquid spray are miconazole. OTC Trade only: Powder 2% 70, 160 g. Spray powder 2% 90, 100, 140 g. Spray liquid 2% 90, 105 mL. Gel 2% 24 g.] ▶L ♀+ ▶? $

NAFTIFINE (*Naftin*) Tinea: Apply daily (cream) or two times per day (gel). [Trade only: Cream 1% 60, 90 g, cream 1% Pump 90 g. Gel 1% 40, 60, 90 g. Cream 2% 45g.] ▶LK ♀B ▶? $$$$$

NYSTATIN—TOPICAL (*Mycostatin,* **← *Nyaderm*)** Candidiasis: Apply two to three times per day. [Generic/Trade: Cream, Ointment 100,000 units/g 15, 30 g. Powder 100,000 units/g 15, 30, 60 g.] ▶Not absorbed ♀C ▶? $

OXICONAZOLE (*Oxistat, Oxizole*) Tinea pedis, cruris, and corporis: Apply one to two times per day. Tinea versicolor (cream only): Apply daily. [Trade only: Cream 1% 15, 30, 60 g. Lotion 1% 30 mL.] ▶? ♀B ▶? $$$

SERTACONAZOLE (*Ertaczo*) Tinea pedis: Apply two times per day. [Trade only: Cream 2% 30, 60 g.] ▶Not absorbed ♀C ▶? $$$

TERBINAFINE—TOPICAL (*Lamisil, Lamisil AT*) Tinea: Apply one to two times per day. [OTC Trade only (Lamisil AT): Cream 1% 12, 24 g. Spray pump soln 1% 30 mL. Gel 1% 6, 12 g.] ▶L ♀B ▶? $

TOLNAFTATE (*Tinactin*) Apply two times per day. [OTC Generic/Trade: Cream 1% 15, 30 g. Soln 1% 10 mL. Powder 1% 45 g. OTC Trade only: Gel 1% 15 g. Powder 1% 90 g. Spray powder 1% 100, 133, 150 g. Spray liquid 1% 100, 113 mL.] ▶? ♀? ▶? $

Antiparasitics (Topical)

A-200 (pyrethrins + piperonyl butoxide, **← *R&C*)** Lice: Apply shampoo, wash after 10 min. Reapply in 5 to 7 days. [OTC Generic/Trade: Shampoo (0.33% pyrethrins, 4% piperonyl butoxide) 60, 120 mL.] ▶L ♀C ▶? $

BENZYL ALCOHOL (*Ulesfia*) Lice: Apply to dry hair to saturate scalp and hair. Rinse after 10 minutes. Reapply in 7 days, if necessary. [Lotion 5% 60 mL and in 2-pack with nit comb.] ▶not absorbed − ♀B ▶? $$$$

CROTAMITON (*Eurax*) Scabies: Apply cream/lotion topically from chin to feet, repeat in 24 h, bathe 48 h later. Pruritus: Massage prn. [Trade only: Cream 10% 60 g. Lotion 10% 60, 480 mL.] ▶? ♀C ▶? $$

LINDANE Other drugs preferred. Scabies: Apply 30 to 60 mL of lotion, wash after 8 to 12 h. Lice: 30 to 60 mL of shampoo, wash off after 4 min. Can cause seizures in epileptics or if overused/misused in children. Not for infants. [Generic only: Lotion 1% 60, 480 mL. Shampoo 1% 60, 480 mL.] ▶L ♀B ▶? $

MALATHION (*Ovide*) Lice: Apply to dry hair, let dry naturally, wash off in 8 to 12 h. Flammable. [Generic/Trade only: Lotion 0.5% 59 mL.] ▶? ♀B ▶? $$$$

PERMETHRIN (*Elimite, Acticin, Nix*, ✦*Kwellada-P*) Scabies: Apply cream from head (avoid mouth/nose/eyes) to soles of feet and wash after 8 to 14 h. 30 g is typical adult dose. Lice: Saturate hair and scalp with 1% rinse, wash after 10 min. Do not use in age younger than 2 mo. May repeat therapy in 7 days, as necessary. [Generic/Trade: Cream (Elimite, Acticin) 5% 60 g. OTC Generic/Trade: Liquid creme rinse (Nix) 1% 60 mL.] ▶L ♀B ▶? $$

RID (*pyrethrins + piperonyl butoxide*) Lice: Apply shampoo/mousse, wash after 10 min. Reapply in 5 to 10 days prn. [OTC Generic/Trade: Shampoo 60, 120, 240 mL. OTC Trade only: Mousse 5.5 oz.] ▶L ♀C ▶? $

SKLICE (*ivermectin*) Lice: Apply to dry hair. Rinse after 10 minutes. Single application only. [Trade: Lotion 0.5%, 120 mL.] ▶minimal absorption − ♀C ▶? $$$$

SPINOSAD (*Natroba*) Lice: Apply to dry hair/scalp to cover. Leave on 10 minutes then rinse. Retreat if live lice seen after 7 days. [Topical susp, 0.9%, 120 mL.] ▶not absorbed − ♀B ▶? $$$$$

Antipsoriatics

ACITRETIN (*Soriatane*) 25 to 50 mg PO daily. Avoid pregnancy during therapy and for 3 years after discontinuation. [Generic/Trade only: Caps 10, 17.5, 25 mg.] ▶L ♀X ▶− $$$$$

ALEFACEPT (*Amevive*) 7.5 mg IV or 15 mg IM once a week for 12 doses. May repeat with 1 additional 12-week course after 12 weeks have elapsed since last dose. ▶? ♀B ▶? $$$$$

ANTHRALIN (*Drithocreme*, ✦*Anthraforte, Anthranol, Anthrascalp*) Apply daily. Short contact periods (ie, 15 to 20 min) followed by removal may be preferred. [Trade only: Cream 0.5, 1% 50 g.] ▶? ♀C ▶− $$$

CALCIPOTRIENE (*Dovonex, Sorilux*) Apply two times per day. [Trade only: Ointment 0.005% 30, 60, 100 g (Dovonex). Cream 0.005% 30, 60, 100 g (Dovonex). Foam for scalp 0.005% 60, 120 g (Sorilux). Generic/Trade: Scalp soln 0.005% 60 mL.] ▶L ♀C ▶? $$$$

TACLONEX (calcipotriene + betamethasone, ✦*Dovobet*) Apply daily for up to 4 weeks. [Calcipotriene 0.005% + betamethasone dipropionate 0.064%. Trade only: Ointment 15, 30, 60, 100 g. Topical susp (Taclonex TS 15, 30, 60 g.] ▶L ♀C ▶? $$$$$

USTEKINUMAB (*Stelara*) Severe plaque psoriasis : Wt less than 100 kg, use 45 mg SC initially and again 4 weeks later, followed by 45 mg SC q 12 weeks. For wt greater than 100 kg, use 90 mg SC initially and again 4 weeks later, followed by 90 mg SC q 12 weeks. [Trade only: 45 and 90 mg prefilled syringe and vial.] ▶L – ♀B ▶? $$$$$

Antivirals (Topical)

ACYCLOVIR—TOPICAL (*Zovirax*) Herpes genitalis : Apply ointment q 3 h (6 times per day) for 7 days. Recurrent herpes labialis : Apply cream 5 times per day for 4 days. [Generic/Trade: Ointment 5% 15, 30g. Trade only: Cream 5% 5 g.] ▶K ♀C ▶? $$$$$

DOCOSANOL (*Abreva*) Oral-facial herpes (cold sores): Apply 5 times per day until healed. [OTC Trade only: Cream 10% 2 g.] ▶Not absorbed ♀B ▶? $

IMIQUIMOD (*Aldara, Zyclara,* ✦ *Vyloma*) Genital/perianal warts: Apply once daily for up to 8 weeks. Wash off after 8 h. Non-hyperkeratotic, non-hypertrophic actinic keratoses on face/scalp in immunocompetent adults: Apply two times per week overnight for 16 weeks (Aldara) or once daily for two 2-week periods separated by a 2-week break (Zyclara). Wash off after 8 h. Primary superficial basal cell carcinoma: Apply 5 times a week for 6 weeks (Aldara). Wash off after 8 h. [Generic/Trade: Cream 5% (Aldara) single-use packets, 3.75% (Zyclara) 7.5 g and 15 g pump, 2.5% 7.5 g and 15 g pump.] ▶Not absorbed ♀C ▶? $$$$$

PENCICLOVIR (*Denavir*) Herpes labialis (cold sores): Apply cream q 2 h while awake for 4 days. [Trade only: Cream 1% tube 1.5 g.] ▶Not absorbed ♀B ▶? $$

PODOFILOX (*Condylox,* ✦ *Condyline, Wartec*) External genital warts (gel and soln) and perianal warts (gel only): Apply two times per day for 3 consecutive days of the week and repeat for up to 4 weeks. [Generic/Trade: Soln 0.5% 3.5 mL. Trade only: Gel 0.5% 3.5 g.] ▶? ♀C ▶? $$$$

PODOPHYLLIN (*Podocon-25, Podofin, Podofilm*) Warts : Apply by physician. [Not to be dispensed to patients. For hospital/clinic use; not intended for outpatient prescribing. Trade only: Liquid 25% 15 mL.] ▶? ♀– ▶– $$$

SINECATECHINS (*Veregen*) Apply three times per day to external genital warts for up to 16 weeks. [Trade only: Ointment 15% 15, 30 g.] ▶Unknown ♀C ▶? $$$$$

Atopic Dermatitis Preparations

NOTE: *Potential risk of cancer. Should only be used as 2nd-line agent for short-term and intermittent treatment of atopic dermatitis in those unresponsive to or intolerant of other treatments.*

PIMECROLIMUS (*Elidel*) Atopic dermatitis: Apply two times per day. [Trade only: Cream 1% 30, 60, 100 g.] ▶L ♀C ▶? $$$$ ∎

TACROLIMUS—TOPICAL (*Protopic*) Atopic dermatitis : Apply two times per day. [Trade only: Ointment 0.03%, 0.1% 30, 60, 100 g.] ▶Minimal absorption ♀C ▶? $$$$$ ∎

CORTICOSTEROIDS—TOPICAL

Potency*	Generic	Trade Name	Forms	Frequency
Low	alclometasone dipropionate	Aclovate	0.05% C/O	bid–tid
Low	clocortolone pivalate	Cloderm	0.1% C	tid
Low	desonide	DesOwen, Tridesilon	0.05% C/L/O	bid–tid
Low	hydrocortisone	Hytone, others	0.5% C/L/O; 1% C/L/O; 2.5% C/L/O	bid–qid
Low	hydrocortisone acetate	Cortaid, Corticaine	0.5% C/O; 1% C/O/Sp	bid–qid
Medium	betamethasone valerate	Luxiq	0.1% C/L/O; 0.12% F (Luxiq)	daily–bid
Medium	desoximetasone‡	Topicort	0.05% C	bid
Medium	fluocinolone	Synalar	0.01% C/S; 0.025% C/O	bid–qid
Medium	flurandrenolide	Cordran	0.025% C/O; 0.05% C/L/O/T	bid–qid
Medium	fluticasone propionate	Cutivate	0.005% O; 0.05% C/L	daily–bid
Medium	hydrocortisone butyrate	Locoid	0.1% C/O/S	bid–tid
Medium	hydrocortisone valerate	Westcort	0.2% C/O	bid–tid
Medium	mometasone furoate	Elocon	0.1% C/L/O	daily
Medium	triamcinolone‡	Aristocort, Kenalog	0.025% C/L/O; 0.1% C/L/O/S	bid–tid
High	amcinonide	Cyclocort	0.1% C/L/O	bid–tid
High	betamethasone dipropionate‡	Maxivate, others	0.05% C/L/O (non-Diprolene)	daily–bid
High	desoximetasone‡	Topicort	0.05% G; 0.25% C/O	bid
High	diflorasone diacetate‡	Maxiflor	0.05% C/O	bid
High	fluocinonide	Lidex	0.05% C/G/O/S	bid–tid
High	halcinonide	Halog	0.1% C/O/S	bid–tid
High	triamcinolone‡	Aristocort, Kenalog	0.5% C/O	bid–tid
Very high	betamethasone dipropionate‡	Diprolene, Diprolene AF	0.05% C/G/L/O	daily–bid
Very high	clobetasol	Temovate, Cormax, Olux	0.05% C/G/O/L/S/Sp/F (Olux)	bid
Very high	diflorasone diacetate‡	Psorcon	0.05% C/O	daily–tid
Very high	halobetasol propionate	Ultravate	0.05% C/O	daily–bid

C.=cream; O.=ointment; L.=lotion; T.=tape; F.=foam; S.=solution; G.=gel; Sp.=spray.
bid=two times per day; tid=three times per day; qid=four times per day.
*Potency based on vasoconstrictive assays, which may not correlate with efficacy. Not all available products are listed, including those lacking potency ratings.
‡These drugs have formulations in more than once potency category.

Corticosteroid/Antimicrobial Combinations

CORTISPORIN (*neomycin + polymyxin + hydrocortisone*) Apply two to four times per day. [Trade only: Cream 7.5 g. Ointment 15 g.] ▶LK ♀C ▶? $$$

FUCIDIN H (*fusidic acid + hydrocortisone*) Canada only. Apply three times per day. [Canada Trade only: Cream (2% fusidic acid, 1% hydrocortisone acetate) 30 g.] ▶L ♀? ▶? $$

LOTRISONE (*clotrimazole + betamethasone,* ✚ *Lotriderm*) Apply two times per day. Do not use for diaper rash. [Generic/Trade: Cream (clotrimazole 1% + betamethasone 0.05%) 15, 45 g. Lotion (clotrimazole 1% + betamethasone 0.05%) 30 mL.] ▶L ♀C ▶? $$$

MYCOLOG II (*nystatin + triamcinolone*) Apply two times per day. [Generic only: Cream, Ointment 15, 30, 60, 120, 454 g.] ▶L ♀C ▶? $

Hemorrhoid Care

DIBUCAINE (*Nupercainal*) Apply three to four times per day prn. [OTC Trade only: Ointment 1% 30, 60 g.] ▶L ♀? ▶? $

PRAMOXINE (*Tucks Hemorrhoidal Ointment, Fleet Pain Relief, ProctoFoam NS*) Apply up to 5 times per day prn. [OTC Trade only: Ointment (Tucks Hemorrhoidal Ointment) 30 g. Pads (Fleet Pain Relief) 100 each. Aerosol foam (ProctoFoam NS) 15 g.] ▶Not absorbed ♀+ ▶+ $

STARCH (*Tucks Suppositories*) 1 suppository up to 6 times per day prn. [OTC Trade only: Suppository (51% topical starch; vegetable oil, tocopheryl acetate) 12, 24 each.] ▶Not absorbed ♀+ ▶+ $

WITCH HAZEL (*Tucks*) Apply to anus/perineum up to 6 times per day prn. [OTC Generic/Trade: Pads 50% 12, 40, 100 ea, generically available in various quantities.] ▶? ♀+ ▶+ $

Other Dermatologic Agents

ALITRETINOIN (*Panretin,* ✚ *Toctino*) Apply two to four times per day to cutaneous Kaposi's lesions. [Trade only: Gel 0.1% 60 g.] ▶Not absorbed ♀D ▶− $$$$$

ALUMINUM CHLORIDE (*Drysol, Certain Dri*) Apply at bedtime. [Rx Trade only: Soln 20% 37.5 mL bottle, 35, 60 mL bottle with applicator. OTC Trade only (Certain Dri): Soln 12.5% 36 mL bottle.] ▶K ♀? ▶? $

BECAPLERMIN (*Regranex*) Diabetic ulcers: Apply daily. [Trade only: Gel 0.01%, 2, 15 g.] ▶Minimal absorption ♀C ▶? $$$$$ ∎

CALAMINE Apply three to four times per day prn for poison ivy/oak or insect bite itching. [OTC Generic only: Lotion 120, 240, 480 mL.] ▶? ♀? ▶? $

CAPSAICIN (*Zostrix, Zostrix-HP, Qutenza*) Arthritis, post-herpetic or diabetic neuralgia: Apply three to four times per day. Post-herpetic neuralgia: 1 patch (Qutenza) applied for 1 h in medical office, may repeat q 3 months. [Rx: Patch 8% (Qutenza). OTC Generic/Trade: Cream 0.025% 60 g, 0.075% (HP) 60 g. OTC Generic only: Lotion 0.025% 59 mL, 0.075% 59 mL.] ▶? ♀? ▶? $

COAL TAR (*Polytar, Tegrin, Cutar, Tarsum*) Apply shampoo for seborrheic dermatitis at least twice a week, or for psoriasis apply one to four times per day. [OTC Generic/Trade: Shampoo, cream, ointment, gel, lotion, liquid, oil, soap.] ▶? ♀? ▶? $

DOXEPIN—TOPICAL (*Zonalon*) Pruritus: Apply four times per day for up to 8 days. [Trade only: Cream 5% 30, 45 g.] ▶L ♀B ▶– $$$$

EFLORNITHINE (*Vaniqa*) Reduction of facial hair: Apply to face two times per day. [Trade only: Cream 13.9% 30 g.] ▶K ♀C ▶? $$$

EMLA (*prilocaine + lidocaine—topical*) Topical anesthesia: Apply 2.5 g cream or 1 disc to region at least 1 h before procedure. Cover with occlusive dressing. [Generic/Trade: Cream (2.5% lidocaine + 2.5% prilocaine) 5, 30 g.] ▶LK ♀B ▶? $$

HYALURONIC ACID (*Bionect, Restylane, Perlane*) Moderate to severe facial wrinkles: Inject into wrinkle/fold (Restylane, Perlane). Protection of dermal ulcers: Apply gel/cream/spray two or three times each day (Bionect). [OTC Trade only: Cream 2% 15, 30 g. Rx Generic/Trade: Soln 3% 30 mL. Gel 4% 30 g. Cream 4% 15, 30, 60 g. Injectable gel 2%.] ▶? ♀? ▶? $$$

HYDROQUINONE (*Eldopaque, Eldoquin, Eldoquin Forte, EpiQuin Micro, Esoterica, Glyquin, Lustra, Melanex, Solaquin, Claripel, ♦Ultraquin*) Hyperpigmentation: Apply two times per day. [OTC Trade only: Cream 2% 15, 30 g. Rx Generic/Trade: Soln 3% 30 mL. Gel 4% 30 g. Cream 4% 15, 30, 60 g.] ▶? ♀C ▶? $

LACTIC ACID (*Lac-Hydrin, AmLactin,*) Apply two times per day. [Trade only: Lotion 12% 150, 360 mL. OTC: Cream 12% 140, 385 g. AmLactin AP is lactic acid (12%) with pramoxine (1%).] ▶? ♀? ▶? $$

LIDOCAINE—TOPICAL (*Xylocaine, Lidoderm, Numby Stuff, LMX, Zingo, ♦Maxilene*) Apply prn. Dose varies with anesthetic procedure, degree of anesthesia required, and individual patient response. Post-herpetic neuralgia: Apply up to 3 patches to affected area at once for up to 12 h within a 24-h period. Apply 30 min prior to painful procedure (ELA-Max 4%). Discomfort with anorectal disorders: Apply prn (ELA-Max 5%). Intradermal powder injection for venipuncture/IV cannulation, 3 to 18 yo (Zingo): 0.5 mg to site 1 to 10 min prior. [For membranes of mouth and pharynx: Spray 10%, Ointment 5%, Liquid 5%, Soln 2%, 4%, Dental patch. For urethral use: Jelly 2%. Patch (Lidoderm $$$$$) 5%. Intradermal powder injection system: 0.5 mg (Zingo). OTC Trade only: Liposomal lidocaine 4% (ELA-Max.).] ▶LK ♀B ▶+ $ – varies by therapy

MINOXIDIL—TOPICAL (*Rogaine, Women's Rogaine, Rogaine Extra Strength, Minoxidil for Men*) Androgenetic alopecia in men or women: 1 mL to dry scalp two times per day. [OTC Generic/Trade: Soln 2% 60 mL (Rogaine, Women's Rogaine). Soln 5% 60 mL (Rogaine Extra Strength, Theroxidil Extra Strength—for men only). Foam 5% 60 g (Rogaine Extra Strength).] ▶K ♀C ▶– $

MONOBENZONE (*Benoquin*) Extensive vitiligo: Apply two to three times per day. [Trade only: Cream 20% 35.4 g.] ▶Minimal absorption ♀C ▶? $$$

OATMEAL (*Aveeno*) Pruritus from poison ivy/oak, varicella: Apply lotion four times per day prn. Also bath packets for tub. [OTC Generic/Trade: Lotion. Bath packets.] ▶Not absorbed ♀? ▶? $

PANAFIL (papain + urea + chlorophyllin copper complex) Debridement of acute or chronic lesions: Apply to clean wound and cover one to two times per day. [Trade only: Ointment 6, 30 g. Spray 33 mL.] ▶? ♀? ▶? $$$

PLIAGIS (tetracaine + lidocaine–topical) Apply 20 to 30 min prior to superficial dermatological procedure (60 min for tattoo removal). [Trade only: Cream lidocaine 7% + tetracaine 7%.] ▶Minimal absorption ♀B ▶?

PRAMOSONE (pramoxine + hydrocortisone, ✦ Pramox HC) Inflammatory and pruritic manifestations of corticosteroid-responsive dermatoses: Apply three to four times per day. [Trade only: 1% pramoxine/1% hydrocortisone: Cream 30, 60 g. Ointment 30 g. Lotion 60, 120, 240 mL. 1% pramoxine/2.5% hydrocortisone acetate: Cream 30, 60 g. Ointment 30 g. Lotion 60, 120 mL.] ▶Not absorbed ♀C ▶? $$$

SELENIUM SULFIDE (Selsun, Exsel, Versel) Dandruff, seborrheic dermatitis: Apply 5 to 10 mL two times per week for 2 weeks then less frequently, thereafter. Tinea versicolor: Apply 2.5% to affected area daily for 7 days. [OTC Generic/Trade: Lotion/Shampoo 1% 120, 210, 240, 325 mL, 2.5% 120 mL. Rx Generic/Trade: Lotion/Shampoo 2.5% 120 mL.] ▶? ♀C ▶? $

SOLAGE (mequinol + tretinoin, ✦ Solage) Canada only: Apply to solar lentigines two times per day. [Trade only: Soln 30 mL (mequinol 2% + tretinoin 0.01%).] ▶Not absorbed ♀X ▶? $$$$

SYNERA (tetracaine + lidocaine—topical) Apply 20 to 30 min prior to superficial dermatological procedure. [Trade only: Topical patch (lidocaine 70 mg + tetracaine 70 mg.] ▶Minimal absorption ♀B ▶? $$

TRI-LUMA (fluocinolone + hydroquinone + tretinoin) Melasma of the face: Apply at bedtime for 4 to 8 weeks. [Trade only: Cream 30 g (fluocinolone 0.01% + hydroquinone 4% + tretinoin 0.05%).] ▶Minimal absorption ♀C ▶? $$$$

VUSION (miconazole—topical + zinc oxide + white petrolatum) Apply to affected diaper area with each change for 7 days. [Trade only: Ointment 50 g.] ▶Minimal absorption ♀C ▶? $$$$$

ENDOCRINE & METABOLIC

Androgens / Anabolic Steroids

NOTE: See OB/GYN section for other hormones.

TESTOSTERONE (***Androderm, AndroGel, Axiron, Delatestryl, Depo-Testosterone, Striant, Testim, Testopel, Testro AQ, ✦ Andriol***) Hypogonadism: Injectable enanthate or cypionate: 50 to 400 mg IM q 2 to 4 weeks. Transdermal: Androderm: Start 4 mg patch to nonscrotal skin at bedtime. AndroGel 1%: Apply 5 g from gel pack or 4 pumps (5 g gel; 50 mg testosterone) from dispenser daily to shoulders/upper arms/abdomen. Androgel 1.62%: Apply 2 pumps (40.5 mg testosterone) from dispenser daily to shoulders or upper arms. Adjust based on serum testosterone concentration q 14 to 28 days. Dose range 1 to 4 pumps daily. Axiron: 60 mg (1 pump of 30 mg to each axilla) once daily. Testim: 1 tube (5 g) daily to shoulders/upper

(cont.)

arms. Pellet: Testopel: 2 to 6 (150 to 450 mg testosterone) pellets SC q 3 to 6 months. Buccal: Striant: 30 mg q 12 h on upper gum above the incisor tooth; alternate sides for each application. [Trade only: Patch 2, 4 mg/24 h (Androderm). Gel 1% 2.5, 5 g packet, 75 g multidose pump (AndroGel 1% 1.25 g gel containing 12.5 mg testosterone per actuation). Gel 1.62%, 20.25 mg testosterone/actuation (AndroGel 1.62%). Gel 1.62% (Androgel 1.62%) 1.25, 2.5 g (package of 30), Gel 1%, 5 g tube (Testim). Solution 90 mL multidose pump (Axiron, 30 mg/actuation). Gel (Fortesta) 10 mg/actuation. Pellet 75 mg (Testopel). Buccal: Blister packs: 30 mg (Striant). Generic/Trade: Injection 100, 200 mg/mL (cypionate), 200 mg/mL (ethanate).] ▶L ♀X ▶?©III $ – varies by therapy ■

Bisphosphonates

ALENDRONATE *(Fosamax, Fosamax Plus D, Binosto, ✦ Fosavance)* Prevention of postmenopausal osteoporosis (Fosamax): 5 mg PO daily or 35 mg PO weekly. Treatment of postmenopausal osteoporosis (Fosamax, Fosamax Plus D, Binosto): 10 mg daily, 70 mg PO weekly, 70 mg/vitamin D3 2800 international units PO weekly, or 70 mg/vitamin D3 5600 international units PO weekly. Treatment of glucocorticoid-induced osteoporosis (Fosamax): 5 mg PO daily in men and women or 10 mg PO daily in postmenopausal women not taking estrogen. Treatment of osteoporosis in men (Fosamax, Fosamax Plus D, Binosto): 10 mg PO daily, 70 mg PO weekly, or 70 mg/vitamin D3 2800 international units PO weekly, or 70 mg/vit D3 5600 international units PO weekly. Paget's disease (Fosamax): 40 mg PO daily for 6 months. [Generic/Trade (Fosamax): Tabs 5, 10, 35, 40, 70 mg. Trade only: Fosamax Plus D: 70 mg + either 2800 or 5600 units of vitamin D3. Binosto: 70 mg effervescent tab.] ▶K ♀C ▶– $

ETIDRONATE *(Didronel)* Paget's disease: 5 to 10 mg/kg PO daily for 6 months or 11 to 20 mg/kg daily for 3 months. [Generic only: Tabs 400 mg. Generic only: Tabs 200 mg.] ▶K ♀C ▶? $$$$$

IBANDRONATE *(Boniva)* Prevention and treatment of postmenopausal osteoporosis: Oral: 150 mg PO once a month. IV: 3 mg IV q 3 months. [Generic/Trade: Tabs 150 mg. Trade only: IV: 3 mg.] ▶K ♀C ▶? $$$$

PAMIDRONATE *(Aredia)* Hypercalcemia of malignancy: 60 to 90 mg IV over 2 to 24 h. Wait at least 7 days before considering retreatment. ▶K ♀D ▶? $$$$$

RISEDRONATE *(Actonel, Atelvia)* Prevention and treatment of postmenopausal osteoporosis: 5 mg PO daily, 35 mg PO weekly, or 150 mg once a month. Treatment of osteoporosis in men: 35 mg PO weekly. Prevention and treatment of glucocorticoid-induced osteoporosis: 5 mg PO daily. Paget's disease: 30 mg PO daily for 2 months. [Trade only: Tabs 5, 30, 35, 150 mg, Delayed-release tab (Atelvia): 35 mg.] ▶K ♀C ▶? $$$$

ZOLEDRONIC ACID *(Reclast, Zometa, ✦ Aclasta)* Treatment of osteoporosis (Reclast): 5 mg once yearly IV infusion over 15 min or longer. Prevention of postmenopausal osteoporosis: (Reclast): 5 mg IV infusion every 2 years.

(cont.)

Prevention and treatment of glucocorticoid-induced osteoporosis (Reclast): 5 mg once a year IV infusion over 15 min or longer. Hypercalcemia (Zometa): 4 mg IV infusion over 15 min or longer. Wait at least 7 days before considering retreatment. Paget's disease (Reclast): 5 mg IV single dose infused over 15 min or longer. Multiple myeloma and metastatic bone lesions from solid tumors (Zometa): 4 mg IV infusion over 15 min or longer q 3 to 4 weeks. [Generic/Trade: 4 mg/5 mL IV (Zometa), 5 mg/100 mL IV (Reclast)] ▶K ♀D ▶? $$$$$

Corticosteroids

NOTE: *See also Dermatology, Ophthalmology.*

BETAMETHASONE (*Celestone, Celestone Soluspan, ✦ Betaject*) Anti-inflammatory/immunosuppressive: 0.6 to 7.2 mg/day PO divided two to four times per day; up to 9 mg/day IM. Fetal lung maturation, maternal antepartum: 12 mg IM q 24 h for 2 doses. [Trade only: Syrup 0.6 mg/5 mL.] ▶L ♀C ▶– $$$$$

CORTISONE (*Cortone*) 25 to 300 mg PO daily. [Generic only: Tabs 25 mg.] ▶L ♀D ▶– $

DEXAMETHASONE (*Decadron, Dexpak, ✦ Dexasone*) Anti-inflammatory/immunosuppressive: 0.5 to 9 mg/day PO/IV/IM, divided two to four times per day. Cerebral edema: 10 to 20 mg IV load, then 4 mg IM q 6 h (off-label IV use common) or 1 to 3 mg PO three times per day. Bronchopulmonary dysplasia in preterm infants: 0.5 mg/kg PO/IV divided q 12 h for 3 days, then taper. Croup: 0.6 mg/kg PO or IM for one dose. Acute asthma: Age older than 2 yo: 0.6 mg/kg to max 16 mg PO daily for 2 days. Fetal lung maturation, maternal antepartum: 6 mg IM q 12 h for 4 doses. Antiemetic, prophylaxis: 8 mg IV or 12 mg PO prior to chemotherapy; 8 mg PO daily for 2 to 4 days. Antiemetic, treatment: 10 to 20 mg PO/IV q 4 to 6 h. [Generic/Trade: Tabs 0.5, 0.75.

(cont.)

CORTICO-STEROIDS	Approximate Equivalent Dose (mg)	Relative Anti-Inflammatory Potency	Relative Mineralocorticoid Potency	Biological Half-life (h)
betamethasone	0.6–0.75	20–30	0	36–54
cortisone	25	0.8	2	8–12
dexamethasone	0.75	20–30	0	36–54
fludrocortisone	n/a	10	125	18–36
hydrocortisone	20	1	2	8–12
methylprednisolone	4	5	0	18–36
prednisolone	5	4	1	18–36
prednisone	5	4	1	18–36
triamcinolone	4	5	0	12–36

n/a, not available.

Generic only: Tabs 0.25, 1.0, 1.5, 2, 4, 6 mg; elixir 0.5 mg/5 mL; Soln 0.5 mg/5 mL, 1 mg/1 mL (concentrate). Trade only: Dexpak 13 day (51 total 1.5 mg tabs for a 13-day taper), Dexpak 10 day (35 total 1.5 mg tabs for 10-day taper), Dexpak 6 days (21 total 1.5 mg tabs for 6-day taper).] ▶L ♀C ▶? $

FLUDROCORTISONE (*Florinef*) Mineralocorticoid activity: 0.1 mg PO 3 times per week to 0.2 mg PO daily. Postural hypotension: 0.05 to 0.4 mg PO daily. [Generic only: Tabs 0.1 mg.] ▶L ♀C ▶? $

HYDROCORTISONE (*Cortef, Cortenema, Solu-Cortef*) Adrenocortical insufficiency: 100 to 500 mg IV/IM q 2 to 6 h prn (sodium succinate) or 20 to 240 mg/day PO divided three to four times per day. Ulcerative colitis: 100 mg retention enema at bedtime (laying on side for 1 h or longer) for 21 days. [Generic/Trade: Tabs 5, 10, 20 mg; Enema 100 mg/60 mL.] ▶L ♀C ▶– $

METHYLPREDNISOLONE (*Solu-Medrol, Medrol, Depo-Medrol*) Anti-inflammatory/immunosuppressive: Oral (Medrol): Dose varies, 4 to 48 mg PO daily. Medrol Dosepak tapers 24 to 0 mg PO over 7 days. IM/Joints (Depo-Medrol): Dose varies, 4 to 120 mg IM q 1 to 2 weeks. Parenteral (Solu-Medrol): Dose varies, 10 to 250 mg IV/IM. Peds: 0.5 to 1.7 mg/kg PO/IV/IM divided q 6 to 12 h. [Trade only: Tabs 2, 16, 32 mg. Generic/Trade: Tabs 4, 8 mg. Medrol Dosepak (4 mg, 21 tabs).] ▶L ♀C ▶– $

PREDNISOLONE (*Flo-Pred, Prelone, Pediapred, Orapred, Orapred ODT*) 5 to 60 mg PO daily. [Generic/Trade: Syrup 15 mg/5 mL (Prelone: wild cherry flavor). Soln 5 mg/5 mL (Pediapred, raspberry flavor), 15 mg/5 mL (Orapred; grape flavor). Trade only: Orally disintegrating tabs 10, 15, 30 mg (Orapred ODT); Susp 5 mg/5 mL, 15 mg/5 mL (Flo-Pred; cherry flavor). Generic only: Tabs 5 mg. Syrup 5 mg/5 mL.] ▶L ♀C ▶+ $$

PREDNISONE (*Rayos, Prednisone Intensol, ✦ Winpred*) 1 to 2 mg/kg or 5 to 60 mg PO daily. [Generic only: Tabs 1, 2.5, 5, 10, 20, 50 mg. Soln 5 mg/5 mL, 5 mg/mL (Prednisone Intensol). Dosepacks (5 mg tabs: Tapers 30 to 5 mg PO over 6 days or 30 to 10 mg over 12 days), Dosepacks Double Strength (10 mg tabs: Tapers 60 to 10 mg over 6 days, or 60 to 20 mg PO over 12 days) taper packs. Trade only: Delayed-release tabs 1, 2, 5 mg.] ▶L ♀C ▶+ $

TRIAMCINOLONE (*Aristospan, Kenalog, Trivaris*) 4 to 48 mg PO/IM daily. Intra-articular 2.5 to 40 mg (Kenalog, Trivaris), 2 to 20 mg (Aristospan). [Trade only: Injection 10 mg/mL, 40 mg/mL (Kenalog), 5 mg/mL, 20 mg/mL (Aristospan), 8 mg (80 mg/mL) syringe (Trivaris).] ▶L ♀C ▶– $

Diabetes-Related—Alpha-Glucosidase Inhibitors

ACARBOSE (*Precose, ✦ Glucobay*) DM, Type 2: Start 25 mg PO three times per day with meals, and gradually increase as tolerated to maintenance, 50 to 100 mg three times per day. [Generic/Trade: Tabs 25, 50, 100 mg.] ▶Gut/K ♀B ▶– $$$

MIGLITOL (*Glyset*) DM, Type 2: Start 25 mg PO three times per day with meals, maintenance 50 to 100 three times per day. [Trade only: Tabs 25, 50, 100 mg.] ▶K ♀B ▶– $$$

Diabetes-Related—Combinations

ACTOPLUS MET, ACTOPLUS MET XR (pioglitazone + metformin) DM, Type 2: 1 tab PO daily or two times per day. If inadequate control with metformin monotherapy, start 15/500 or 15/850 PO one to two times per day. If inadequate control with pioglitazone monotherapy, start 15/500 two times per day or 15/850 daily. Max 45/2550 mg/day. Extended-release, start 1 tab (15/100 mg or 30/1000 mg) daily with evening meal. Max: 45/2000 mg/day. Obtain LFTs before therapy and periodically thereafter. [Generic/Trade: Tabs 15/500, 15/850 mg Trade only: Extended-release (Actoplus Met XR), tabs: 15/1000 mg, 30/1000 mg.] ▶LK ♀C ▶? $$$$$ ■

AVANDAMET (rosiglitazone + metformin) DM, Type 2, initial therapy (drug-naive): Start 2/500 mg PO one or two times per day. If inadequate control with metformin alone, select tab strength based on adding 4 mg/day rosiglitazone to existing metformin dose. If inadequate control with rosiglitazone alone, select tab strength based on adding 1000 mg/day metformin to existing rosiglitazone dose. Max 8/2000 mg/day. Obtain LFTs before therapy and periodically thereafter. Due to potential for elevated cardiovascular risks, rosiglitazone products restricted by FDA to use in patients where other medications cannot control Type 2 DM. [Trade only: Tabs 2/500, 4/500, 2/1000, 4/1000 mg.] ▶KL ♀C ▶? $$$$$ ■

AVANDARYL (rosiglitazone + glimepiride) DM, Type 2, initial therapy (drug-naive): Start 4/1 mg PO daily. If switching from monotherapy with a sulfonylurea or glitazone, consider 4/2 mg PO daily. Max 8/4 mg/day. Obtain LFTs before therapy and periodically thereafter. Due to potential for elevated cardiovascular risks, rosiglitazone products restricted by FDA to use in patients where other medications cannot control Type 2 diabetes. [Trade only (restricted access): Tabs 4/1, 4/2, 4/4, 8/2, 8/4 mg rosiglitazone/glimepiride.] ▶LK ♀C ▶? $$$$ ■

DUETACT (pioglitazone + glimepiride) DM, Type 2: Start 30/2 mg PO daily. Start up to 30/4 mg PO daily if prior glimepiride therapy, or 30/2 mg PO daily if prior pioglitazone therapy; max 30/4 mg/day. Obtain LFTs before therapy and periodically thereafter. [Generic/Trade: Tabs 30/2, 30/4 mg pioglitazone/glimepiride.] ▶LK ♀C ▶− $$$$$ ■

GLUCOVANCE (glyburide + metformin) DM, Type 2, Initial therapy (drug-naive): Start 1.25/250 mg PO daily or two times per day with meals; max 10/2000 mg daily. Inadequate control with a sulfonylurea or metformin alone: Start 2.5/500 or 5/500 mg PO two times per day with meals; max 20/2000 mg daily. [Generic/Trade: Tabs 1.25/250, 2.5/500, 5/500 mg.] ▶KL ♀B ▶? $$$ ■

JANUMET, JANUMET XR (sitagliptin + metformin) DM, Type 2: Individualize based on patient's current therapy. Immediate-release: 1 tab PO two times per day. Extended-release: 1 tab PO daily. If inadequate control with metformin monotherapy: Immediate-release: Start 50/500 or 50/1000 two times per day based on current metformin dose. Extended-release: Start 100 mg sitagliptin daily plus current daily metformin. If inadequate control on

(cont.)

sitagliptin: Immediate-release: Start 50/500 two times per day. Extended-release: Start 100/1000 daily. Max 100/2000 mg/day. Give with meals. [Trade only: Immediate-release tabs 50/500, 50/1000 mg, extended-release tabs 100/1000, 50/500, 50,1000 mg sitagliptin/metformin.] ▶K ♀B ▶? $$$$$ ■

JENTADUETO (linagliptin + metformin) DM, Type 2: If prior metformin, start 2.5 mg linagliptin and current metformin dose two times per day. If no prior metformin, start 2.5/5 mg PO two times per day. If current linagliptin/metformin, start at current doses. Max 2.5/1000 mg. [Trade only: 2.5/500, 2.5/850, 2.5/1000 mg.] ▶KL − ♀B ▶? $$$$$ ■

JUVISYNC (sitagliptin + simvastatin) DM, Type 2 with hyperlipidemia: 100/40 (sitagliptin/simvatatin) mg PO once daily in evening. [Trade only: Tabs 100/10, 100/20, 100/40 mg sitagliptin/simvastain.] ▶KL − ♀X ▶? $$$$$

KAZANO (alogliptin + metformin) DM, Type 2: Individualize based on patient's current therapy. 1 tab PO two times per day. Max 25/2000 mg/day. Give with meals. [Trade only: 12.5/500, 12.5/1000 mg alogliptin/metformin.] ▶K − ♀B ▶? $$$$$

KOMBIGLYZE XR (saxagliptin + metformin, ✦ Komboglyze) DM, Type 2: If inadequately controlled on metformin alone, start 2.5 to 5 mg of saxagliptin plus current dose of metformin; give once daily with evening meal. If inadequately controlled on saxagliptin, start 5/500 mg once daily with evening meal. Max: 5/2000 mg/day. [Trade only: Tabs 5/500, 2.5/1000, 5/1000 mg.] ♀B ▶? $$$$$ ■

METAGLIP (glipizide + metformin) DM, Type 2, Initial therapy (drug-naive): Start 2.5/250 mg PO daily to 2.5/500 mg PO two times per day with meals; max 10/2000 mg daily. Inadequate control with a sulfonylurea or metformin alone: Start 2.5/500 or 5/500 mg PO two times per day with meals; max 20/2000 mg daily. [Generic/Trade: Tabs 2.5/250, 2.5/500, 5/500 mg.] ▶KL ♀C ▶? $$$ ■

OSENI (alogliptin + pioglitazone) DM, Type 2: Individualize based on patient's current therapy. 1 tab PO two times per day. Max 25/45 mg/day Obtain LFTs before therapy and periodically thereafter. [Trade only: Tabs 12.5/15, 12.5/30, 12.5/45, 25/15, 25/30, 25/45 alogliptin/pioglitazone.] ▶KL − ♀C ▶? $$$$$ ■

PRANDIMET (repaglinide + metformin) DM, Type 2, Initial therapy (drug-naive): Start 1/500 mg PO daily before meals; max 10/2500 mg daily or 4/1000 mg/meal. May start higher if already taking higher coadministered doses of repaglinide and metformin. [Trade: Tabs 1/500, 2/500 mg.] ▶KL ♀C ▶? $$$ ■

Diabetes-Related—DPP-4 Inhibitors

ALOGLIPTIN (Nesina) DM, Type 2: 25 mg PO daily. [Trade only: Tabs 6.25, 12.5, 25 mg.] ▶K − ♀B ▶? $$$$$

LINAGLIPTIN (Tradjenta, ✦ Trajenta) DM, Type 2: 5 mg PO once daily. [Trade only: Tab 5 mg.] ▶L − ♀B ▶? $$$$$

SAXAGLIPTIN (Onglyza) DM, Type 2: 2.5 or 5 mg PO daily. [Trade only: Tabs 2.5, 5 mg.] ▶LK ♀B ▶? $$$$$

A1C Reduction in Type 2 Diabetes

Intervention	Expected A1C Reduction with Monotherapy
Alpha-glucosidase inhibitors	0.5-0.8%
Canagliflozin	0.7-1%
DPP-4 Inhibitors (Gliptins)	0.5-0.8%
GLP-1 agonists	0.5-1%
Insulin	1.5-3.5%
Lifestyle modifications	1-2%
Meglitinides	0.5-1.5%
Metformin	1-2%
Pramlintide	0.5-1%
Sulfonylureas	1-2%
Thiazolidinediones	0.5-1.4%

References: *Diabetes Care* 2009; 32:195. *Diabetes Obes Metab* 2013;15:372-82.▨

SITAGLIPTIN (*Januvia*) DM, Type 2: 100 mg PO daily. [Trade only: Tabs 25, 50, 100 mg.] ▶K ♀B ▶? $$$$$

Diabetes-Related—GLP-1 Agonists

EXENATIDE (*Byetta, Bydureon*) DM, Type 2, adjunctive therapy: Immediate-release: 5 mcg SC two times per day (within 1 h before the morning and evening meals, or 1 h before the two main meals of the day at least 6 h apart). May increase to 10 mcg SC two times per day after 1 month. Extended-release: 2 mg SC once weekly. [Trade only: Byetta, prefilled pen (60 doses each) 5 mcg/dose, 1.2 mL; 10 mcg/dose, 2.4 mL. Bydureon (extended-release): 2 mg/vial.] ▶K ♀C ▶? $$$$$ ■

LIRAGLUTIDE (*Victoza*) DM, Type 2: Start 0.6 mg SC daily for 1 week, then increase to 1.2 mg SC daily. May increase to 1.8 mg SC daily. [Trade only: Multidose pen (18 mg/3 mL) delivers doses of 0.6 mg, 1.2 mg or 1.8 mg.] ♀C ▶? $$$$$ ■

Diabetes-Related—Insulins

INSULIN—INJECTABLE COMBINATIONS (*Humalog Mix 75/25, Humalog Mix 50/50, Humulin 70/30, Novolin 70/30, Novolog Mix 70/30*)) Diabetes: Doses vary, but typically total insulin 0.3 to 1 unit/kg/day SC in divided doses (Type 1), and 0.5 to 1.5 unit/kg/day SC in divided doses (Type 2). Administer rapid-acting insulin mixtures (Humalog, NovoLog) within 15 min before or immediately after a meal. Administer regular insulin mixtures 30 min before meals. [Trade only: Insulin lispro protamine susp/insulin lispro (Humalog Mix 75/25, Humalog Mix 50/50). Insulin aspart protamine/insulin aspart (Novolog Mix 70/30). NPH and regular mixtures (Humulin 70/30, Novolin 70/30). Insulin

(cont.)

DIABETES NUMBERS*

Criteria for diagnosis	Self-monitoring glucose goals
<u>Pre-diabetes:</u> Fasting glucose 100–125 mg/dL or A1C 5.7–6.4% or 140–199 mg/dL 2 h after 75 g oral glucose load	<u>Preprandial:</u> 70–130 mg/dL <u>Postprandial:</u> < 180 mg/dL
<u>Diabetes:</u>[†] A1C ≥ 6.5% Fasting glucose ≥ 126 mg/dL. Random glucose with symptoms: ≥ 200 mg/dL, or ≥ 200 mg/dL 2 h after 75 g oral glucose load	<u>A1C goal:</u> < 7% for most non-pregnant adults, individualize based on age, comorbid conditions, microvascular complications, known cardiovascular disease hypoglycemia, and other patient-specific factors.

<u>Hospitalized patients:</u> may consider more stringent goal if safely achievable without hypoglycemia

<u>Critically ill glucose goal:</u> 140–180 mg/day

<u>Non-critically ill glucose goal (hospitalized patients):</u> premeal blood glucose < 140 mg/dL, random < 180 mg/dL

<u>Estimated average glucose (eAG):</u> eAG (mg/dL) = (28.7 × A1C) − 46.7

<u>Complications prevention and management:</u> ASA[‡] (75–162 mg/day) in Type 1 and 2 adults for primary prevention if 10-year cardiovascular risk > 10% (includes most men older than 50 yo or women older than 60 yo with at least one other major risk factor) and secondary prevention (those with vascular disease); statin therapy to achieve goal LDL regardless of baseline LDL (for those with vascular disease, those older than 40 yo and additional risk factor, or those younger than 40 yo but LDL > 100 mg/dL); ACE inhibitor or ARB if hypertensive or micro-/macro-albuminuria; pneumococcal vaccine (revaccinate one time if 65 yo or older and previously received vaccine when younger than 65 or older and more than 5 years ago); hepatitis B vaccine if previously unvaccinated and 19 to 59 yo; consider if age 60 yo or older.

<u>Every visit:</u> Measure wt and BP (goal < 140/80 mm Hg[♥]); visual foot exam; review self-monitoring glucose record; review/adjust meds; review self-mgmt skills, dietary needs, and physical activity; smoking cessation counseling.

<u>Twice a year:</u> A1C in those meeting treatment goals with stable glycemia (quarterly if not); dental exam.

<u>Annually:</u> Fasting lipid profile** [goal LDL < 100 mg/dL, cardiovascular disease consider LDL < 70 mg/dL; HDL > 40 mg/dL (> 50 mg/dL in women), TG < 150 mg/dL], q 2 years with low-risk lipid values; creatinine; albumin to creatinine ratio spot collection; dilated eye exam; flu vaccine.

*See recommendations at: http://care.diabetesjournals.org. Reference: *Diabetes Care* 2013;36(Suppl 1):S11-66. Glucose values are plasma.

[†] In the absence of symptoms, confirm diagnosis with glucose testing on subsequent day.

[‡] Avoid ASA if younger than 21 yo due to Reye's Syndrome risk; use if younger than 30 yo has not been studied.

[♥] Lower systolic targets (< 130 mmHg) may be considered on a patient-specific basis if treatment goals can be met without excessive treatment burden.

**LDL is primary target of therapy, consider 30 to 40% LDL reduction from baseline as alternate goal if unable to reach targets on maximal tolerated statin.

INJECTABLE INSULINS*

		Onset (h)	Peak (h)	Duration (h)
Rapid-/short-acting	Insulin aspart (NovoLog)	< 0.2	1–3	3–5
	Insulin glulisine (Apidra)	0.30–0.4	1	4–5
	Insulin lispro (Humalog)	0.25–0.5	0.5–2.5	≤ 5
	Regular (Novolin R, Humulin R)	0.5–1	2–3	3–6
Intermediate-/long acting	NPH (Novolin N, Humulin N)	2–4	4–10	10–16
	Insulin detemir (Levemir)	n.a.	flat action profile	up to 23†
	Insulin glargine (Lantus)	2–4	peakless	24
Mixtures	Insulin aspart protamine susp/aspart (NovoLog Mix 70/30)	0.25	1–4 (biphasic)	up to 24
	Insulin lispro protamine susp/insulin lispro (Humalog Mix 75/25, Humalog Mix 50/50)	< 0.25	1–3 (biphasic)	10–20
	NPH/Reg (Humulin 70/30, Novolin 70/30)	0.5–1	2–10 (biphasic)	10–20

*These are general guidelines, as onset, peak, and duration of activity are affected by the site of injection, physical activity, body temperature, and blood supply.
†Dose-dependent duration of action, range from 6 to 23 h.
n.a.= not available.

available in pen form: Novolin 70/30 InnoLet, Novolog Mix 70/30 FlexPen, Humulin 70/30, Humalog Mix 75/25 KwikPen, Humalog Mix 50/50 KwikPen.] ▶LK ♀B/C ▶+ $$$$

INSULIN—INJECTABLE INTERMEDIATE-/LONG-ACTING (*Novolin N, Humulin N, Lantus, Levemir*) Diabetes : Doses vary, but typically total insulin 0.3 to 0.5 unit/kg/day SC in divided doses (Type 1), and 1 to 1.5 unit/kg/day SC in divided doses (Type 2). Generally, 50 to 70% of insulin requirements are provided by rapid- or short-acting insulin and the remainder as intermediate- or long-acting insulin. Lantus : Start 10 units SC daily (same time everyday) in insulin-naive patients. Levemir, Type 2 DM (inadequately controlled on oral meds): Start 0.1 to 0.2 units/kg once daily in evening or 10 units SC daily or two times per day. [Trade only: Injection NPH (Novolin N, Humulin N). Insulin glargine (Lantus). Insulin detemir (Levemir). Insulin available in pen form: Novolin N InnoLet, Humulin N Pen, Lantus SoloStar Levemir FlexPen. Premixed preparations of NPH and regular insulin also available.] ▶LK ♀B/C ▶+ $$$$

INSULIN—INJECTABLE SHORT-/RAPID-ACTING (*Apidra, Novolin R, NovoLog, Humulin R, Humalog, ✦ NovoRapid*) Diabetes: Doses vary, but typically total insulin 0.3 to 0.5 unit/kg/day SC in divided doses (Type 1), and 1 to 1.5 unit/kg/day SC in divided doses (Type 2). Generally, 50 to 70% of insulin requirements are provided by rapid- or short-acting insulin and the remainder from intermediate- or long-acting insulin. Administer rapid-acting insulin (Humalog, NovoLog, Apidra) within 15 min before or immediately after a meal. Administer regular insulin 30 min before meals. Severe hyperkalemia: 5 to 10 units regular insulin plus concurrent dextrose IV. Profound hyperglycemia (eg, DKA): 0.1 unit regular/kg IV bolus, then initial infusion 100 units regular in 100 mL NS (1 unit/mL), at 0.1 units/kg/h. [Trade only: Injection regular 100 units/mL (Novolin R, Humulin R). Injection regular 500 units/mL (Humulin U-500, concentrated). Insulin glulisine (Apidra). Insulin lispro (Humalog). Insulin aspart (NovoLog). Insulin available in pen form: Novolin R InnoLet, Humulin R, Apidra Solostar, Humalog KwikPen, Novolog FlexPen.] ▶LK ♀B/C ▶+ $$$

Diabetes-Related—Meglitinides

NATEGLINIDE (*Starlix*) DM, Type 2: 120 mg PO three times per day within 30 min before meals; use 60 mg PO three times per day in patients who are near goal A1C. [Generic/Trade: Tabs 60, 120 mg.] ▶L ♀C ▶? $$$

REPAGLINIDE (*Prandin, ✦ Gluconorm*) DM, Type 2: Start 0.5 to 2 mg PO three times per day before meals, maintenance 0.5 to 4 mg three to four times per day, max 16 mg/day. [Trade only: Tabs 0.5, 1, 2 mg.] ▶L ♀C ▶? $$$$$

Diabetes-Related—Sulfonylureas—2nd Generation

GLICLAZIDE (✦ *Diamicron, Diamicron MR*) Canada only. DM, Type 2, immediate-release: Start 80 to 160 mg PO daily, max 320 mg/day (160 mg or more per day should be in divided doses). Modified-release: Start 30 mg PO daily, max 120 mg daily. [Generic/Trade: Tabs 80 mg (Diamicron). Trade only: Tabs, modified-release 30 mg (Diamicron MR).] ▶KL ♀C ▶? $

GLIMEPIRIDE (*Amaryl*) DM, Type 2: Start 1 to 2 mg PO daily, usual 1 to 4 mg/day, max 8 mg/day. [Generic/Trade: Tabs 1, 2, 4 mg. Generic only: Tabs 3, 6, 8 mg.] ▶LK ♀C ▶— $$

GLIPIZIDE (*Glucotrol, Glucotrol XL*) DM, Type 2: Start 5 mg PO daily, usual 10 to 20 mg/day, max 40 mg/day (divide two times per day if more than 15 mg/day). Extended-release: Start 5 mg PO daily, usual 5 to 10 mg/day, max 20 mg/day. [Generic/Trade: Tabs 5, 10 mg; Extended-release tabs 2.5, 5, 10 mg.] ▶LK ♀C ▶? $

GLYBURIDE (*DiaBeta, Glynase PresTab, ✦ Euglucon*) DM, Type 2: Start 1.25 to 5 mg PO daily, usual 1.25 to 20 mg daily or divided two times per day, max 20 mg/day. Micronized tabs: Start 1.5 to 3 mg PO daily, usual 0.75 to 12 mg/day divided two times per day, max 12 mg/day. [Generic/Trade: Tabs (scored) 1.25, 2.5, 5 mg. Micronized Tabs (scored) 1.5, 3, 4.5, 6 mg.] ▶LK ♀B ▶? $

Diabetes-Related—Thiazolidinediones

PIOGLITAZONE (*Actos*) DM, Type 2: Start 15 to 30 mg PO daily, max 45 mg/day. Monitor LFTs. [Generic/Trade: Tabs 15, 30, 45 mg.] ▶L ♀C ▶– $ ■

ROSIGLITAZONE (*Avandia*) DM, Type 2 monotherapy or in combination with metformin or sulfonylurea: Start 4 mg PO daily or divided two times per day, max 8 mg/day. Obtain LFTs before therapy and periodically thereafter. Due to potential for elevated cardiovascular risks, rosiglitazone products restricted by FDA to use in patients where other medications cannot control Type 2 DM. [Trade only (restricted access): Tabs 2, 4, 8 mg.] ▶L ♀C ▶– $$$$ ■

Diabetes-Related—Other

CANAGLIFLOZIN (*Invokana*) DM, Type 2: 100 mg PO daily before first meal of the day. If tolerated and needed for glycemic control, may increase to 300 mg PO daily if CrCl>60 mL/min. [Trade only: Tabs 100, 300 mg.] ▶LK - ♀C ▶? $$$$$

DEXTROSE (*Glutose, B-D Glucose, Insta-Glucose, Dex-4*) Hypoglycemia: 0.5 to 1 g/kg (1 to 2 mL/kg) up to 25 g (50 mL) of 50% soln IV. Dilute to 25% for pediatric administration. [OTC Generic/Trade: Chewable tabs 4 g (Dex-4), 5 g (Glutose). Trade only: Oral gel 40%.] ▶L ♀C ▶? $

GLUCAGON (*GlucaGen*) Hypoglycemia: 1 mg IV/IM/SC, onset 5 to 20 min. Diagnostic aid: 1 mg IV/IM/SC. [Trade only: Injection 1 mg.] ▶LK ♀B ▶? $$$

METFORMIN (*Glucophage, Glucophage XR, Glumetza, Fortamet, Riomet*) DM, type 2: Immediate-release: Start 500 mg PO one to two times per day or 850 mg PO daily with meals, may gradually increase to max 2550 mg/day. Extended-release: Glucophage XR: 500 mg PO daily with evening meal; increase by 500 mg once a week to max 2000 mg/day (may divide two times per day). Glumetza: 1000 mg PO daily with evening meal; increase by 500 mg once a week to max 2000 mg/day (may divide two times per day). Fortamet: 500 to 1000 mg daily with evening meal; increase by 500 mg once a week to max 2500 mg/day. Polycystic ovary syndrome (unapproved, immediate-release): 500 mg PO three times per day. DM prevention, Type 2 (with lifestyle modifications, unapproved): 850 mg PO daily for 1 month, then increase to 850 mg PO two times per day. All products started at low doses to improve GI tolerability, gradually increase as tolerated. [Generic/Trade: Tabs 500, 850, 1000 mg, extended-release 500, 750 mg. Trade only, extended-release: Fortamet 500, 1000 mg; Glumetza 500, 1000 mg. Trade only: Oral soln 500 mg/5 mL (Riomet).] ▶K ♀B ▶? $ ■

PRAMLINTIDE (*Symlin, Symlinpen*) DM, Type 1 with mealtime insulin therapy: Initiate 15 mcg SC immediately before major meals and titrate by 15-mcg increments (if significant nausea has not occurred for at least 3 days) to maintenance 30 to 60 mcg as tolerated. DM, Type 2 with mealtime insulin therapy: Initiate 60 mcg SC immediately before major meals and increase to 120 mcg as tolerated (if significant nausea has not occurred for 3 to 7 days). Decrease initial premeal short-acting insulin doses by 50% including fixed-mix insulin (ie, 70/30). [Trade only: 600 mcg/mL in 5 mL vials, 1000 mcg/mL pen injector (Symlinpen) 1.5, 2.7 mL.] ▶K ♀C ▶? $$$$ ■

Diagnostic Agents

COSYNTROPIN (*Cortrosyn*, ✦ *Synacthen Depot*) Rapid screen for adrenocortical insufficiency: 0.25 mg IM/IV over 2 min; measure serum cortisol before and 30 to 60 min after. ▶L ♀C ▶? $

Gout-Related

ALLOPURINOL (*Aloprim, Zyloprim*) Mild gout or recurrent calcium oxalate stones: 200 to 300 mg PO daily to two times per day, max 800 mg/day. [Generic/Trade: Tabs 100, 300 mg.] ▶K ♀C ▶+ $

COLBENEMID (colchicine + probenecid) Gout: 1 tab PO daily for 1 week, then 1 tab two times per day. [Generic only: Tabs 0.5 mg colchicine + 500 mg probenecid.] ▶KL ♀C ▶? $

COLCHICINE (*Colcrys*) Rapid treatment of acute gouty arthritis: 1.2 mg (2 tab) PO at signs of attack then 0.6 mg (1 tab) 1 h after initial administration. Gout prophylaxis: 0.6 mg PO two times per day if CrCl is 50 mL/min or greater, 0.6 mg PO daily if CrCl is 35 to 49 mL/min, 0.6 mg PO q 2 to 3 days if CrCl is 10 to 34 mL/min. Familial Mediterranean Fever: 1.2 to 2.4 mg PO daily or divided two times per day. [Trade: Tabs 0.6 mg.] ▶L ♀C ▶? $$$$

FEBUXOSTAT (*Uloric*) Hyperuricemia with gout: Start 40 mg PO daily, max 80 mg daily. [Trade only: Tabs 40, 80 mg.] ▶LK ♀C ▶? $$$$

PEGLOTICASE (*Krystexxa*) Chronic gout (refractory): 8 mg IV infusion q 2 weeks. [Trade only: Single-use vial (8 mg/mL)] ▶NA ♀C ▶? $$$$$ ■

PROBENECID Gout: 250 mg PO two times per day for 7 days, then 500 mg two times per day. Adjunct to penicillin injection: 1 to 2 g PO in divided doses. [Generic only: Tabs 500 mg.] ▶KL ♀B ▶? $

Minerals

CALCIUM ACETATE (*PhosLo, Eliphos, Phoslyra*) Phosphate binder to reduce serum phosphorous in end-stage renal disease: Initially 2 tabs/caps or 10 mL of soln PO with each meal. [Generic/Trade: Gelcaps 667 mg (169 mg elem Ca). Tab 667 mg (169 mg elem Ca). Trade only: Solution (Phoslyra): 667mg (169 mg elemental calcium)/5 mL.] ▶K ♀C ▶? $

CALCIUM CARBONATE (*Caltrate, Mylanta Children's, Os-Cal, Oyst-Cal, Tums, Surpass, Viactiv*) Supplement: 1 to 2 g elemental Ca/day or more PO with meals divided two to four times per day. Antacid: 1000 to 3000 mg PO q 2 h prn or 1 to 2 pieces gum chewed prn, max 7000 mg/day. [OTC Generic/Trade: Tabs 500, 650, 750, 1000, 1250, 1500 mg, Chewable tabs 400, 500, 750, 850, 1000, 1177, 1250 mg, Caps 1250 mg, Gum 300, 450 mg, Susp 1250 mg/5 mL. Calcium carbonate is 40% elem Ca and contains 20 mEq of elem Ca/g calcium carbonate. Not more than 500 to 600 mg elemental Ca/dose. Available in combination with sodium fluoride, vitamin D, and/or vitamin K. Trade examples: Caltrate 600 + D = 600 mg elemental Ca/200 units vitamin D, Os-Cal 500 + D = 500 mg elemental Ca/200 units vitamin D, Os-Cal Extra D = 500 mg elemental Ca/400 units vitamin D, Tums (regular strength) = 200

(cont.)

mg elemental Ca, Tums (ultra) = 400 mg elemental Ca, Viactiv (chewable) 500 mg elemental Ca+ 100 units vitamin D + 40 mcg vitamin K.] ▶K ♀+ (? 1st trimester) ▶? $

CALCIUM CHLORIDE 500 to 1000 mg slow IV q 1 to 3 days. [Generic only: Injectable 10% (1000 mg/10 mL) 10 mL ampules, vials, syringes.] ▶K ♀+ ▶+ $

CALCIUM CITRATE (*Citracal*) 1 to 2 g elemental Ca/day or more PO with meals divided two to four times per day. [OTC Trade/Generic (mg elem Ca/units vitamin D): 200/250, 250/200, 315/250, 600/500 (slow release); some products available with magnesium and/or phosphorous. Chewable gummies: 250 mg with 250 units vitamin D.] ▶K ♀+ ▶+ $

CALCIUM GLUCONATE 2.25 to 14 mEq slow IV. 500 to 2000 mg PO two to four times per day. [Generic only: Injectable 10% (1000 mg/10 mL, 4.65 mEq/10 mL) 1, 10, 50, 100, 200 mL. OTC Generic only: Tabs 50, 500, 650, 975, 1000 mg. Chewable tabs 650 mg.] ▶K ♀+ ▶+ $

FERRIC GLUCONATE COMPLEX (*Ferrlecit*) 125 mg elemental iron IV over 10 min or diluted in 100 mL NS IV over 1 h. Peds age 6 yo or older: 1.5 mg/kg (max 125 mg) elemental iron diluted in 25 mL NS and administered IV over 1 h. ▶KL ♀B ▶? $$$$$

FERROUS GLUCONATE (*Fergon*) 800 to 1600 mg ferrous gluconate PO divided three times per day. [OTC Generic/Trade: Tabs (ferrous gluconate) 240 mg (27 mg elemental iron). Generic only: Tabs 324, 325 mg.] ▶K ♀+ ▶+ $

FERROUS SULFATE (*Fer-in-Sol, Feosol, Slow FE, ✦ Ferodan, Slow-Fe*) 500 to 1000 mg ferrous sulfate (100 to 200 mg elemental iron) PO divided tid. [OTC Generic/Trade (mg ferrous sulfate): Tabs extended-release 160 mg. Tabs 200, 324, 325 mg. OTC Generic only (mg ferrous sulfate): Soln 75 mg/0.6 mL, Elixir 220 mg/5 mL.] ▶K ♀+ ▶+ $

FERUMOXYTOL (*Feraheme*) Iron deficiency in chronic kidney disease: Give 510 mg IV push, followed by 510 mg IV push once given 3 to 8 days after initial injection. ▶KL ♀C ▶? $$$$$

FLUORIDE (*Luride, ✦ Fluor-A-Day*) Adult dose: 10 mL of topical rinse swish and spit daily. Peds daily dose based on fluoride content of drinking water (see table). [Generic only: Chewable tabs 0.5, 1 mg; Tabs 1 mg, gtts 0.125 mg, 0.25 mg, and 0.5 mg/dropperful, Lozenges 1 mg, Soln 0.2 mg/mL, Gel 0.1%, 0.5%, 1.23%, Rinse (sodium fluoride) 0.05, 0.1, 0.2%).] ▶K ♀? ▶? $

FLUORIDE SUPPLEMENTATION

Age	<0.3 ppm in drinking water	0.3–0.6 ppm in drinking water	>0.6 ppm in drinking water
0–6 mo	none	none	none
6 mo–3 yo	0.25 mg PO daily	none	none
3–6 yo	0.5 mg PO daily	0.25 mg PO daily	none
6–16 yo	1 mg PO daily	0.5 mg PO daily	none

JADA 2010;141:1480-1489

IV SOLUTIONS

Solution	Dextrose	Calories/Liter	Na*	Ca*	Lactate*	Osm*
0.9 NS	0 g/L	0	154	0	0	310
LR	0 g/L	9	130	3	28	273
D5 W	50 g/L	170	0	0	0	253
D5 0.2 NS	50 g/L	170	34	0	0	320
D5 0.45 NS	50 g/L	170	77	0	0	405
D5 0.9 NS	50 g/L	170	154	0	0	560
D5 LR	50 g/L	179	130	2.7	28	527

* All given in mEq/L

IRON DEXTRAN *(InFed, DexFerrum, ◆ Dexiron, Infufer)* 25 to 100 mg IM daily prn. Equations available to calculate IV dose based on wt and Hb. ▶KL ♀C ▶? $$$$ ■

IRON POLYSACCHARIDE *(Niferex, Niferex-150, Nu-Iron 150, Ferrex 150)* 50 to 200 mg PO divided one to three times per day. [OTC Trade only: Caps 60 mg (Niferex). OTC Generic/Trade: Caps 150 mg (Niferex-150, Nu-Iron 150, Ferrex-150), Elixir 100 mg/5 mL (Niferex). 1 mg iron polysaccharide = 1 mg elemental iron.] ▶K ♀+ ▶+ $$ ■

IRON SUCROSE *(Venofer)* Iron deficiency with hemodialysis: 5 mL (100 mg elemental iron) IV over 5 min or diluted in 100 mL NS IV over 15 min or longer. Iron deficiency in nondialysis dependent chronic kidney disease: 10 mL (200 mg elemental iron) IV over 5 min. ▶KL ♀B ▶? $$$$$

MAGNESIUM CHLORIDE *(Slow-Mag)* 2 tabs PO daily. [OTC Trade only: Enteric coated tab 64 mg. 64 mg tab Slow-Mag = 64 mg elemental magnesium.] ▶K ♀A ▶+ $

MAGNESIUM GLUCONATE *(Almora, Magtrate, Maganate, ◆ Maglucate)* 500 to 1000 mg PO divided three times per day. [OTC Generic only: Tabs 500 mg (27 mg elemental Mg), liquid 54 mg elemental Mg/5 mL.] ▶K ♀A ▶+ $

MAGNESIUM OXIDE *(Mag-200, Mag-Ox 400)* 400 to 800 mg PO daily. [OTC Generic/Trade: Caps: 140 (84.5 mg elemental Mg), 250 (elemental), 400 (240 mg elemental Mg), 420 (253 mg elemental Mg), 500 mg (elemental).] ▶K ♀A ▶+ $

MAGNESIUM SULFATE Hypomagnesemia: 1 g of 20% soln IM q 6 h for 4 doses, or 2 g IV over 1 h (monitor for hypotension). Peds: 25 to 50 mg/kg IV/IM q 4 to 6 h for 3 to 4 doses, max single dose 2 g. Eclampsia: 4 to 6 g IV over 30 min, then 1 to 2 g/h. Drip: 5 g in 250 mL D5W (20 mg/mL), 2 g/h is a rate of 100 mL/h. Preterm labor: 6 g IV over 20 min, then 1 to 3 g/h titrated to decrease contractions. Monitor respirations and reflexes. If needed, may reverse toxic effects with calcium gluconate 1 g IV. Torsades de pointes: 1 to 2 g IV in D5W over 5 to 60 min. ▶K ♀A/C/D ▶+ $

PHOSPHORUS *(Neutra-Phos, K-Phos)* 1 cap/packet PO four times per day. 1 to 2 tabs PO four times per day. Severe hypophosphatemia (eg, less than 1 mg/dL): 0.08 to 0.16 mmol/kg IV over 6 h. [OTC Trade only: (Neutra-Phos,

(cont.)

POTASSIUM (oral forms)*

Effervescent Granules	
20 mEq	Klorvess Effervescent, K-vescent
Effervescent Tabs	
10 mEq	Effer-K
20 mEq	Effer-K
25 mEq	Effer-K, K+Care ET, K-Lyte, K-Lyte/Cl, Klor-Con/EF
50 mEq	K-Lyte DS, K-Lyte/Cl 50
Liquids	
20 mEq/15 mL	Cena-K, Kaochlor S-F, K-G Elixir, Kaochlor 10%, Kay Ciel, Kaon, Kaylixir, Kolyum, Potasalan, Twin-K
30 mEq/15 mL	Rum-K
40 mEq/15 mL	Cena-K, Kaon-Cl 20%
45 mEq/15 mL	Tri-K
Powders	
15 mEq/pack	K+Care
20 mEq/pack	Gen-K, K+Care, Kay Ciel, K-Lor, Klor-Con
25 mEq/pack	K+Care, Klor-Con 25
Tabs/Caps	
8 mEq	K+8, Klor-Con 8, Slow-K, Micro-K
10 mEq	K+10, K-Norm, Kaon-Cl 10, Klor-Con M10 Klotrix, K-Tab, K-Dur 10, Micro-K 10
20 mEq	Klor-Con M20, K-Dur 20

*Table provides examples and is not intended to be all inclusive.

Neutra-Phos K) tab/cap/packet 250 mg (8 mmol) phosphorus. Rx: Trade only: (K-Phos) tab 250 mg (8 mmol) phosphorus.] ▶K ♀C ▮? $

POTASSIUM (*Cena-K, Effer-K, K+8, K+10, Kaochlor, Kaon, Kaon Cl, Kay Ciel, Kaylixir, K+Care, K+Care ET, K-Dur, K-G Elixir, K-Lease, K-Lor, Klor-con, Klorvess Effervescent, Klotrix, K-Lyte, K-Lyte Cl, K-Norm, Kolyum, K-Tab, K-vescent, Micro-K, Micro-K LS, Sl*) IV infusion 10 mEq/h (diluted). 20 to 40 mEq PO one or two times per day. Use IV or immediate-release PO if rapid replacement needed. [Injectable, many different products in a variety of salt forms (ie, chloride, bicarbonate, citrate, acetate, gluconate), available in tabs, caps, liquids, effervescent tabs, packets. Potassium gluconate is available OTC. See table.] ▶K ♀C ▮? $

ZINC ACETATE (*Galzin*) Dietary supplement : 8 to 12 mg (elemental) daily. Zinc deficiency : 25 to 50 mg (elemental) daily. Wilson's disease : 25 to 50 mg (elemental) PO three times per day. [Trade only: Caps 25, 50 mg elemental zinc.] ▶Minimal absorption ♀A ▮– $$$

ZINC SULFATE (*Orazinc, Zincate*) Dietary supplement: 8 to 12 mg (elemental) daily. Zinc deficiency: 25 to 50 mg (elemental) PO daily. [OTC Generic/Trade: Tabs 66, 110, 200 mg. Rx Generic/Trade: Caps 220 mg.] ▶Minimal absorption ♀A ▶− $

Nutritionals

BANANA BAG Alcoholic malnutrition (example formula): Add thiamine 100 mg + folic acid 1 mg + IV multivitamins to 1 liter NS and infuse over 4 h. Magnesium sulfate 2 g may be added. "Banana bag" and "rally pack" are jargon and not valid drug orders. Specify individual components. ▶KL ♀+▶+ $

FAT EMULSION (*Intralipid, Liposyn, ✦ Clinoleic*) Dosage varies. ▶L ♀C ▶? $$$$$

LEVOCARNITINE (*Carnitor*) 10 to 20 mg/kg IV at each dialysis session. [Generic/Trade: Tabs 330 mg, Oral soln 1 g/10 mL.] ▶KL ♀B ▶? $$$$$

Phosphate Binders

LANTHANUM CARBONATE (*Fosrenol*) Hyperphosphatemia in end-stage renal disease: Start 1500 mg/day PO in divided doses with meals. Titrate dose q 2 to 3 weeks in increments of 750 mg/day until acceptable serum phosphate is reached. Most will require 1500 to 3000 mg/day to reduce phosphate less than 6.0 mg/dL. Chew or crush tabs completely before swallowing; not to be swallowed whole. [Trade only: Chewable tabs 500, 750, 1000 mg.] ▶Not absorbed ♀C ▶? $$$$$

SEVELAMER (*Renagel, Renvela*) Hyperphosphatemia: 800 to 1600 mg PO three times per day with meals. [Trade only (Renagel—sevelamer hydrochloride): Tabs 400, 800 mg. (Renvela—sevelamer carbonate): Tabs 800 mg; Powder: 800, 2400 mg packets.] ▶Not absorbed ♀C ▶? $$$$$

Thyroid Agents

LEVOTHYROXINE (*Levothroid, Levoxyl, Synthroid, Tirosint, Unithroid, T4, ✦ Eltroxin, Euthyrox*) Start 100 to 200 mcg PO daily (healthy adults) or 12.5 to 50 mcg PO daily (elderly or CV disease), increase by 12.5 to 25 mcg daily at 3- to 8-week intervals. Usual maintenance dose 100 to 200 mcg/day, max 300 mcg/day. [Generic/Trade: Tabs 25, 50, 75, 88, 100, 112, 125, 137, 150, 175, 200, 300 mcg. Trade only (Tirosint): 13, 25, 50, 75, 88, 100, 112, 125, 137, 150 mcg.] ▶L ♀A ▶+ $ ■

LIOTHYRONINE (*T3, Cytomel, Triostat*) Start 25 mcg PO daily, max 100 mcg/day. [Generic/Trade: Tabs 5, 25, 50 mcg.] ▶L ♀A ▶? $$ ■

METHIMAZOLE (*Tapazole*) Start 5 to 20 mg PO three times per day or 10 to 30 mg PO daily, then adjust. [Generic/Trade: Tabs 5, 10. Generic only: Tabs 15, 20 mg.] ▶L ♀D ▶+ $$$

PROPYLTHIOURACIL (*PTU, ✦ Propyl Thyracil*) Hyperthyroidism: Start 100 mg PO three times per day, then adjust. Thyroid storm: 200 to 300 mg PO four times per day, then adjust. [Generic only: Tabs 50 mg.] ▶L ♀D (but preferred over methimazole in first trimester) ▶+ $ ■

Vitamins

ASCORBIC ACID (vitamin C, **✦Redoxon**) 70 to 1000 mg PO daily. [OTC Generic only: Tabs 25, 50, 100, 250, 500, 1000 mg, Chewable tabs 100, 250, 500 mg, Timed-release tabs 500, 1000, 1500 mg, Timed-release caps 500 mg, Lozenges 60 mg, Liquid 35 mg/0.6 mL, Oral soln 100 mg/mL, Syrup 500 mg/5 mL.] ▶K ♀C ▶? $

CALCITRIOL (*Rocaltrol, Calcijex*) 0.25 to 2 mcg PO daily. Hypocalcemia and/or secondary hyperparathyroidism in chronic renal dialysis IV: 1 to 2 mcg, 3 times a week; increase dose by 0.5 to 1 mcg q 2 to 4 weeks. Adjust based on PTH. [Generic/Trade: Caps 0.25, 0.5 mcg. Oral soln 1 mcg/mL. Injection 1, 2 mcg/mL.] ▶L ♀C ▶? $$

CYANOCOBALAMIN (vitamin B12, *CaloMist, Nascobal*) Deficiency states: 100 to 200 mcg IM once a month or 1000 to 2000 mcg PO daily for 1 to 2 weeks followed by 1000 mcg PO daily, 500 mcg intranasal weekly (Nascobal: 1 spray 1 nostril once a week), or 50 to 100 mcg intranasal daily (CaloMist: 1 to 2 sprays each nostril daily). [OTC Generic only: Tabs 100, 500, 1000, 5000 mcg; Lozenges 100, 250, 500 mcg. Rx Trade only: Nasal spray 500 mcg/spray (Nascobal 2.3 mL), 25 mcg/spray (CaloMist, 18 mL).] ▶K ♀C ▶+ $

DOXERCALCIFEROL (*Hectorol*) Secondary hyperparathyroidism on dialysis: Oral: 10 mcg PO 3 times a week. May increase q 8 weeks by 2.5 mcg/dose; max 60 mcg/week. IV: 4 mcg IV 3 times a week. May increase dose q 8 weeks by 1 to 2 mcg/dose; max 18 mcg/week. Secondary hyperparathyroidism not on dialysis: Start 1 mcg PO daily, may increase by 0.5 mcg/dose q 2 weeks. Max 3.5 mcg/day. [Generic/Trade: Caps 0.5 mcg. Trade only: Caps 2.5 mcg.] ▶L ♀B ▶? $$$$$

ERGOCALCIFEROL (vitamin D2, *Calciferol, Drisdol*) Osteoporosis prevention and treatment (age 50 yo or older): 800 to 1000 units daily. Familial hypophosphatemia (vitamin D–resistant Rickets): 12,000 to 500,000 units PO daily. Hypoparathyroidism: 50,000 to 200,000 units PO daily. Vitamin D deficiency: 50,000 units PO weekly or biweekly for 8 to 12 weeks. Adequate daily intake: 1 to 70 yo: 600 units (15 mcg); older than 70 yo: 800 units (20 mcg). [OTC Generic only: Caps 400, 1000, 5000 units, Soln 8000 units/mL (Calciferol). Rx Generic/Trade: Caps 50,000 units. Rx Generic only: Caps 25,000 units.] ▶L ♀A (C if exceed RDA) ▶+ $

FOLIC ACID (folate, *Folvite*) 0.4 to 1 mg IV/IM/PO/SC daily. [OTC Generic only: Tabs 0.4, 0.8 mg. Rx Generic 1 mg] ▶K ♀A ▶+ $

MULTIVITAMINS (MVI) Dose varies with product. Tabs come with and without iron. [OTC and Rx: Many different brands and forms available with and without iron (tabs, caps, chewable tabs, gtts, liquid).] ▶LK ♀+ ▶+ $

NEPHROCAP (ascorbic acid + folic acid + niacin + thiamine + riboflavin + pyridoxine + pantothenic acid + biotin + cyanocobalamin) 1 cap PO daily. If on dialysis, take after treatment. [Generic/Trade: Vitamin C 100 mg/folic acid 1 mg/niacin 20 mg/thiamine 1.5 mg/riboflavin 1.7 mg/pyridoxine 10 mg/pantothenic acid 5 mg/biotin 150 mcg/cyanocobalamin 6 mcg.] ▶K ♀? ▶? $

NEPHROVITE (ascorbic acid + folic acid + niacin + thiamine + riboflavin + pyridoxine + pantothenic acid + biotin + cyanocobalamin) 1 tab PO daily. If on dialysis, take after treatment. [Generic/Trade: Vitamin C 60 mg/folic acid 1 mg/niacin 20 mg/thiamine 1.5 mg/riboflavin 1.7 mg/pyridoxine 10 mg/pantothenic acid 10 mg/biotin 300 mcg/cyanocobalamin 6 mcg.] ▶K ♀? ▶? $

NIACIN (vitamin B3, nicotinic acid, *Niacor, Nicolar, Slo-Niacin, Niaspan*) Niacin deficiency: 10 to 500 mg PO daily. Hyperlipidemia: Start 50 to 100 mg PO two to three times per day with meals, increase slowly, usual maintenance range 1.5 to 3 g/day, max 6 g/day. Extended-release (Niaspan): Start 500 mg at bedtime, increase monthly up to max 2000 mg. Extended-release formulations not listed here may have greater hepatotoxicity. Start with low doses and increase slowly to minimize flushing; 325 mg aspirin (non-EC) 30 to 60 min prior to niacin ingestion will minimize flush. [OTC Generic only: Tabs 50, 100, 250, 500 mg; Timed-release caps 125, 250, 400 mg; Timed-release tabs 250, 500 mg; Liquid 50 mg/5 mL. Trade only: 250, 500, 750 mg (Slo-Niacin). Rx: Trade only: Tabs 500 mg (Niacor), Timed-release caps 500 mg, Timed-release tabs 500, 750, 1000 mg (Niaspan, $$$$).] ▶K ♀C ▶? $

PARICALCITOL (*Zemplar*) Prevention/treatment of secondary hyperparathyroidism with renal insufficiency: 1 to 2 mcg PO daily or 2 to 4 mcg PO three times per week; increase dose by 1 mcg/day or 2 mcg/week until desired PTH level is achieved. Prevention/treatment of secondary hyperparathyroidism with renal failure (CrCl less than 15 mL/min): PO: To calculate initial dose, divide baseline iPTH by 80 and then administer this dose in mcg three times per week. To titrate dose based on response, divide recent iPTH by 80 then administer this dose in mcg three times per week. IV: 0.04 to 0.1 mcg/kg (2.8 to 7 mcg) IV three times per week at dialysis; increase dose by 2 to 4 mcg q 2 to 4 weeks until desired PTH level is achieved. Max dose 0.24 mcg/kg (16.8 mcg). [Trade only: Caps 1, 2, 4 mcg.] ▶L ♀C ▶? $$$$$

PHYTONADIONE (vitamin K, *Mephyton, AquaMephyton*) Single dose of 0.5 to 1 mg IM within 1 h after birth. Excessive oral anticoagulation: Dose varies based on INR. INR 4.5–10: 2012 CHEST guidelines recommend AGAINST routine vitamin K administration; INR greater than 10 with no bleeding: 2012 CHEST guidelines recommend giving vitamin K, but do not specify a dose, 2008 guidelines previously recommended 5 to 10 mg PO; serious bleeding and elevated INR: 5 to 10 mg slow IV infusion. Adequate daily intake: 120 mcg (males) and 90 mcg (females). [Trade only: Tabs 5 mg.] ▶L ♀C ▶+ $ ■

PYRIDOXINE (vitamin B6) 10 to 200 mg PO daily. Prevention of deficiency due to isoniazid in high-risk patients: 10 to 25 mg PO daily. Treatment of neuropathies due to isoniazid: 50 to 200 mg PO daily. Hyperemesis of pregnancy: 10 to 50 mg PO q 8 h. [OTC Generic only: Tabs 25, 50, 100 mg; Timed-release tabs 100 mg.] ▶K ♀A ▶+ $

RIBOFLAVIN (vitamin B2) 5 to 25 mg PO daily. [OTC Generic only: Tabs 25, 50, 100 mg.] ▶K ♀A ▶+ $

THIAMINE (vitamin B1) 10 to 100 mg IV/IM/PO daily. [OTC Generic only: Tabs 50, 100, 250, 500 mg; Enteric-coated tabs 20 mg.] ▶K ♀A ▶+ $

VITAMIN A RDA : 900 mcg RE (retinol equivalents) (males), 700 mcg RE (females). Treatment of deficiency : 100,000 units IM daily for 3 days, then 50,000 units IM daily for 2 weeks. 1 RE is equivalent to 1 mcg retinol or 6 mcg beta-carotene. Max recommended daily dose 3000 mcg. [OTC Generic only: Caps 10,000, 15,000 units. Trade only: Tabs 5000 units. Rx: Generic: 25,000 units. Trade only: Soln 50,000 units/mL.] ▶L ♀A (C if exceed RDA, X in high doses) ▶+ $

VITAMIN D3 (**cholecalciferol, DDrops**) Osteoporosis prevention and treatment (age 50 or older): 800 to 1000 units daily. Familial hypophosphatemia (Vitamin D–resistant Rickets): 12,000 to 500,000 units PO daily. Hypoparathyroidism : 50,000 to 200,000 units PO daily. Adequate daily intake : 1 to 70 yo: 600 units; older than 70 yo: 800 units. [OTC Generic: 200 units, 400 units, 800 units, 1000 units, 2000 units (cap/tab). Trade only: Soln 400 units/drop, 1000 units/drop, 2000 units/drop.] ▶L – ▶+ $

VITAMIN E (**tocopherol, ✦ Aquasol E**) RDA: 22 units (natural, d-alpha-tocopherol) or 33 units (synthetic, d,l-alpha-tocopherol) or 15 mg (alpha-tocopherol). Max recommended 1000 mg alpha-tocopherol (1500 units) daily. [OTC Generic only: Tabs 200, 400 units. Caps 73.5, 100, 147, 165, 200, 330, 400, 500, 600, 1000 units; Gtts 50 mg/mL.] ▶L ♀A ▶? $

Other

BROMOCRIPTINE (**Cycloset, Parlodel**) Type 2 DM: 0.8 mg PO q am (within 2 h of waking), may increase weekly by 0.8 mg to max tolerated dose of 1.6 to 4.8 mg. Hyperprolactinemia : Start 1.25 to 2.5 mg PO at bedtime, then increase q 3 to 7 days to usual effective dose of 2.5 to 15 mg/day, max 40 mg/day. Acromegaly : Usual effective dose is 20 to 30 mg/day, max 100 mg/day. Doses greater than 20 mg/day can be divided two times per day. Also approved for Parkinson's disease, but rarely used. Take with food to minimize dizziness and nausea. [Generic/Trade: Tabs 2.5 mg. Caps 5 mg. Trade only: Tabs 0.8 mg (Cycloset).] ▶L ♀B ▶– $$$$$

CABERGOLINE (**Dostinex**) Hyperprolactinemia: 0.25 to 1 mg PO two times per week. [Generic/Trade: Tabs 0.5 mg.] ▶L ♀B ▶– $$$$$

CALCITONIN (**Miacalcin, Fortical, ✦ Calcimar, Caltine**) Osteoporosis: 100 units SC/IM every other day or 200 units (1 spray) intranasal daily (alternate nostrils). Paget's disease : 50 to 100 units SC/IM daily. Hypercalcemia : 4 units/kg SC/IM q 12 h. May increase after 2 days to max of 8 units/kg q 6 h. Skin test before using injectable product: 1 unit intradermally and observe for local reaction. Acute osteoporotic vertebral fracture pain (unapproved use): 100 units SC/IM daily or 200 units intranasal daily (alternate nostrils). [Generic/Trade: Nasal spray 200 units/activation in 3.7 mL bottle (minimum of 30 doses/bottle).] ▶Plasma ♀C ▶? $$$$

DENOSUMAB (**Xgeva, ✦ Prolia**) Postmenopausal osteoporosis: 60 mg SC q 6 months. Increase bone mass in men receiving androgen deprivation therapy for nonmetastatic prostate cancer : 60 mg SC q 6 months. Increase bone mass in women receiving adjuvant aromatase inhibitor therapy for breast cancer at high risk of fracture : 60 mg SC q 6 months. [Trade only: 60 mg/1 mL vial, prefilled syringe.] ▶? ♀X ▶? $$$$

DESMOPRESSIN (*DDAVP*, *Stimate*, ✦ *Minirin*, *Octostim*) Diabetes insipidus: 10 to 40 mcg intranasally daily or divided two to three times per day, 0.05 to 1.2 mg/day PO or divided two to three times per day, or 0.5 to 1 mL/day SC/IV in 2 divided doses. Hemophilia A, von Willebrand's disease: 0.3 mcg/kg IV over 15 to 30 min, or 150 to 300 mcg intranasally. Enuresis: 0.2 to 0.6 mg PO at bedtime. Not for children younger than 6 yo. [Trade only: Stimate nasal spray 150 mcg/0.1 mL (1 spray), 2.5 mL bottle (25 sprays). Generic/Trade (DDAVP nasal spray): 10 mcg/0.1 mL (1 spray), 5 mL bottle (50 sprays). Note difference in concentration of nasal soln. Rhinal Tube: 2.5 mL bottle with 2 flexible plastic tube applicators with graduation marks for dosing. Generic only: Tabs 0.1, 0.2 mg.] ▶LK ♀B ▶? $$$$

SODIUM POLYSTYRENE SULFONATE (*Kayexalate*) Hyperkalemia: 15 g PO one to four times per day or 30 to 50 g retention enema (in sorbitol) q 6 h prn. Retain for 30 min to several hours. Irrigate with tap water after enema to prevent necrosis. [Generic only: Susp 15 g/60 mL. Powdered resin.] ▶Fecal excretion ♀C ▶? $$$$

SOMATROPIN (**human growth hormone**, *Genotropin*, *Humatrope*, *Norditropin*, *Norditropin NordiFlex*, *Nutropin*, *Nutropin AQ*, *Nutropin Depot*, *Omnitrope*, *Protropin*, *Serostim*, *Serostim LQ*, *Saizen*, *Tev-Tropin*, *Valtropin*, *Zorbtive*) Dosages vary by indication and product. [Single-dose vials (powder for injection with diluent). Tev-Tropin: 5 mg vial (powder for injection with diluent, stable for 14 days when refrigerated). Genotropin: 1.5, 5.8, 13.8 mg cartridges. Humatrope: 6, 12, 24 mg pen cartridges; 5 mg vial (powder for injection with diluent, stable for 14 days when refrigerated). Nutropin AQ: 10 mg multidose vial, 5, 10, 20 mg/pen cartridges. Norditropin: 5, 10, 15 mg pen cartridges. Norditropin NordiFlex: 5, 10, 15 mg prefilled pens. Omnitrope: 1.5, 5.8 mg vial (powder for injection with diluent). Saizen: Preassembled reconstitution device with autoinjector pen. Serostim: 4, 5, 6 mg single-dose vials; 4, 8.8 mg multidose vials; and 8.8 mg cartridges for autoinjector. Valtropin: 5 mg single-dose vials, 5 mg prefilled syringe. Zorbtive: 8.8 mg vial (powder for injection with diluent, stable for 14 days when refrigerated).] ▶LK ♀B/C ▶? $$$$$

TERIPARATIDE (*Forteo*) Treatment of postmenopausal osteoporosis, treatment of men and women with glucocorticoid-induced osteoporosis, or to increase bone mass in men with primary or hypogonadal osteoporosis and high risk for fracture: 20 mcg SC daily in thigh or abdomen for no longer than 2 years. [Trade only: 28 dose pen injector (20 mcg/dose).] ▶LK ♀C ▶− $$$$$ ■

VASOPRESSIN (*Pitressin*, **ADH**, ✦ *Pressyn AR*) Diabetes insipidus: 5 to 10 units IM/SC two to four times per day prn. Cardiac arrest: 40 units IV; may repeat if no response after 3 min. Septic shock: 0.01 to 0.04 units/min. Variceal bleeding: 0.2 to 0.4 units/min initially (max 0.8 units/min). ▶LK ♀C ▶? $$$$$

ENT

Antihistamines—Non-Sedating

DESLORATADINE *(Clarinex, ♦ Aerius)* 5 mg PO daily for age older than 12 yo. Peds: 2 mL (1 mg) PO daily for age 6 to 11 mo, ½ teaspoonful (1.25 mg) PO daily for age 12 mo to 5 yo, 1 teaspoonful (2.5 mg) PO daily for age 6 to 11 yo. [Generic/Trade: Tabs 5 mg. Orally disintegrating tabs 2.5, 5 mg. Trade only: Syrup 0.5 mg/mL.] ▶LK ♀C ▶+ $$$$

FEXOFENADINE *(Allegra)* 60 mg PO two times per day or 180 mg daily. Peds: 30 mg PO two times per day for age 2 to 11 yo. [OTC Generic/Trade: Tabs 30, 60, 180 mg, Caps 60 mg. Trade only: Susp 30 mg/5 mL, Orally disintegrating tabs 30 mg.] ▶LK ♀C ▶+ $$$

LORATADINE *(Claritin, Claritin Hives Relief, Claritin RediTabs, Alavert, Tavist ND)* 10 mg PO daily for age older than 6 yo, 5 mg PO daily for age 2 to 5 yo. [OTC Generic/Trade: Tabs 10 mg. Fast-dissolve tabs (Alavert, Claritin RediTabs) 5, 10 mg. Syrup 1 mg/mL. Rx Trade only (Claritin): Chewable tabs 5 mg, Liqui-gel caps 10 mg.] ▶LK ♀B ▶+ $

Antihistamines—Other

NOTE: *Antihistamines ineffective when treating the common cold. Contraindicated in narrow-angle glaucoma, BPH, stenosing peptic ulcer disease, and bladder obstruction. Use half the normal dose in the elderly. May cause drowsiness and/or sedation, which may be enhanced with alcohol, sedatives, and other CNS depressants. Deaths have occurred in children younger than 2 yo attributed to toxicity from cough and cold medications; the FDA does not recommend their use in this age group.*

CETIRIZINE *(Zyrtec, ♦ Reactine, Aller-Relief)* 5 to 10 mg PO daily for age older than 6 yo. Peds: Give 2.5 mg PO daily for age 6 to 23 mo, give 2.5 mg PO daily to two times per day for age 2 to 5 yo. [OTC Generic/Trade: Tabs 5, 10 mg. Syrup 5 mg/5 mL. Chewable tabs, grape flavored 5, 10 mg.] ▶LK ♀B ▶–$$$

CHLORPHENIRAMINE *(Chlor-Trimeton, Aller-Chlor)* 4 mg PO q 4 to 6 h. Max 24 mg/day. Peds: Give 2 mg PO q 4 to 6 h for age 6 to 11 yo. Max 12 mg/day. [OTC Trade only: Tabs, extended-release 12 mg. Generic/Trade: Tabs 4 mg. Syrup 2 mg/5 mL. Tabs, extended-release 8 mg.] ▶LK ♀B ▶–$

CLEMASTINE *(Tavist-1)* 1.34 mg PO two times per day. Max 8.04 mg/day. [OTC Generic/Trade: Tabs 1.34 mg. Rx: Generic/Trade: Tabs 2.68 mg, Syrup 0.67 mg/5 mL. Rx: Generic only: Syrup 0.5 mg/5 mL.] ▶LK ♀B ▶–$

CYPROHEPTADINE *(Periactin)* Start 4 mg PO three times per day. Max 32 mg/day. [Generic only: Tabs 4 mg. Syrup 2 mg/5 mL.] ▶LK ♀B ▶–$

DEXCHLORPHENIRAMINE *(Polaramine)* 2 mg PO q 4 to 6 h. Timed-release tabs: 4 or 6 mg PO at bedtime or q 8 to 10 h. [Generic only: Tabs, immediate-release 2 mg, timed-release 4, 6 mg. Syrup 2 mg/5 mL.] ▶LK ♀? ▶–$$

DIPHENHYDRAMINE *(Benadryl, Banophen, Allermax, Diphen, Diphenhist, Dytan, Siladryl, Sominex, ♦ Allerdryl, Nytol)* Allergic rhinitis, urticaria, hypersensitivity reactions: 25 to 50 mg IV/IM/PO q 4 to 6 h. Peds: 5 mg/kg/

(cont.)

ENT COMBINATIONS (selected)	Decon-gestant	Antihist-amine	Anti-tussive	Typical Adult Doses
OTC				
Actifed Cold & Allergy	PE	CH	–	1 tab q 4–6 h
Actifed Cold & Sinus†	PS	CH	–	2 tabs q 6 h
Allerfrim, Aprodine	PS	TR	–	1 tab or 10 mL q 4–6 h
Benadryl Allergy/Cold†	PE	DPH	–	2 tabs q 4 h
Benadryl-D Allergy/Sinus Tablets	PE	DPH	–	1 tab q 4 h
Claritin-D 12-h, Alavert D-12	PS	LO	–	1 tab q 12 h
Claritin-D 24-h	PS	LO	–	1 tab daily
Dimetapp Cold & Allergy Elixir	PE	BR	–	20 mL q 4 h
Dimetapp DM Cold & Cough	PE	BR	DM	20 mL q 4 h
Drixoral Cold & Allergy	PS	DBR	–	1 tab q 12 h
Mucinex-DM Extended-Release	–	–	GU, DM	1–2 tabs q 12 h
Robitussin CF	PE	–	GU, DM	10 mL q 4 h*
Robitussin DM, Mytussin DM	–	–	GU, DM	10 mL q 4 h*
Robitussin PE, Guiatuss PE	PE	–	GU	10 mL q 4 h*
Triaminic Cold & Allergy	PE	CH	–	10 mL q 4 h
Rx Only				
Allegra-D 12-h	PS	FE	–	1 tab q 12 h
Allegra-D 24-h	PS	FE	–	1 tab daily
Bromfenex	PS	BR	–	1 cap q 12 h
Clarinex-D 24-h	PS	DL	–	1 tab daily
Deconamine	PS	CH	–	1 tab or 10 mL tid–qid
Deconamine SR, Chlordrine SR	PS	CH	–	1 tab q 12 h
Deconsal I	PE	–	GU	1–2 tabs q 12 h
Dimetane-DX	PS	BR	DM	10 mL PO q 4 h
Duratuss	PE	–	GU	1 tab q 12 h
Duratuss HD©III	PE	–	GU, HY	5-10 mL q 4–6 h
Entex PSE, Guaifenex PSE 120	PS	–	GU	1 tab q 12 h
Histussin D ©III	PS	–	HY	5 mL qid
Histussin HC ©III	PE	CH	HY	10 mL q 4 h
Humibid DM	–	–	GU, DM	1 tab q 12 h
Hycotuss ©III	–	–	GU, HY	5 mL after meals & at bedtime
Phenergan/Dextromethorphan	–	PR	DM	5 mL q 4–6 h
Phenergan VC	PE	PR	–	5 mL q 4–6 h
Phenergan VC w/codeine ©V	PE	PR	CO	5 mL q 4–6 h
Robitussin AC ©V (generic only)	–	–	GU, CO	10 mL q 4 h*
Robitussin DAC ©V (generic only)	PS	–	GU, CO	10 mL q 4 h*
Rondec Syrup	PE	CH	–	5 mL qid†
Rondec DM Syrup	PE	CH	DM	5 mL qid†
Rondec Oral Drops	PE	CH	–	0.75 to 1 mL qid
Rondec DM Oral Drops	PE	CH	DM	0.75 to 1 mL qid
Rynatan	PE	CH	–	1–2 tabs q 12 h
Rynatan-P Pediatric	PE	CH	–	2.5–5 mL q 12 h*
Semprex-D	PS	AC	–	1 c ap q 4–6 h
Tanafed (generic only)	PS	CH	–	10–20 mL q 12 h*
Tussionex ©III	–	CH	HY	5 mL q 12 h

tid=three times per day; qid=four times per day
©=class

AC=acrivastine	DL=desloratadine	FE=fexofenadine	PE=phenylephrine
BR=brompheniramine	DM=dextromethorphan	GU=guaifenesin	PR=promethazine
CH=chlorpheniramine	DBR=dexbrompheniramine	HY=hydrocodone	PS=pseudoephedrine
CO=codeine	DPH=diphenhydramine	LO=loratadine	TR=triprolidine

*5 mL/dose if 6–11 yo. 2.5 mL if 2–5 yo.
†2.5 mL/dose if 6–11 yo. 1.25 mL if 2–5 yo.
‡Also contains acetaminophen.

day divided q 4 to 6 h. EPS: 25 to 50 mg PO three to four times per day or 10 to 50 mg IV/IM three to four times per day. Insomnia: 25 to 50 mg PO at bedtime. [OTC Trade only: Tabs 25, 50 mg, Chewable tabs 12.5 mg. OTC and Rx: Generic only: Caps 25, 50 mg, softgel cap 25 mg. OTC Generic/Trade: Soln 6.25 or 12.5 mg per 5 mL. Rx: Trade only: (Dytan) Susp 25 mg/mL, Chewable tabs 25 mg.] ▶LK ♀B ▶– $

HYDROXYZINE (*Atarax, Vistaril*) 25 to 100 mg IM/PO one to four times per day or prn. [Generic only: Tabs 10, 25, 50, 100 mg; Caps 100 mg; Syrup 10 mg/5 mL. Generic/Trade: Caps 25, 50 mg, Susp 25 mg/5 mL (Vistaril). (Caps = Vistaril, Tabs = Atarax).] ▶L ♀C ▶– $$

LEVOCETIRIZINE (*Xyzal*) 5 mg PO daily for age 12 yo or older. Peds: Give 2.5 mg PO daily for age 6 to 11 yo. [Generic/Trade: Tabs, scored 5 mg; Oral soln 2.5 mg/5 mL (148 mL).] ▶K ♀B ▶– $$$

MECLIZINE (*Antivert, Bonine, Medivert, Meclicot, Meni-D, ✦Bonamine*) Motion sickness: 25 to 50 mg PO 1 h prior to travel, then 25 to 50 mg PO daily. Vertigo: 25 mg PO q 6 h prn. [Rx/OTC/Generic/Trade: Tabs 12.5, 25 mg; Chewable tabs 25 mg. Rx/Trade only: Tabs 50 mg.] ▶L ♀B ▶? $

Antitussives / Expectorants

BENZONATATE (*Tessalon, Tessalon Perles*) 100 to 200 mg PO three times per day. Swallow whole. Do not chew. Numbs mouth; possible choking hazard. [Generic/Trade: Softgel caps: 100, 200 mg.] ▶L ♀C ▶? $$

DEXTROMETHORPHAN (*Benylin, Delsym, DexAlone, Robitussin Cough, Vick's 44 Cough*) 10 to 20 mg PO q 4 h or 30 mg PO q 6 to 8 h. Sustained action liquid 60 mg PO q 12 h. [OTC Trade only: Caps 15 mg (Robitussin), 30 mg (DexAlone), Susp, extended-release 30 mg/5 mL (Delsym). Generic/Trade: Syrup 5, 7.5, 10, 15 mg/5 mL. Generic only: Lozenges 5, 10 mg.] ▶L ♀+ ▶+ $

GUAIFENESIN (*Robitussin, Hytuss, Guiatuss, Mucinex*) 100 to 400 mg PO q 4 h. 600 to 1200 mg PO q 12 h (extended-release). Peds: 50 to 100 mg/dose for age 2 to 5 yo, give 100 to 200 mg/dose for age 6 to 11 yo. [Rx Generic/Trade: Extended-release tabs 600, 1200 mg. OTC Generic/Trade: Liquid, Syrup 100 mg/5 mL. OTC Trade only: Susp 200 mg (Hytuss), Extended-release tabs 600 mg (Mucinex). OTC Generic only: Tabs 100, 200, 400 mg.] ▶L ♀C ▶+ $

Decongestants

NOTE: *See ENT—Nasal Preparations for nasal spray decongestants (oxymetazoline, phenylephrine). Deaths have occurred in children younger than 2 yo attributed to toxicity from cough and cold medications; the FDA does not recommend their use in this age group.*

PHENYLEPHRINE (*Sudafed PE*) 10 mg PO q 4 h. [OTC Trade only: Tabs 10 mg.] ▶L ♀C ▶+ $

PSEUDOEPHEDRINE (*Sudafed, Sudafed 12 Hour, Efidac/24, Dimetapp Decongestant Infant Drops, PediaCare Infants' Decongestant Drops, Triaminic Oral Infant Drops, ✦Pseudofrin*) Adult: 60 mg PO q 4 to 6 h.

(cont.)

Extended-release tabs: 120 mg PO two times per day or 240 mg PO daily. Peds: Give 15 mg PO q 4 to 6 h for age 2 to 5 yo, give 30 mg PO q 4 to 6 h for age 6 to 12 yo. [OTC Generic/Trade: Tabs 30, 60 mg, Tabs, extended-release 120 mg (12 h), Soln 15, 30 mg/5 mL. Trade only: Chewable tabs 15 mg, Tabs, extended-release 240 mg (24 h). Rx only in some states.] ▶L ♀C ▶+ $

Ear Preparations

AURALGAN (benzocaine + antipyrine) 2 to 4 gtts in ear's three to four times per day prn. [Generic/Trade: Otic soln 10, 15 mL.] ▶Not absorbed ♀C ▶? $

CARBAMIDE PEROXIDE (*Debrox, Murine Ear*) 5 to 10 gtts in ear(s) two times per day for 4 days. [OTC Generic/Trade: Otic soln 6.5%, 15, 30 mL.] ▶Not absorbed ♀? ▶? $

CIPRO HC OTIC (ciprofloxacin + hydrocortisone) 3 gtts in ear(s) two times per day for 7 days for age 1 yo to adult. [Trade only: Otic susp 10 mL.] ▶Not absorbed ♀C ▶– $$$$

CIPRODEX OTIC (ciprofloxacin + dexamethasone) 4 gtts in ear(s) two times per day for 7 days for age 6 mo to adult. [Trade only: Otic susp 5, 7.5 mL.] ▶Not absorbed ♀C ▶– $$$$

CIPROFLOXACIN (*Cetraxal*) 1 single-use container in ear(s) two times per day for 7 days for age 1 yo to adult. [Trade only: 0.25 mL single-use containers with 0.2% ciprofloxacin soln, #14.] ▶Not absorbed ♀C ▶– $$$$

CORTISPORIN OTIC (hydrocortisone + polymyxin + neomycin, *Pediotic*) 4 gtts in ear(s) three to four times per day up to 10 days or soln or susp. Peds: 3 gtts in ear(s) three to four times per day up to 10 days. Caution with perforated TMs or tympanostomy tubes as this increases the risk of neomycin ototoxicity, especially if use prolonged or repeated. Use susp rather than acidic soln. [Generic only: Otic soln or susp 7.5, 10 mL.] ▶Not absorbed ♀? ▶? $

CORTISPORIN TC OTIC (hydrocortisone + neomycin + thonzonium + colistin) 4 to 5 gtts in ear(s) three to four times per day up to 10 days. [Trade only: Otic susp, 10 mL.] ▶Not absorbed ♀? ▶? $$$

DOMEBORO OTIC (acetic acid + aluminum acetate) 4 to 6 gtts in ear(s) q 2 to 3 h. Peds: 2 to 3 gtts in ear(s) q 3 to 4 h. [Generic only: Otic soln 60 mL.] ▶Not absorbed ♀? ▶? $

FLUOCINOLONE—OTIC (*DermOtic*) 5 gtts in affected ear(s) two times per day for 7 to 14 days for age 2 yo to adult. [Trade only: Otic oil 0.01% 20 mL.] ▶L ♀C ▶? $$

OFLOXACIN—OTIC (*Floxin Otic*) Otitis externa : 5 gtts in ear(s) daily for age 1 to 12 yo, 10 gtts in ear(s) daily for age 12 yo or older. [Generic/Trade: Otic soln 0.3% 5, 10 mL. Trade only: "Singles": Single-dispensing containers 0.25 mL (5 gtts), 2 per foil pouch.] ▶Not absorbed ♀C ▶– $$$

SWIM-EAR (isopropyl alcohol + anhydrous glycerins) 4 to 5 gtts in ears after swimming. [OTC Trade only: Otic soln 30 mL.] ▶Not absorbed ♀? ▶? $

VOSOL HC (acetic acid + propylene glycol + hydrocortisone) 5 gtts in ear(s) three to four times per day. Peds age older than 3 yo: 3 to 4 gtts in ear(s) three to four times per day. [Generic/Trade: Otic soln 2%/3%/1% 10 mL.] ▶Not absorbed ♀? ▶? $

Mouth and Lip Preparations

AMLEXANOX (*Aphthasol, OraDisc A*) Aphthous ulcers: Apply ¼ inch paste or mucoadhesive patch to affected area four times per day after oral hygiene for up to 10 days. Up to 3 patches may be applied at one time. [Trade only: Oral paste 5% (Aphthasol), 3, 5 g tube. Mucoadhesive patch (OraDisc) 2 mg, #20.] ▶LK ♀B ▶? $

CEVIMELINE (*Evoxac*) Dry mouth due to Sjögren's syndrome: 30 mg PO three times per day. [Trade only: Caps 30 mg.] ▶L ♀C ▶– $$$$$

CHLORHEXIDINE GLUCONATE (*Peridex, Periogard, ✦ Denticare*) Rinse with 15 mL of undiluted soln for 30 sec two times per day. Do not swallow. Spit after rinsing. [Generic/Trade: Oral rinse 0.12% 473 to 480 mL bottles.] ▶Fecal excretion ♀B ▶? $

DEBACTEROL (sulfuric acid + sulfonated phenolics) Aphthous stomatitis, mucositis: Apply to dry ulcer. Rinse with water. [Trade only: 1 mL prefilled, single-use applicator.] ▶Not absorbed ♀C ▶+ $$

GELCLAIR (maltodextrin + propylene glycol) Aphthous ulcers, mucositis, stomatitis: Rinse mouth with 1 packet three times per day or prn. Do not eat or drink for 1 h after treatment. [Trade only: 21 packets/box.] ▶Not absorbed ♀+ ▶+ $$$

LIDOCAINE—VISCOUS (*Xylocaine*) Mouth or lip pain in adults only: 15 to 20 mL topically or swish and spit q 3 h. [Generic/Trade: Soln 2%, 20 mL unit dose, 100 mL bottle.] ▶LK ♀B ▶+ $

MAGIC MOUTHWASH (diphenhydramine + Mylanta + sucralfate) 5 mL PO swish and spit or swish and swallow three times per day before meals and prn. [Compounded susp. A standard mixture is 30 mL diphenhydramine liquid (12.5 mg/5 mL)/60 mL Mylanta or Maalox/4 g Carafate.] ▶LK ▶– $$$

PILOCARPINE (*Salagen*) Dry mouth due to radiation of head and neck or Sjögren's syndrome: 5 mg PO three to four times per day. [Generic/Trade: Tabs 5, 7.5 mg.] ▶L ♀C ▶– $$$$

Nasal Preparations—Corticosteroids

BECLOMETHASONE (*Beconase AQ, Qnas, Vancenase*) Vancenase: 1 spray per nostril two to four times per day. Beconase AQ: 1 to 2 spray(s) per nostril two times per day. Vancenase AQ Double Strength: 1 to 2 spray(s) per nostril daily. Qnasl: 1 to 2 spray(s) per nostril daily. [Trade only: Beconase AQ 42 mcg/spray, 200 sprays/bottle. Qnasl: 80 mcg/spray, 120 sprays/bottle.] ▶L ♀C ▶? $$$$

BUDESONIDE—NASAL (*Rhinocort Aqua*) 1 to 4 sprays per nostril daily. [Trade only: Nasal inhaler 120 sprays/bottle.] ▶L ♀B ▶? $$$$

CICLESONIDE (*Omnaris, Zetonna*) Omnaris: 2 sprays per nostril daily. Zetonna: 1 actuation per nostril daily. [Trade only: Nasal spray, 50 mcg/spray, 120 sprays/bottle (Omnaris). Nasal aerosol, 37 mcg/actuation, 60 actuations/cannister (Zetonna).] ▶L ♀C ▶? $$$

FLUNISOLIDE (*Nasalide, ✦ Rhinalar*) Start 2 sprays per nostril two times per day. Max 8 sprays/nostril/day. [Generic only: Nasal soln 0.025%] ▶L ♀C ▶? $$$

FLUTICASONE—NASAL *(Flonase, Veramyst, ✦ Avamys)* 2 sprays per nostril daily. [Generic/Trade: Flonase: Nasal spray 0.05%, 120 sprays/bottle. Trade only: (Veramyst): Nasal spray susp: 27.5 mcg/spray, 120 sprays/bottle.] ▶L ♀C ▶? $$$

MOMETASONE—NASAL *(Nasonex)* Adult: 2 sprays/nostril daily. Peds 2 to 11 yo: 1 spray/nostril daily. [Trade only: Nasal spray, 120 sprays/bottle.] ▶L ♀C ▶? $$$$

TRIAMCINOLONE—NASAL *(Nasacort AQ, Nasacort HFA, Tri-Nasal, AllerNaze)* Nasacort HFA, Tri-Nasal, AllerNaze: 2 sprays per nostril daily to two times per day. Max 4 sprays/nostril/day. Nasacort AQ: 1 to 2 sprays per nostril daily. [Trade only: Nasal inhaler 55 mcg/spray, 100 sprays/bottle (Nasacort HFA). Nasal spray, 55 mcg/spray, 120 sprays/bottle (Nasacort AQ). Nasal spray 50 mcg/spray, 120 sprays/bottle (Tri-Nasal, AllerNaze).] ▶L ♀C ▶– $$$$

Nasal Preparations—Other

AZELASTINE—NASAL *(Astelin, Astepro)* 1 to 2 sprays per nostril two times per day. [Generic/Trade: Nasal spray, 200 sprays/bottle. Trade only: Astepro 0.15% nasal spray 200 sprays/bottle] ▶L ♀C ▶? $$$$

CETACAINE **(benzocaine + tetracaine + butamben)** Topical anesthesia of mucous membranes : Spray: Apply for no more than 1 sec. Liquid or gel: Apply with cotton applicator directly to site. [Trade only: (14%/2%/2%) Spray 56 mL. Topical liquid 56 mL. Topical gel 5, 29 g.] ▶LK ♀C ▶? $$

CROMOLYN—NASAL *(NasalCrom)* 1 spray per nostril three to four times per day. [OTC Generic/Trade: Nasal inhaler 200 sprays/bottle 13, 26 mL.] ▶LK ♀B ▶+ $

DYMISTA **(azelastine + fluticasone)** 1 spray per nostril 2 times per day. [Trade only: Nasal spray: 137 mcg azelastine/50 mcg fluticasone/spray, 120 sprays/bottle.] ▶L – ♀C ▶? $$$$

IPRATROPIUM—NASAL *(Atrovent Nasal Spray)* 2 sprays per nostril two to four times per day. [Generic/Trade: Nasal spray 0.03%, 345 sprays/bottle, 0.06%, 165 sprays/bottle.] ▶L ♀B ▶? $$

✦ LEVOCABASTINE—NASAL *(Livostin)* Canada only. 2 sprays per nostril two times per day, increase prn to three to four times per day. [Trade only: Nasal spray 0.5 mg/mL, plastic bottles of 15 mL. 50 mcg/spray.] ▶L (but minimal absorption) ♀C ▶– $$

OLOPATADINE—NASAL *(Patanase)* 2 sprays per nostril two times per day. [Trade only: Nasal spray, 240 sprays/bottle.] ▶L ♀C ▶? $$$

OXYMETAZOLINE *(Afrin, Dristan 12 Hr Nasal, Nostrilla, Vicks Sinex 12 Hr)* 2 to 3 gtts/sprays per nostril two times per day prn nasal congestion for no more than 3 days. [OTC Generic/Trade: Nasal spray 0.05% 15, 30 mL; Nose gtts 0.025%, 0.05% 20 mL with dropper.] ▶L ♀C ▶? $

PHENYLEPHRINE—NASAL *(Neo-Synephrine, Vicks Sinex)* 2 to 3 sprays or gtts per nostril q 4 h prn for 3 days. [OTC Generic/Trade: Nasal gtts/spray 0.25, 0.5, 1% (15 mL).] ▶L ♀C ▶? $

SALINE NASAL SPRAY *(SeaMist, Entsol, Pretz, NaSal, Ocean, ✦ HydraSense)* Nasal dryness : 1 to 3 sprays or gtts per nostril prn. [Generic/Trade: Nasal spray 0.4, 0.5, 0.65, 0.75%, Nasal gtts 0.4, 0.65%. Trade only: Preservative-free nasal spray 3% (Entsol).] ▶Not metabolized ♀A ▶+ $

GASTROENTEROLOGY

Antidiarrheals

BISMUTH SUBSALICYLATE (*Pepto-Bismol, Kaopectate*) 2 tabs or caplets or 30 mL (262 mg/15 mL) PO q 30 min to 1 h up to 8 doses per day for up to 2 days. Peds: 5 mL (262 mg/15 mL) or ⅓ tab, chew tab, or cap PO for age 3 to 6 yo, 10 mL (262 mg/15 mL) or ⅔ tab, chew tab, or cap PO for age 6 to 9 yo. Risk of Reye's syndrome in children. [OTC Generic/Trade: Chewable tabs 262 mg. Susp 262, 525, 750 mg/15 mL. OTC Trade only: Caplets 262 mg (Pepto-Bismol). Susp 87 mg/5 mL (Kaopectate Children's Liquid).] ▶K ♀D ▶? $

IMODIUM MULTI-SYMPTOM RELIEF (loperamide + simethicone) 2 tabs or caplets PO initially, then 1 tab or caplet PO after each unformed stool to a max of 4 tabs/caplets per day. Peds: 1 tab or caplet PO initially, then ½ caplet PO after each unformed stool (up to 2 tabs or caplets PO per day for age 6 to 8 yo or wt 48 to 59 lbs or up to 3 tabs or caplets PO per day for age 9 to 11 yo or wt 60 to 95 lbs). [OTC Generic/Trade: Caplets, Chewable tabs 2 mg loperamide/125 mg simethicone.] ▶L ♀C ▶– $

LOMOTIL (diphenoxylate + atropine) 2 tabs or 10 mL PO four times per day. [Generic/Trade: Oral soln or tab 2.5 mg/0.025 mg diphenoxylate/atropine per 5 mL or tab.] ▶L ♀C ▶–©V $

LOPERAMIDE (*Imodium, Imodium AD, ✦Loperacap, Diarr-eze*) 4 mg PO initially, then 2 mg PO after each unformed stool to a maximum of 16 mg per day. Peds: 1 mg PO three times per day for wt 13 to 20 kg, 2 mg PO two times per day for wt 21 to 30 kg, 2 mg PO three times per day for wt greater than 30 kg. [OTC Generic/Trade: Tabs 2 mg. Oral soln 1 mg/5 mL. Oral soln 1 mg/7.5 mL.] ▶L ♀C ▶+ $

MOTOFEN (difenoxin + atropine) 2 tabs PO initially, then 1 tab after each loose stool q 3 to 4 h prn (up to 8 tabs per day). [Trade only: Tabs difenoxin 1 mg + atropine 0.025 mg.] ▶L ♀C ▶–©IV $$

OPIUM (opium tincture, paregoric) Paregoric: 5 to 10 mL PO daily (up to four times). Opium tincture: 0.6 mL (range 0.3 to 1 mL) PO q 2 to 6 h, prn, to a max of 6 mL per day. Opium tincture contains 25 times more morphine than paregoric. [Trade only: Opium tincture 10% (deodorized opium tincture, 10 mg morphine equivalent/mL). Generic only: Paregoric (camphorated opium tincture, 2 mg morphine equivalent/5 mL).] ▶L ♀B (D with long-term use) ▶?©II (opium tincture), III (paregoric) $$

Antiemetics—5-HT3 Receptor Antagonists

DOLASETRON (*Anzemet*) Nausea with chemo: 1.8 mg/kg (up to 100 mg) PO single dose. Postop nausea: 12.5 mg IV in adults and 0.35 mg/kg IV in children as single dose. Alternative for prevention: 100 mg (adults) PO or 1.2 mg/kg (children) PO 2 h before surgery. [Trade only: Tabs 50, 100 mg. Injectable no longer available in Canada.] ▶LK ♀B ▶? $$$

GRANISETRON (*Sancuso*, ✦ *Kytril*) Nausea with chemo: Transdermal (Sancuso): 1 patch to upper outer arm at least 24 h (but up to 48 h) before chemotherapy. Remove 24 h after completion of chemotherapy. Can be worn up to 7 days depending on the duration of chemo. [Trade only: Transdermal patch (Sancuso) 34.3 mg of granisetron delivering 3.1 mg/24 h.] ▶L ♀B ▶? $$$$

ONDANSETRON (*Zofran*) Nausea with chemo: IV: 0.15 mg/kg dose (max 16 mg) 30 min prior to chemo and repeated at 4 and 8 h after 1st dose for age 6 mo or older. PO: 4 mg PO 30 min prior to chemo and repeat at 4 and 8 h for age 4 to 11 yo, 8 mg PO and repeated 8 h later for age 12 yo or older. Prevention of postop N/V: 4 mg IV over 2 to 5 min or 4 mg IM or 16 mg PO 1 h before anesthesia. Give 0.1 mg/kg IV over 2 to 5 min as a single dose for age 1 mo to 12 yo if wt 40 kg or less; 4 mg IV over 2 to 5 min as a single dose if wt greater than 40 kg. Prevention of N/V associated with radiotherapy: 8 mg PO three times per day. [Generic/Trade: Tabs 4, 8, 24 mg. Orally disintegrating tabs 4, 8 mg. Oral soln 4 mg/5 mL. Generic only: Tabs 16 mg.] ▶L ♀B ▶? $$$$$

PALONOSETRON (*Aloxi*) Nausea with chemo: 0.25 mg IV over 30 sec, 30 min prior to chemo. Prevention of postop N/V: 0.075 mg IV over 10 sec just prior to anesthesia. [Trade only: injectable.] ▶L ♀B ▶? $$$$$

Antiemetics—Other

APREPITANT (*Emend, fosaprepitant*) Prevention of nausea with moderately to highly emetogenic chemo, in combination with a corticosteroid and a 5-HT3 antagonist: 125 mg PO on day 1 (1 h prior to chemo), then 80 mg PO q am on days 2 and 3. Alternative for 1st dose only is 115 mg IV (fosaprepitant) over 15 min given 30 min prior to chemo. Alternatively, single dose of 150 mg IV (fosaprepitant) over 20 to 30 minutes, with a corticosteroid and a 5-HT3 antagonist. Prevention of postop N/V: 40 mg PO within 3 h prior to anesthesia. [Trade only (aprepitant): Caps 40, 80, 125 mg. IV prodrug form is fosaprepitant.] ▶L ♀B ▶? $$$$$

DICLEGIS (*doxylamine + pyridoxine*) N/V due to pregnancy: 2 tabs PO at bedtime. If not controlled, can increase to a maximum of 4 tabs daily (2 tabs PO q am, 1 tab PO mid-afternoon, 2 tabs PO at bedtime). [Trade: Tabs, doxylamine 10 mg and pyridoxine 10 mg.] ▶LK – ♀A ▶– $$$$$

DIMENHYDRINATE (*Dramamine*, ✦ *Gravol*) 50 to 100 mg PO/IM/IV q 4 to 6 h prn (max 400 mg/24 h PO, 600 mg/day IV/IM). Canada only: 50 to 100 mg/dose PR q 4 to 6 h prn. [OTC Generic/Trade: Tabs 50 mg. Trade only: Chewable tabs 25, 50 mg. Generic only: Oral soln 12.5 mg/5 mL. Canada only: Supp 25, 50, 100 mg.] ▶LK ♀B ▶– $

DOMPERIDONE Canada only. Postprandial dyspepsia: 10 to 20 mg PO three to four times per day, 30 min before a meal. N/V: 20 mg PO three to four times per day. [Canada only. Trade/Generic: Tabs 10, 20 mg.] ▶L ♀? ▶– $$

DOXYLAMINE (*Unisom Nighttime Sleep Aid, others*) N/V associated with pregnancy: 12.5 mg PO two to four times per day; often used in combination with pyridoxine. [OTC, Generic/Trade: Tabs 25 mg.] ▶L ♀A ▶? $

DRONABINOL (*Marinol*) Nausea with chemo: 5 mg/m^2 PO 1 to 3 h before chemo then 5 mg/m^2/dose q 2 to 4 h after chemo for 4 to 6 doses/day. Anorexia associated with AIDS: Initially 2.5 mg PO two times per day before lunch and dinner. If indicated and tolerated, increase to 20 mg/day. [Generic/Trade: Caps 2.5, 5, 10 mg.] ▶L ♀C ▶–©III $$$$$

DROPERIDOL (*Inapsine*) 0.625 to 2.5 mg IV or 2.5 mg IM. May cause fatal QT prolongation, even in patients with no risk factors. Monitor ECG before. ▶L ♀C ▶? $

METOCLOPRAMIDE (*Reglan, Metozolv ODT, ✦Maxeran*) GERD/diabetic gastroparesis: 10 mg IV/IM q 2 to 3 h prn. 10 to 15 mg PO four times per day, 30 min before meals and at bedtime. Caution with long-term (more than 3 months) use. Prevention of postop nausea: 10 to 20 mg IM/IV near end of surgical procedure, may repeat q 3 to 4 h prn. [Generic/Trade: Tabs 5, 10 mg. Trade: Orally disintegrating tabs 5, 10 mg (Metozolv). Generic only: Oral soln 5 mg/5 mL.] ▶K ♀B ▶? $

NABILONE (*Cesamet*) 1 to 2 mg PO two times per day, 1 to 3 h before chemotherapy. [Trade only: Caps 1 mg.] ▶L ♀C ▶–©II $$$$$

PHOSPHORATED CARBOHYDRATES (*Emetrol*) 15 to 30 mL PO q 15 min prn, max 5 doses. Peds: 5 to 10 mL per dose. [OTC Generic/Trade: Soln containing dextrose, fructose, and phosphoric acid.] ▶L ♀A ▶+ $

PROCHLORPERAZINE (*Compazine, ✦Stemetil*) 5 to 10 mg IV over at least 2 min. 5 to 10 mg PO/IM three to four times per day. 25 mg PR q 12 h. Sustained-release: 15 mg PO q am or 10 mg PO q 12 h. Peds: 0.1 mg/kg/dose PO/PR three to four times per day or 0.1 to 0.15 mg/kg/dose IM three to four times per day. [Generic only: Tabs 5, 10, 25 mg. Supp 25 mg.] ▶LK ♀C ▶? $

PROMETHAZINE (*Phenergan*) Adults: 12.5 to 25 mg PO/IM/PR q 4 to 6 h. Peds: 0.25 to 1 mg/kg PO/IM/PR q 4 to 6 h. Contraindicated if age younger than 2 yo; caution in older children. IV use common but not approved. [Generic only: Tab/Supp 12.5, 25, 50 mg. Syrup 6.25 mg/5 mL.] ▶LK ♀C ▶– $

SCOPOLAMINE (*Transderm-Scop, Scopace, ✦Transderm-V*) Motion sickness: Apply 1 disc (1.5 mg) behind ear 4 h prior to event; replace q 3 days. Tabs: 0.4 to 0.8 mg PO 1 h before travel and q 8 h prn. [Trade only: Topical disc 1.5 mg/72 h, box of 4. Oral tabs 0.4 mg.] ▶L ♀C ▶+ $$

TRIMETHOBENZAMIDE (*Tigan*) 300 mg PO q 6 to 8 h, 200 mg IM q 6 to 8 h. [Generic/Trade: Cap 300 mg.] ▶LK ♀C ▶? $

Antiulcer—Antacids

ALKA-SELTZER (acetylsalicylic acid + citrate + bicarbonate) 2 regular-strength tabs in 4 oz water q 4 h PO prn (up to 8 tabs daily for age younger than 60 yo, up to 4 tabs daily for age 60 yo or older) or 2 extra-strength tabs in 4 oz water q 6 h PO prn (up to 7 tabs daily for age younger than 60 yo, up to 3 tabs daily for age 60 yo or older). [OTC Trade only: Regular-strength, original: aspirin 325 mg + citric acid 1000 mg + sodium bicarbonate 1916 mg. Regular-strength lemon lime and cherry: 325 mg + 1000 mg + 1700 mg. Extra-strength: 500 mg + 1000 mg + 1985 mg. Not all forms of Alka-Seltzer contain aspirin (eg, Alka-Seltzer Heartburn Relief).] ▶LK ♀? (– 3rd trimester) ▶? $

ALUMINUM HYDROXIDE (*Alternagel, Amphojel, Alu-Tab, Alu-Cap, ♣ Basalgel, Mucaine*) 5 to 10 mL or 300 to 600 mg PO up to 6 times per day. Constipating. [OTC Generic/Trade: Susp 320, 600 mg/ 5 mL.] ▶K ♀C ▶? $

GAVISCON (aluminum hydroxide + magnesium carbonate) 2 to 4 tabs or 15 to 30 mL (regular-strength) or 10 mL (extra-strength) PO four times per day prn. [OTC Trade only: Tabs: Regular-strength (Al hydroxide 80 mg + Mg carbonate 20 mg), Extra-strength (Al hydroxide 160 mg + Mg carbonate 105 mg). Liquid: Regular-strength (Al hydroxide 95 mg + Mg carbonate 358 mg per 15 mL), Extra-strength (Al hydroxide 254 mg + Mg carbonate 237.5 mg per 5 mL).] ▶K ♀? ▶? $

MAALOX (aluminum hydroxide + magnesium hydroxide) 10 to 20 mL or 1 to 2 tabs PO prn. [OTC Generic/Trade: Regular-strength chewable tabs (Al hydroxide + Mg hydroxide 200/200 mg), susp (225/200 mg per 5 mL). Other strengths available.] ▶K ♀C ▶? $

MAGALDRATE (*Riopan*) 5 to 10 mL PO prn. [OTC Trade/generic: Susp 540/20 mg/5 mL.] ▶K ♀C ▶? $

MYLANTA (aluminum hydroxide + magnesium hydroxide + simethicone) 10 to 20 mL PO between meals and at bedtime prn. [OTC Generic/Trade: Liquid (various concentrations—regular-strength, maximum-strength, supreme, etc.).] ▶K ♀C ▶? $

ROLAIDS (calcium carbonate + magnesium hydroxide) 2 to 4 tabs PO q 1 h prn, max 12 tabs/day (regular-strength) or 10 tabs/day (extra-strength). [OTC Trade only: Tabs, regular-strength (Ca carbonate 550 mg, Mg hydroxide 110 mg), extra-strength (Ca carbonate 675 mg, Mg hydroxide 135 mg).] ▶K ♀? ▶? $

Antiulcer—H2 Antagonists

CIMETIDINE (*Tagamet, Tagamet HB*) 300 mg IV/IM/PO q 6 to 8 h, 400 mg PO two times per day, or 400 to 800 mg PO at bedtime. Erosive esophagitis: 800 mg PO two times per day or 400 mg PO four times per day. Continuous IV infusion 37.5 to 50 mg/h (900 to 1200 mg/day). [Tabs 200, 300, 400, 800 mg. Rx Generic only: Oral soln 300 mg/5 mL. OTC Generic/Trade: Tabs 200 mg.] ▶LK ♀B ▶+ $

FAMOTIDINE (*Pepcid, Pepcid AC, Maximum Strength Pepcid AC*) 20 mg IV q 12 h, 20 to 40 mg PO at bedtime, or 20 mg PO two times per day. [Generic/Trade: Tabs 10 mg (OTC, Pepcid AC Acid Controller), 20 mg (Rx and OTC, Maximum Strength Pepcid AC), 40 mg. Rx Generic/Trade: Susp 40 mg/5 mL.] ▶LK ♀B ▶? $

NIZATIDINE (*Axid, Axid AR*) 150 to 300 mg PO at bedtime, or 150 mg PO two times per day. [OTC (Axid AR): Tabs 75 mg. Rx Generic: Caps 150 mg. Oral soln 15 mg/mL (120, 480 mL). Caps 300 mg.] ▶K ♀B ▶? $$$$

PEPCID COMPLETE (famotidine + calcium carbonate + magnesium hydroxide) 1 tab PO prn. Max 2 tabs/day. [OTC trade/generic: Chewable tab, famotidine 10 mg with calcium carbonate 800 mg and magnesium hydroxide 165 mg.] ▶LK ♀B ▶? $

RANITIDINE (*Zantac, Zantac Efferdose, Zantac 75, Zantac 150, Peptic Relief*) 150 mg PO two times per day or 300 mg PO at bedtime. 50 mg IV/IM q 8 h, or continuous infusion 6.25 mg/h (150 mg/day). [Generic/Trade: Tabs 75 mg (OTC: Zantac 75), 150 mg (OTC and Rx: Zantac 150), 300 mg. Syrup 75 mg/5 mL. Rx Trade only: Effervescent tabs 25 mg. Rx Generic only: Caps 150, 300 mg.] ▶K ♀B ▶? \$\$\$

Antiulcer—Helicobacter pylori *Treatment*

HELIDAC (bismuth subsalicylate + metronidazole + tetracycline) 1 dose PO four times per day for 2 weeks. To be given with an H2 antagonist. [Trade only: Each dose consists of: bismuth subsalicylate 524 mg (2 × 262 mg) chewable tab + metronidazole 250 mg tab + tetracycline 500 mg cap.] ▶LK ♀D ▶− \$\$\$\$\$

PREVPAC (lansoprazole + amoxicillin + clarithromycin, ◆HP-Pac) 1 dose PO two times per day for 10 to 14 days. [Trade only: Each dose consists of lansoprazole 30 mg cap + amoxicillin 1 g (2 × 500 mg cap), + clarithromycin 500 mg tab.] ▶LK ♀C ▶? \$\$\$\$\$

PYLERA (bismuth subcitrate potassium + metronidazole + tetracycline) 3 caps PO four times per day (after meals and at bedtime) for 10 days. Use with omeprazole 20 mg PO two times per day. [Trade only: Each cap contains bismuth subcitrate potassium 140 mg + metronidazole 125 mg + tetracycline 125 mg.] ▶LK ♀D ▶− \$\$\$\$\$

Antiulcer—Proton Pump Inhibitors

ESOMEPRAZOLE (*Nexium*) Erosive esophagitis: 20 to 40 mg PO daily for 4 to 8 weeks. Maintenance of erosive esophagitis: 20 mg PO daily. Zollinger-Ellison: 40 mg PO two times per day GERD: 20 mg PO daily for 4 weeks. GERD with esophagitis: 20 to 40 mg IV daily for 10 days until taking PO. Prevention of NSAID-associated gastric ulcer: 20 to 40 mg PO daily for up to 6 months. *H. pylori* eradication: 40 mg PO daily with amoxicillin 1000 mg PO two times per day and clarithromycin 500 mg PO two times per day for 10 days. [Trade only: Caps, delayed-release 20, 40 mg. Delayed-release granules for oral susp 2.5, 5, 10, 20, 40 mg per packet.] ▶L ♀B ▶? \$\$\$\$\$

HELICOBACTER PYLORI THERAPY

- Triple therapy PO for 10 to 14 days: clarithromycin 500 mg two times per day plus amoxicillin 1 g two times per day (or metronidazole 500 mg two times per day) plus PPI*
- Quadruple therapy PO for 14 days: bismuth subsalicylate 525 mg (or 30 mL) three to four times per day plus metronidazole 500 mg three to four times per day plus tetracycline 500 mg three to four times per day plus a PPI* or an H2 blocker†
- PPI or H2 blocker may need to be continued past 14 days to heal the ulcer.

*PPIs include esomeprazole 40 mg daily, lansoprazole 30 mg two times per day, omeprazole 20 mg two times per day, pantoprazole 40 mg two times per day, rabeprazole 20 mg two times per day.
†H2 blockers include cimetidine 400 mg two times per day, famotidine 20 mg two times per day, nizatidine 150 mg two times per day, ranitidine 150 mg two times per day. Adapted from *Medical Letter Treatment Guidelines* 2008:55.

LANSOPRAZOLE (*Prevacid*) Heartburn : 15 mg PO daily. Duodenal ulcer or maintenance therapy after healing of duodenal ulcer : 15 mg PO daily for up to 12 months. NSAID–induced gastric ulcer : 30 mg PO daily for 8 weeks (treatment), 15 mg PO daily for up to 12 weeks (prevention). GERD : 15 mg PO daily. Gastric ulcer : 30 mg PO daily. Erosive esophagitis : 30 mg PO daily for up to 8 weeks or 30 mg IV daily for 7 days or until taking PO. [OTC Generic/Trade : Caps 15 mg. Rx Generic/Trade: 15, 30 mg. Rx Trade only: Orally disintegrating tab 15, 30 mg.] ▶L ♀B ▶? $$$$

OMEPRAZOLE (*Prilosec*, ✦ *Losec*) GERD, duodenal ulcer, erosive esophagitis : 20 mg PO daily. Heartburn (OTC): 20 mg PO daily for 14 days. Gastric ulcer : 40 mg PO daily. Hypersecretory conditions : 60 mg PO daily. [Rx Generic/Trade: Caps 10, 20, 40 mg. Trade only: Granules for oral susp 2.5 mg, 10 mg. OTC Trade only: Cap 20 mg.] ▶L ♀C ▶? OTC $, Rx $$$$

PANTOPRAZOLE (*Protonix*, ✦ *Pantoloc, Tecta*) Treatment of erosive esophagitis associated with GERD : 40 mg PO daily. Maintenance of erosive esophagitis: 40 mg PO once daily. Zollinger-Ellison syndrome : 40 mg PO twice daily or 80 mg IV q 8 to 12 h for 7 days until taking PO. [Generic/Trade: Tabs 20, 40 mg. Trade only: Granules for susp 40 mg/packet.] ▶L ♀B ▶? $

RABEPRAZOLE (*AcipHex*, ✦ *Pariet*) GERD, duodenal ulcer, erosive esophagitis: 20 mg PO daily. [Trade: Tabs 20 mg. Sprinkle caps (open and sprinkle on soft food or liquid) 5 mg and 10 mg.] ▶L ♀B ▶? $$$$

ZEGERID (omeprazole + bicarbonate) Duodenal ulcer, GERD, erosive esophagitis : 20 mg PO daily for 4 to 8 weeks. Maintenance of erosive esophagitis: 20 mg PO daily. Gastric ulcer : 40 mg PO once daily for 4 to 8 weeks. Reduction of risk of upper GI bleed in critically ill (susp only): 40 mg PO, then 40 mg 6 to 8 h later, then 40 mg once daily thereafter for up to 14 days. [OTC Trade only: omeprazole/sodium bicarbonate caps 20 mg/1.1 g. Rx Generic/Trade: Caps 20 mg/1.1 g and 40 mg/1.1 g. Trade only: Powder packets for susp 20 mg/1.1 g and 40 mg/1.68 g.] ▶L ♀C ▶? $$$$$

Antiulcer—Other

DICYCLOMINE (*Bentyl*, ✦ *Bentylol*) 10 to 20 mg PO/IM four times per day up to 40 mg PO four times per day. [Generic/Trade: Tabs 20 mg. Caps 10 mg.] ▶LK ♀B ▶– $

DONNATAL (phenobarbital + hyoscyamine + atropine + scopolamine) 1 to 2 tabs/caps or 5 to 10 mL PO three to four times per day. 1 extended-release tab PO q 8 to 12 h. [Generic/trade: Phenobarbital 16.2 mg + hyoscyamine 0.1 mg + atropine 0.02 mg + scopolamine 6.5 mcg in each tab or 5 mL. Trade only: Extended-release tab 48.6 + 0.3111 + 0.0582 + 0.0195 mg.] ▶LK ♀C ▶– $$$

GI COCKTAIL (*green goddess*) Acute GI upset: Mixture of Maalox/Mylanta 30 mL + viscous lidocaine (2%) 10 mL + Donnatal 10 mL administered PO in a single dose. ▶LK ♀See individual ▶See individual $

HYOSCINE (✦ *Buscopan*) Canada: GI or bladder spasm: 10 to 20 mg PO/IV up to 60 mg daily (PO) or 100 mg daily (IV). [Canada Trade only: Tabs 10 mg.] ▶LK ♀C ▶? $$

HYOSCYAMINE (*Anaspaz, A-spaz, Cystospaz, ED Spaz, Hyosol, Hyospaz, Levbid, Levsin, Levsinex, Medispaz, NuLev, Spacol, Spasdel, Symax*) Bladder spasm, control gastric secretion, GI hypermotility, irritable bowel syndrome: 0.125 to 0.25 mg PO/SL q 4 h or prn. Extended-release: 0.375 to 0.75 mg PO q 12 h. Max 1.5 mg/day. [Generic/Trade: Tabs 0.125. Sublingual tabs 0.125 mg. Chewable tabs 0.125 mg. Extended-release tabs 0.375 mg. Elixir 0.125 mg/5 mL. Gtts 0.125 mg/1 mL.] ▶LK ♀C ▶– $

MISOPROSTOL (*PGE1, Cytotec*) Prevention of NSAID–induced gastric ulcers: Start 100 mcg PO two times per day, then titrate as tolerated up to 200 mcg PO four times per day. Cervical ripening: 25 mcg intravaginally q 3 to 6 h (or 50 mcg q 6 h). First trimester pregnancy failure: 800 mcg intravaginally, repeat on day 3 if expulsion incomplete. [Generic/Trade: Oral tabs 100, 200 mcg.] ▶LK ♀X ▶– $$$$

PROPANTHELINE (*Pro-Banthine*) 7.5 to 15 mg PO 30 min after meals and 30 mg at bedtime. [Generic only: Tabs 15 mg.] ▶LK ♀C ▶– $$$

SIMETHICONE (*Mylicon, Gas-X, Phazyme, ✦ Ovol*) 40 to 360 mg PO four times per day prn, max 500 mg/day. Infants: 20 mg PO four times per day prn. [OTC Generic/Trade: Chewable tabs 80, 125 mg. Gtts 40 mg/0.6 mL. Trade only: Softgels 166 mg (Gas-X) 180 mg (Phazyme). Strips, oral (Gas-X) 62.5 mg (adults), 40 mg (children).] ▶Not absorbed ♀C but + ▶? $

SUCRALFATE (*Carafate, ✦ Sulcrate*) 1 g PO 1 h before meals (2 h before other medications) and at bedtime. [Generic/Trade: Tabs 1 g. Susp 1 g/10 mL.] ▶Not absorbed ♀B ▶? $$

Laxatives—Bulk-Forming

METHYLCELLULOSE (*Citrucel*) 1 heaping tablespoon in 8 oz water or 2 caplets PO daily (up to three times per day). [OTC Trade only: Regular and sugar-free packets and multiple-use canisters, Clear-mix soln, Caplets 500 mg.] ▶Not absorbed ♀+ ▶? $

POLYCARBOPHIL (*FiberCon, Konsyl Fiber, Equalactin*) Laxative: 2 tabs (1250 mg) PO four times per day prn. Diarrhea: 2 tabs (1250 mg) PO q 30 min. Max daily dose 6 g. [OTC Generic/Trade: Tabs/Caps 625 mg. OTC Trade only: Chewable tabs 625 mg (Equalactin).] ▶Not absorbed ♀+ ▶? $

PSYLLIUM (*Metamucil, Fiberall, Konsyl, Hydrocil*) 1 teaspoon in liquid, 1 packet in liquid, or 1 to 2 wafers with liquid PO daily (up to three times per day). [OTC Generic/Trade: Regular and sugar-free powder, Granules, Caps, Wafers, including various flavors and various amounts of psyllium.] ▶Not absorbed ♀+ ▶? $

Laxatives—Osmotic

GLYCERIN (*Fleet*) 1 adult or infant supp or 5 mL to 15 mL as an enema PR prn. [OTC Generic/Trade: Supp infant and adult, Soln (Fleet Babylax) 4 mL/applicator.] ▶Not absorbed ♀C ▶? $

LACTULOSE (*Enulose, Kristalose*) Constipation: 15 to 30 mL (syrup) or 10 to 20 g (powder for oral soln) PO daily. Hepatic encephalopathy: 30 to 45 mL

(cont.)

(syrup) PO three to four times per day, or 300 mL retention enema. [Generic/Trade: Syrup 10 g/15 mL. Trade only (Kristalose): 10, 20 g packets for oral soln.] ▶Not absorbed ♀B ▶? $$

MAGNESIUM CITRATE   150 to 300 mL PO once or in divided doses. 2 to 4 mL/kg/day once or in divided doses for age younger than 6 yo. [OTC Generic only: Soln 300 mL/bottle. Low-sodium and sugar-free available.] ▶K ♀B ▶? $

MAGNESIUM HYDROXIDE   (*Milk of Magnesia*) Laxative: 30 to 60 mL regular-strength (400 mg per 5 mL) liquid PO. Antacid: 5 to 15 mL regular-strength liquid or 622 to 1244 mg PO four times per day prn. [OTC Generic/Trade: Susp 400 mg/5 mL. Trade only: Chewable tabs 311, 400 mg. Generic only: Susp 800 mg/5 mL, (concentrated) 1200 mg/5 mL, sugar-free 400 mg/5 mL.] ▶K ♀+ ▶? $

POLYETHYLENE GLYCOL   (*MiraLax, GlycoLax*) 17 g (1 heaping tablespoon) in 4 to 8 oz water, juice, soda, coffee, or tea PO daily. [OTC Generic/Trade: Powder for oral soln 17 g/scoop. Rx Generic/Trade: Powder for oral soln 17 g/scoop.] ▶Not absorbed ♀C ▶? $

POLYETHYLENE GLYCOL WITH ELECTROLYTES   (*GoLytely, Colyte, Suclear, Suprep, TriLyte, NuLytely, Moviprep, HalfLytely, Bisacodyl Tablet Kit, ♣ Klean-Prep, Electropeg, Peg-Lyte*) Bowel prep: 240 mL q 10 min PO or 20 to 30 mL/min per NG until 4 L are consumed. Moviprep, Suclear, Suprep: Follow specific instructions. [Generic/Trade: Powder for oral soln in disposable jug 4 L or 2 L (Moviprep). Also, as a kit of 2 L bottle of polyethylene glycol with electrolytes and 2 or 4 bisacodyl tabs 5 mg (HalfLytely and Bisacodyl Tablet Kit). Trade only GoLytely: Packet for oral soln to make 3.785 L. Suclear: Dose 1 (16 oz) and Dose 2 (2 L bottle) for reconstitution. Suprep: Two 6 oz bottles.] ▶Not absorbed ♀C ▶? $

PREPOPIK   (*sodium picosulfate, magnesiu oxide, citric acid*) Preferred method: 1 packet (diluted in 5 oz of water) evening before the colonoscopy and 2nd packet (diluted in 5 oz of water) morning prior to colonoscopy. Alternatively, 1st dose during afternoon or early evening before the colonoscopy and 2nd dose 6 h later in evening before colonoscopy. Additional clear liquids should be consumed. [Trade: 2 packets of 16 g powder for reconstitution.] ▶minimal absorption − ♀B ▶? $

SODIUM PHOSPHATE   (*Fleet enema, Fleet Phospho-Soda, Fleet EZ-Prep, Accu-Prep, Osmoprep, Visicol, ♣ Enemol, Phoslax*) Constipation: 1 adult or pediatric enema PR or 20 to 30 mL of oral soln PO prn (max 45 mL/24 h). Prep prior to colonoscopy: Visicol: Evening before colonoscopy: 3 tabs with 8 oz clear liquid q 15 min until 20 tabs are consumed. Day of colonoscopy: Starting 3 to 5 h before procedure, 3 tabs with 8 oz clear liquid q 15 min until 20 tabs are consumed. Osmoprep: 32 tabs PO with total of 2 quarts clear liquids as follows: Evening before procedure: 4 tabs PO with 8 oz of clear liquids q 15 min for a total of 20 tabs; day of procedure: 3 to 5 h before procedure, 4 tabs with 8 oz of clear liquids q 15 min for a total of 12 tabs. [OTC Generic/Trade: Adult enema, oral soln. OTC Trade only: Pediatric enema, bowel prep. Rx Trade only: Visicol, Osmoprep tab ($$$$) 1.5 g.] ▶Not absorbed ♀C ▶? $ ■

SORBITOL   30 to 150 mL (of 70% soln) PO or 120 mL (of 25 to 30% soln) PR as a single dose. Cathartic: 4.3 mL/kg PO. [Generic only: Soln 70%.] ▶Not absorbed ♀C ▶? $

SUPREP (sodium sulfate + potassium sulfate + magnesium sulfate) Evening before colonoscopy: Dilute 1 bottle to 16 oz with water and drink, then drink 32 oz water over next hour. Next morning, repeat both steps. Compete 1 h before colonoscopy. [Trade: Two 6 oz bottles for dilution.] ▶not absorbed ♀C ▶? $

Laxatives—Stimulant

BISACODYL (*Correctol, Dulcolax, Feen-a-Mint, Fleet*) 5 to 15 mg PO prn, 10 mg PR prn if 2 to 11 yo. [OTC Generic/Trade: Tabs 5 mg, supp 10 mg. OTC Trade only: Enema, 10 mg/30 mL.] ▶L ♀C ▶? $

CASCARA 325 mg PO at bedtime prn or 5 mL of aromatic fluid extract PO at bedtime prn. [OTC Generic only: Tabs 325 mg, liquid aromatic fluid extract.] ▶L ♀C ▶+ $

CASTOR OIL Children: 5 to 15 mL/dose of castor oil PO or 7.5 to 30 mL emulsified castor oil PO once a day. Adult: 15 to 60 mL of castor oil or 30 to 60 mL emulsified castor oil PO once a day. [OTC Generic only: Oil 60, 120, 180, 480 mL.] ▶Not absorbed ♀– ▶? $

SENNA (*Senokot, SenokotXTRA, Ex-Lax, Fletcher's Castoria*) 2 tabs or 1 teaspoon granules or 10 to 15 mL syrup PO. Max 8 tabs, 4 teaspoon granules, 30 mL syrup/day. Take granules with full glass of water. [OTC Generic/Trade (All dosing is based on sennosides content; 1 mg sennosides is equivalent to 21.7 mg standardized senna concentrate): Syrup 8.8 mg/5 mL, Liquid 33.3 mg senna concentrate/mL (Fletcher's Castoria), Tabs 8.6, 15, 17, 25 mg, Chewable tabs 10, 15 mg.] ▶L ♀C ▶+ $

Laxatives—Stool Softener

DOCUSATE (*Colace, Docu-Soft, DOK, Dulcolax, Docu-Liquid, Enemeez, Fleet Sof-Lax, Octycine, Silace*) Constipation: Docusate calcium: 240 mg PO daily. Docusate sodium: 50 to 500 mg/day PO divided in 1 to 4 doses. Peds: 10 to 40 mg/day for age younger than 3 yo, give 20 to 60 mg/day for age 3 to 6 yo, give 40 to 150 mg/day for age 6 to 12 yo. In all cases doses are divided up to four times per day. Cerumen impaction: 1 mL in affected ear. [Docusate calcium OTC Generic/Trade: Caps 240 mg. Docusate sodium OTC Generic/Trade: Caps 50, 100, 250 mg. Liquid 50 mg/5 mL. Syrup 20 mg/5 mL. Docusate sodium OTC Trade only (Enemeez): Enema, rectal 283 mg/5 mL.] ▶L ♀C ▶? $

Laxatives—Other or Combinations

LUBIPROSTONE (*Amitiza*) Chronic idiopathic constipation: 24 mcg PO two times per day with food and water. Irritable bowel syndrome with constipation in women age 18 yo or older: 8 mcg PO two times per day. Opioid-induced constipation in adults with chronic, non-cancer pain: 24 mcg PO two times per day with food and water. [Trade only: Caps 8, 24 mcg.] ▶Gut ♀C ▶? $$$$$

MINERAL OIL (*Kondremul, Fleet Mineral Oil Enema, Liqui-Doss, ✦ Lansoyl*) 15 to 45 mL PO. Peds: 5 to 15 mL/dose PO. Mineral oil enema: 60 to 150 mL PR. Peds: 30 to 60 mL PR. [OTC Generic/Trade: Oil (30, 480 mL), Enema (Fleet). OTC only: Oral liquid (Liqui-Doss) 13.5 mg/15 mL. Oral microemulsion (Kondremul) 2.5 mg/5 mL.] ▶Not absorbed ♀C ▶? $

PERI-COLACE (*docusate + sennosides*) 2 to 4 tabs PO once daily or in divided doses prn. [OTC Generic/Trade: Tabs 50 mg docusate + 8.6 mg sennosides.] ▶L ♀C ▶? $

SENOKOT-S (*senna + docusate*) 2 tabs PO daily. [OTC Generic/Trade: Tabs 8.6 mg senna concentrate + 50 mg docusate.] ▶L ♀C ▶+ $

Ulcerative Colitis

BALSALAZIDE (*Colazal, Giazo*) Active mild to moderate ulcerative colitis: 2.25 g PO three times per day (Colazal) for 8 to 12 weeks or 1.1 g PO twice per day (Giazo) for 8 weeks. [Generic/Trade (Colazal): Caps 750 mg. Trade (Giazo): Tabs 1.1 g.] ▶Minimal absorption ♀B ▶? $$$$$

MESALAMINE (*5-aminosalicylic acid, Apriso, 5-Aspirin, Asacol, Lialda, Pentasa, Canasa, Rowasa, Delzicol, ✦ Mesasal, Mezavant, Salofalk*) Apriso: 1.5 g (4 caps) PO q am. Asacol: 800 to 1600 mg PO three times per day. Delzicol: 800 mg PO three times a day (treatment) or 800 mg PO twice a day (maintenance). Pentasa: 1000 mg PO four times per day. Lialda: 2.4 to 4.8 g PO daily with a meal. Canasa: 500 mg PR two to three times per day or 1000 mg PR at bedtime. Susp: 4 g enema PR at bedtime (retain 8 h) for 3 to 6 weeks. [Trade only: Delayed-release tabs 400 mg (Asacol), 800 mg (Asacol HD). Delayed-release caps (Delizol) 400 mg. Controlled-release caps 250, 500 mg (Pentasa). Delayed-release tabs 1200 mg (Lialda). Rectal supp 1000 mg (Canasa). Controlled-release caps 0.375 g (Apriso). Generic/Trade: Rectal susp 4 g/60 mL (Rowasa).] ▶Gut ♀C ▶? $$$$$

OLSALAZINE (*Dipentum*) Ulcerative colitis: 500 mg PO two times per day with food. [Trade only: Caps 250 mg.] ▶L ♀C ▶– $$$$$

SULFASALAZINE (*Azulfidine, Azulfidine EN-tabs, ✦ Salazopyrin En-tabs*) Ulcerative colitis: 500 to 1000 mg PO four times per day. Peds: 30 to 60 mg/kg/day PO divided q 4 to 6 h. RA: 500 mg PO two times per day after meals up to 1 g PO two times per day. May turn body fluids, contact lenses, or skin orange-yellow. [Generic/Trade: Tabs 500 mg, scored. Enteric-coated, delayed-release (EN-tabs) 500 mg.] ▶L ♀D ▶? $$

Other GI Agents

ALOSETRON (*Lotronex*) Prescribers must be certified to prescribe. Diarrhea-predominant irritable bowel syndrome in women who have failed conventional therapy: 0.5 mg PO two times per day for 4 weeks; discontinue in patients who become constipated. If well tolerated and symptoms not controlled after 4 weeks, may increase to 1 mg PO two times per day. Discontinue if symptoms not controlled in 4 weeks on 1 mg PO two times per day. [Trade only: Tabs 0.5, 1 mg.] ▶L ♀B ▶? $$$$$ ■

ALPHA-GALACTOSIDASE (*Beano*) 5 gtts or 1 tab per ½ cup gassy food, 2 to 3 tabs PO (chew, swallow, crumble) or 1 melt-away tab or 10 gtts per typical meal. [OTC Trade only: Oral gtts, tabs, melt-away tabs.] ▶Minimal absorption ♀? ▶? $

ALVIMOPAN (*Entereg*) Short-term (up to 15 doses) in hospitalized patients undergoing partial large or small bowel resection surgery with primary anastomosis; 12 mg PO 30 min to 5 h prior to surgery, then 12 mg PO two times per day starting the day after surgery for up to 7 days. [Trade only: Caps 12 mg.] ▶Intestinal flora ♀B ▶? ?

BUDESONIDE (*Entocort EC, Uceris*) 9 mg PO daily for up to 8 weeks (remission induction), Crohn's, ulcerative colitis or 6 mg PO daily for 3 months (maintenance, Entocort only). [Generic/Trade: Caps 3 mg Trade only: Extended-release Tabs (Uceris for ulcerative colitis only) 9 mg.] ▶L ♀C ▶? $$$$$

CERTOLIZUMAB (*Cimzia*) Crohn's: 400 mg SC at 0, 2, and 4 weeks. If response occurs, then 400 mg SC q 4 weeks. Rheumatoid arthritis: 400 mg SC at 0, 2, and 4 weeks. [Trade only: 400 mg kit (two 200 mg/mL pre-filled syringes). 1200 mg Starter Kit (six 200 mg/mL pre-filled syringes)] ▶Plasma, K ♀B ▶? $$$$$

CHLORDIAZEPOXIDE—CLIDINIUM (✚*Librax*)1 cap PO three to four times per day. [Generic: Caps, chlordiazepoxide 5 mg + clidinium 2.5 mg.] ▶K ♀D ▶– $$$

CROFELEMER (*Fulyzaq*) Non infectious AIDS diarrhea: 125 mg PO twice daily. [Trade: Delayed-release tabs 125 mg.] ▶Na – ♀C ▶? $$$$$

GLYCOPYRROLATE (*Robinul, Robinul Forte, Cuvposa*) Peptic ulcer disease: 1 to 2 mg PO two to three times per day. Chronic drooling in children (Cuvposa): 0.02 mg/kg PO three times per day. [Trade: Solution 1 mg/5 mL (480 mL, Cuvposa). Generic/Trade: Tabs 1, 2 mg.] ▶K ♀B ▶? $$$$

LACTASE (*Lactaid*) Swallow or chew 3 caplets (Original-strength), 2 tabs/caplets (Extra-strength), 1 caplet (Ultra) with first bite of dairy foods. Adjust dose based on response. [OTC Generic/Trade: Caplets, Chewable tabs.] ▶Not absorbed ♀+ ▶+ $

LINACLOTIDE (*Linzess*) IBS: 290 mcg PO daily. Chronic idiopathic constipation: 145 mcg PO once daily. Contraindicated in children 6 yo or younger. [Trade: Cap 145, 290 mcg.] ▶gut – ♀C ▶? $$$$$ ■

LORCASERIN (*Belviq*) Obesity or overweight with comorbidities: 10 mg PO once daily. [Trade: Tab 10 mg.] ▶L – ♀X ▶– $$$

METHYLNALTREXONE (*Relistor*) Opioid-induced constipation: Less than 38 kg: 0.15 mg/kg SC every other day; 38 kg to 61 kg: 8 mg SC every other day; 62 kg to 114 kg: 12 mg SC every other day; 115 kg or greater: 0.15 mg/kg SC every other day. [Injectable soln 12 mg/0.6 mL.] ▶unchanged ♀B ▶? $$$$$

NEOMYCIN—ORAL (*Neo-Fradin*) Hepatic encephalopathy: 4 to 12 g/day PO divided q 4 to 6 h. Peds: 50 to 100 mg/kg/day PO divided q 6 to 8 h. [Generic only: Tabs 500 mg. Trade only: Soln 125 mg/5 mL.] ▶Minimally absorbed ♀D ▶? $$$

OCTREOTIDE (*Sandostatin, Sandostatin LAR*) Variceal bleeding: Bolus 25 to 50 mcg IV followed by infusion 25 to 50 mcg/h. AIDS diarrhea: 25 to 250 mcg SC three times per day. [Generic/Trade: Injection vials 0.05, 0.1, 0.2, 0.5, 1 mg. Trade only: Long-acting injectable susp (Sandostatin LAR) 10, 20, 30 mg.] ▶LK ♀B ▶? $$$$$

ORLISTAT (*Alli, Xenical*) Weight loss: 60 to 120 mg PO three times per day with meals. [OTC Trade only (Alli): Caps 60 mg. Rx Trade only (Xenical): Caps 120 mg.] ▶Gut ♀X ▶? $$$

PANCREATIN (*Creon, Ku-Zyme,* ✦ *Entozyme*) 8000 to 24,000 units lipase (1 to 2 tabs/caps) PO with meals and snacks. [Tabs, Caps with varying amounts of lipase, amylase, and protease.] ▶Gut ♀C ▶? $$$

PANCRELIPASE (*Creon, Pancreaze, Viokase, Pancrease, Pancrecarb, Cotazym, Ku-Zyme HP, Ultresa, Viokace, Zenpep*) Varies by wt. Initial infant dose 2000 to 4000 lipase units PO per 120 mL formula or breast milk. 12 mo or older to younger than 4 yo: 1000 lipase units/kg PO. 4 yo or older: 500 lipase units/kg per meal PO, max 2500 lipase units/kg per meal. [Tabs, Caps, Powder with varying amounts of lipase, amylase, and protease.] ▶Gut ♀C ▶? $$$

✦ **PINAVERIUM** (*Dicetel*) 50 to 100 mg PO three times per day. [Trade only: tabs 50, 100 mg.] ▶? ♀C ▶− $$$

QSYMIA (**phentermine and topiramate**) Obesity or overweight with comorbidities: 3.75 mg/23 mg PO once daily for 14 days, then increase to 7.5 mg/46 mg PO once daily. Max dose 15 mg/92 mg PO daily. [Trade: Tab 3.75/23, 7.5/46, 11.25/69, 15/92 mg (phentermine/topiramate).] ▶KL − ♀X ▶−⊙IV $$$$ ■

RECTIV (**nitroglycerin**) Painful chronic anal fissures: Apply 1 inch intra-anally q 12 h for up to 3 weeks. [Ointment 0.4% 30 g.] ▶L − ♀C ▶? $$$$$

SECRETIN (*SecreFlo, ChiRhoStim*) Test dose 0.2 mcg IV. If tolerated, 0.2 to 0.4 mcg/kg IV over 1 min. ▶Serum ♀C ▶? $$$$$

TEDUGLUTIDE (*Gattex*) Short bowel syndrome patients receiving IV TPN: 0.05 mg/kg (max 3.8 mg) SC daily. [Trade only: 5 mg/vial, powder for reconstitution.] ▶endogenous − ♀B ▶? $$$$$

URSODIOL (*Actigall, URSO, URSO Forte*) Gallstone solution (Actigall): 8 to 10 mg/kg/day PO divided two to three times per day. Prevention of gallstones associated with rapid wt loss (Actigall): 300 mg PO two times per day. Primary biliary cirrhosis (URSO): 13 to 15 mg/kg/day PO divided in 2 to 4 doses. [Generic/Trade: Caps 300 mg, Tabs 250, 500 mg.] ▶Bile ♀B ▶? $$$$

HEMATOLOGY

Anticoagulants—Direct Thrombin Inhibitors

NOTE: *See Cardiovascular section for antiplatelet drugs and thrombolytics.*

ARGATROBAN HIT: Start 2 mcg/kg/min IV infusion. Get PTT at baseline and 2 h after starting infusion. Adjust dose (max dose: 10 mcg/kg/min) until PTT is 1.5 to 3 times baseline (not more than 100 sec). ACCP recommends starting at max of 2 mcg/kg/min with lower doses of 0.5 to 1.2 mcg/kg/min in patients with heart failure, multi-organ failure, anasarca, or post-cardiac surgery. ▶L ♀B ▶− $$$$$

BIVALIRUDIN (*Angiomax*) Anticoagulation during PCI (patients with or at risk of HIT): 0.75 mg/kg IV bolus prior to intervention, then 1.75 mg/kg/h for duration of procedure (with provisional GPIIb/IIIa inhibition). For CrCl less

(cont.)

than 30 mL/min, reduce infusion dose to 1 mg/kg/h after bolus. For patients on dialysis, reduce infusion to 0.25 mg/kg/h after bolus. Use with aspirin 300 to 325 mg PO daily. Additional bolus of 0.3 mg/kg if activated clotting time is less than 225 sec. ▶proteolysis/K ♀B ▶? $$$$$ ■

DABIGATRAN (*Pradaxa*) Stroke prevention in atrial fibrillation: CrCl greater than 30 mL/min: 150 mg PO two times per day; CrCl between 15 and 30 mL/min: 75 mg PO two times per day; CrCl less than 15 mL/min: contraindicated. Per ACCP CHEST guidelines, not recommended if CrCl < 30 mL/min. [Trade only: Caps 75, 150 mg.] ▶K ♀C ▶? $$$$$ ■

DESIRUDIN (*Iprivask*) DVT prophylaxis (hip replacement surgery): 15 mg SC q 12 h. (If CrCl is 31 to 60 mL/min, give 5 mg SC q 12 h; if CrCl < 31 mL/min, give 1.7 mg SC q 12 h.) ▶K ♀C ▶? $$$$$ ■

Anticoagulants—Factor Xa Inhibitors

APIXABAN (*Eliquis*) Nonvalvular atrial fibrillation: 5 mg PO two times per day. If at least two of the following characteristics: Age 80 y or older, wt 60 kg or less, serum creatnine 1.5 mg/dL or greater, then decrease dose to 2.5 mg PO two times daily. [Trade only: Tabs 2.5, 5 mg.] ♀B ▶? $$$$$ ■

FONDAPARINUX (*Arixtra*) DVT prophylaxis, hip/knee replacement or hip fracture surgery, abdominal surgery: 2.5 mg SC daily starting 6 to 8 h postop. DVT/PE treatment based on Wt: wt less than 50 kg: 5 mg SC daily; wt between 50 and 100 kg: 7.5 mg SC daily; wt greater than 100 kg: 10 mg SC daily for at least 5 days and therapeutic oral anticoagulation. [Generic/Trade: Prefilled syringes 2.5 mg/0.5 mL, 5 mg/0.4 mL, 7.5 mg/0.6 mL, 10 mg/0.8 mL.] ▶K ♀B ▶? $$$$$ ■

RIVAROXABAN (*Xarelto*) DVT prophylaxis in knee or hip replacement: 10 mg PO daily, if CrCl < 30 mL/min avoid use. Nonvalvular atrial fibrillation: 20 mg PO daily if CrCl > 50 mL/min; reduce dose to 15 mg PO daily if CrCl is 15 to 50 mL/min, avoid use if CrCl < 15 mL/min. DVT/PE treatment and to reduce risk of DVT/PE recurrence: 15 mg PO two times daily with food for 21 days, then 20 mg PO daily with food. If CrCl is 30 to 49 mL/min: 15 mg PO twice daily with food for 3 weeks, then 15 mg PO daily with food. [Trade only: Tabs 10, 15, 20 mg.] ▶K – ♀C ▶? $$$$$ ■

Anticoagulants—Low Molecular Weight Heparins (LWMH)

DALTEPARIN (*Fragmin*) DVT prophylaxis, acute medical illness with restricted mobility: 5000 units SC daily. DVT prophylaxis, abdominal surgery: 2500 units SC 1 to 2 h preop and daily postop. DVT prophylaxis, abdominal surgery in patients with malignancy: 5000 units SC evening before surgery and daily postop, or 2500 units 1 to 2 h preop and 12 h later, then 5000 units daily. DVT prophylaxis, hip replacement: Preop start (day of surgery): 2500 units SC given 2 h preop, 4 to 8 h postop, then 5000 units daily starting at least 6 h after 2nd dose, or 5000 units 10 to 14 h preop, 4 to 8 h postop, then daily (approximately 24 h between doses). Preop start (evening before

(cont.)

surgery): 5000 units SC given evening before surgery then 5000 units daily starting at least 4 to 8 h postop (approximately 24 h between doses). Postop start: 2500 units 4 to 8 h postop, then 5000 units daily starting at least 6 h after 1st dose. Treatment of DVT/PE in cancer: 200 units/kg SC daily for 1 month, then 150 units/kg SC daily for 5 months; max 18,000 units/day. Unstable angina or non-Q-wave MI: 120 units/kg up to 10,000 units SC q 12 h with aspirin (75 to 165 mg/day PO) until clinically stable. [Trade only: Single-dose syringes 2500, 5000 units/0.2 mL, 7500 units/0.3 mL, 10,000 units/1 mL, 12,500 units/0.5 mL, 15,000 units/0.6 mL, 18,000 units/0.72 mL; multidose vial 10,000 units/mL, 9.5 mL and 25,000 units/mL, 3.8 mL.] ▶KL ♀B ▶+ $$$$$ ■

ENOXAPARIN (*Lovenox*) See table. [Generic/Trade: Syringes 30, 40 mg; graduated syringes 60, 80, 100, 120, 150 mg. Concentration is 100 mg/mL except for 120, 150 mg, which are 150 mg/mL. All strengths also available preservative free. Trade only: Multidose vial 300 mg.] ▶KL ♀B ▶+ $$$$$ ■

Enoxaparin Adult Dosing

Indication	Dose	Dosing in Renal Impairment (CrCl less than 30 mL/min)*
DVT prophylaxis		
Abdominal surgery	40 mg SC once daily	30 mg SC once daily
Knee replacement	30 mg SC q 12 h	30 mg SC once daily
Hip replacement	30 mg SC q 12 h or 40 mg SC once daily	30 mg SC once daily
Medical patients	40 mg SC once daily	30 mg SC once daily
Acute DVT		
Inpatient treatment with or without PE	1 mg/kg SC q 12 h or 1.5 mg/kg SC once daily	1 mg/kg once daily
Outpatient treatment without PE	1 mg/kg SC q 12 h	1 mg/kg once daily
Acute coronary syndrome		
Unstable angina and non-Q-wave MI with aspirin	1 mg/kg SC q 12 h with aspirin	1 mg/kg once daily
Acute STEMI in patients younger than 75 yo with aspirin†	30 mg IV bolus with 1 mg/kg SC dose, then 1 mg/kg SC q 12 h (max 100 mg/dose for the 1 two doses)	30 mg IV bolus with 1 mg/kg SC dose, then 1 mg/kg SC once daily
Acute STEMI in patients 75 yo or older with aspirin†	No IV bolus, 0.75 mg/kg SC q 12 h (max 75 mg/dose for the 1 two doses)	No IV bolus, 1 mg/kg SC once daily

DVT=Deep vein thrombosis, PE=pulmonary embolism.

*Not FDA-approved in dialysis.

†If used with thrombolytics, SC dose should be started between 15 min before and 30 min after thrombolytic dose.

Anticoagulants—Other

HEPARIN Venous thrombosis/pulmonary embolus treatment: Load 80 units/kg IV, then initiate infusion at 18 units/kg/h. Adjust based on coagulation testing (PTT)—see table. DVT prophylaxis: 5000 units SC q 8 to 12 h. Acute coronary syndromes with or without PCI: 60 units/kg IV, then 12 units/kg/h infusion, adjust according to aPTT or antiXa. See table. Peds: Load 50 units/kg IV, then infuse 25 units/kg/h. [Generic only: 1000, 5000, 10,000, 20,000 units/mL in various vial and syringe sizes.] ▶Reticuloendothelial system ♀C but + ▶+ $$ ■

WARFARIN (*Coumadin, Jantoven*) Individualize dosing. Start 2 to 5 mg PO daily for 1 to 2 days, then adjust dose to maintain therapeutic INR. For healthy outpatients, 2012 ACCP CHEST guidelines recommend starting at 10 mg PO daily for 2 days, then adjust dose to maintain therapeutic INR. See product information if CYP2C9 or VKOR1C genotypes are known. [Generic/Trade: Tabs 1, 2, 2.5, 3, 4, 5, 6, 7.5, 10 mg.] ▶L ♀X, (D for mechanical heart valve replacement) ▶+ $ ■

HEPARIN DOSING FOR ACUTE CORONARY SYNDROME (ACS)

ST elevation myocardial infarction (STEMI)	Adjunct to thrombolytics: For use with alteplase, reteplase, or tenecteplase: Bolus 60 units/kg IV load (max 4000 units), then initial infusion 12 units/kg/h (max 1000 units/h) adjusted to achieve goal PTT 1.5 to 2 × control.
Unstable angina/Non-ST elevation myocardial infarction (UA/NSTEMI)	Initial treatment: Bolus 60 units/kg IV load (max 4000 units), then initiate infusion at 12 to 15 units/kg/h (max 1000 units) and adjust to achieve goal PTT 1.5 to 2.5 × control.
Percutaneous coronary intervention (PCI)	With prior anticoagulant therapy but *without* concurrent GPIIb/IIIa inhibitor planned: additional heparin as needed (2000 to 5000 units) to achieve target ACT 250–300 seconds for HemoTec or 300–350 seconds for Hemochron.
	With prior anticoagulant therapy and *with* planned concurrent GPIIb/IIIa inhibitor: additional heparin as needed (2000 to 5000 units) to achieve target 200–250 seconds.
	Without prior anticoagulant therapy and *without* concurrent GPIIb/IIIa inhibitor planned: Bolus 70–100 units/kg with target ACT 250–300 seconds for HemoTec or 300–350 seconds for Hemochron.
	Without prior anticoagulant therapy and *with* planned concurrent GPIIb/IIIa inhibitor: Bolus 50–70 units/kg with target ACT 200–250 seconds.

References: *J Am Coll Cardiol* 2011;57:1946. *Circulation* 2011;124:e608. *Circulation* 2004;110;e82-292. *J Am Coll Cardiol* 2009;54:2235.

WEIGHT-BASED HEPARIN DOSING FOR DVT/PE*

Initial dose	80 units/kg IV bolus, then 18 units/kg/h; check PTT in 6 h
PTT less than 35 sec (less than 1.2 × control)	80 units/kg IV bolus, then increase infusion rate by 4 units/kg/h
PTT 35–45 sec (1.2–1.5 × control)	40 units/kg IV bolus, then increase infusion by 2 units/kg/h
PTT 46–70 sec (1.5–2.3 × control)	No change
PTT 71–90 sec (2.3–3 × control)	Decrease infusion rate by 2 units/kg/h
PTT greater than 90 sec (greater than 3 × control)	Hold infusion for 1 h, then decrease infusion rate by 3 units/kg/h

*PTT = Activated partial thromboplastin time. Reagent-specific target PTT may differ; use institutional nomogram when available. Consider establishing a max bolus dose/max initial infusion rate or use an adjusted body wt in obesity. Monitor PTT 6 h after heparin initiation and 6 h after each dosage adjustment. When PTT is stable within therapeutic range, monitor every morning. Therapeutic PTT range corresponds to anti-factor Xa activity of 0.3–0.7 units/mL. Check platelets between days 3 and 5. Can begin warfarin on 1 day of heparin; continue heparin for at least 4 to 5 days of combined therapy. Adapted from *Ann Intern Med* 1993;119:874. *Chest* 2012;141:e28S, e154S. *Circulation* 2001;103:2994.

THERAPEUTIC GOALS FOR ANTICOAGULATION

INR Range*	Indication
2.0–3.0	Atrial fibrillation, deep venous thrombosis, pulmonary embolism, bioprosthetic heart valve (mitral position), mechanical prosthetic heart valve (aortic position)
2.5–3.5	Mechanical prosthetic heart valve (mitral position)

*Aim for an INR in the middle of the INR range (eg, 2.5 for range of 2 to 3 and 3.0 for range of 2.5 to 3.5). Adapted from: *Chest* 2012; 141:e422S, e425S, e533S, e578S; see these guidelines for additional information and other indications.

Colony-Stimulating Factors

DARBEPOETIN   (*Aranesp, NESP*) Anemia of chronic renal failure: 0.45 mcg/kg IV/SC once a week, or 0.75 mcg/kg q 2 weeks in some nondialysis patients. Cancer chemo anemia: 2.25 mcg/kg SC weekly, or 500 mcg SC q 3 weeks. Adjust dose based on Hb. [Trade only: All forms are available with or without albumin. Single-dose vials: 25, 40, 60, 100, 200, 300, 500 mcg/1 mL, and 150 mcg/0.75 mL. Single-dose prefilled syringes or autoinjectors: 25 mcg/0.42 mL, 40 mcg/0.4 mL, 60 mcg/0.3 mL, 100 mcg/0.5 mL, 150 mcg/0.3 mL, 200 mcg/0.4 mL, 300 mcg/0.6 mL, 500 mcg/1 mL.]   ▶cellular sialidases, L ♀C ▶? $$$$$ ■

EPOETIN ALFA   (*Epogen, Procrit*, erythropoietin alpha, *Eprex*) Anemia: 1 dose IV/SC 3 times a week. Initial dose if renal failure is 50 to 100 units/kg: Zidovudine-induced anemia is 100 units/kg, or chemo-associated anemia is 150 units/kg. Alternate for chemo-associated anemia: 40,000 units SC once a week. Adjust dose based on Hb. [Trade only: Single-dose 1-mL vials 2000, 3000, 4000, 10,000, 40,000 units/mL. Multidose vials 10,000 units/mL 2 mL, 20,000 units/mL 1 mL.]   ▶L ♀C ▶? $$$$$ ■

FILGRASTIM (**G-CSF, *Neupogen*)** Neutropenia: 5 mcg/kg SC/IV daily. Bone marrow transplant: 10 mcg/kg/day SC/IV infusion. [Trade only: Single-dose vials: 300 mcg/1 mL, 480 mcg/1.6 mL. Single-dose syringes: 300 mcg/0.5 mL, 480 mcg/0.8 mL.] ▶L ♀C ▶? $$$$$

OPRELVEKIN (***Neumega***) Chemotherapy-induced thrombocytopenia in adults: 50 mcg/kg SC daily. [Trade only: 5 mg single-dose vials with diluent.] ▶K ♀C ▶? $$$$$ ■

PEGFILGRASTIM (***Neulasta***) 6 mg SC once each chemo cycle. [Trade only: Single-dose syringes 6 mg/0.6 mL.] ▶Plasma ♀C ▶? $$$$$

SARGRAMOSTIM (**GM-CSF, *Leukine***) Specialized dosing for bone marrow transplant. ▶L ♀C ▶? $$$$$

Other Hematological Agents

AMINOCAPROIC ACID (***Amicar***) Hemostasis: 4 to 5 g PO/IV over 1 h, then 1 g/h prn. [Generic/Trade: Syrup 250 mg/mL, Tabs 500 mg. Trade only: Tabs 1000 mg.] ▶K ♀D ▶? $ IV $$$$$ Oral

ANAGRELIDE (***Agrylin***) Thrombocythemia due to myeloproliferative disorders: Start 0.5 mg PO four times per day or 1 mg PO two times per day, then after 1 week adjust to lowest effective dose. Max 10 mg/day. [Generic/Trade: Caps 0.5 mg. Generic only: Caps 1 mg.] ▶LK ♀C ▶? $$$$$

DEFERASIROX (***Exjade***) Chronic iron overload due to blood transfusions: 20 mg/kg PO daily; adjust dose q 3 to 6 months based on ferritin trends. Max 40 mg/kg/day. Chronic iron overload in non-transfusion-dependent thalassemia syndromes: 10mg/kg PO daily; adjust dose based on ferritin and liver iron concentration. Max 20 mg/kg/day. [Trade only: Tabs for dissolving into oral susp 125, 250, 500 mg.] ▶LK ♀C ▶? $$$$$ ■

HYDROXYUREA (***Hydrea, Droxia***) Sickle cell anemia (Droxia): Start 15 mg/kg PO daily while monitoring CBC q 2 weeks. If no marrow depression, then increase dose q 12 weeks by 5 mg/kg/day (max 35 mg/kg/day). Solid tumors (Hydrea): Intermittent therapy: 80 mg/kg PO for a single dose q 3 days. Continuous therapy: 20 to 30 mg/kg PO daily. Head and neck cancer with radiation (Hydrea): 80 mg/kg PO for a single dose q 3 days. Resistant chronic myelocytic leukemia: 20 to 30 mg/kg PO daily. Give concomitant folic acid. [Generic/Trade: Caps 500 mg. Trade only: (Droxia) Caps 200, 300, 400 mg.] ▶LK ♀D ▶– $ varies by therapy ■

PROTAMINE Reversal of heparin: Within 30 minutes of IV heparin: 1 mg antagonizes about 100 units heparin. If greater than 30 minutes since IV heparin: 0.5 mg antagonizes about 100 units heparin. Due to short half-life of heparin (60 to 90 min), use IV heparin doses only from last several hours to calculate dose of protamine. SC heparin may require prolonged administration of protamine. Reversal of low-molecular-weight heparin: If within 8 h of LMWH dose: Give 1 mg protamine per 100 anti-Xa units of dalteparin or 1 mg protamine per 1 mg enoxaparin. Smaller doses advised if more than 8 h since LMWH administration. Give IV (max 50 mg) over 10 min. May cause allergy/anaphylaxis. ▶Plasma ♀C ▶? $ ■

HERBAL & ALTERNATIVE THERAPIES

Herbal & Alternative Therapies

NOTE: *In the United States, herbal and alternative therapy products are regulated as dietary supplements, not drugs. Premarketing evaluation and FDA approval are not required unless specific therapeutic claims are made. Because these products are not required to demonstrate efficacy, it is unclear whether many of them have health benefits. In addition, there may be considerable variability in content from lot to lot or between products.*

ALOE VERA (**acemannan, burn plant**) Topical: Efficacy unclear for seborrheic dermatitis, psoriasis, genital herpes, skin burns. Do not apply to surgical incisions; impaired healing reported. Oral: Efficacy unclear for mild to moderate active ulcerative colitis, type 2 diabetes. OTC laxatives containing aloe latex were removed from US market due to possible increased risk of colon cancer. [Not by prescription.]   ▶LK ♀oral− topical+? ▶oral− topical+? $

ALPHA LIPOIC ACID (**lipoic acid**) Peripheral neuropathy: Usual dose is 600 mg daily [Not by prescription.]   ▶gut − ♀? ▶? $

ARTICHOKE LEAF EXTRACT (*Cynara scolymus*) May reduce total cholesterol, but clinical significance is unclear. Possibly effective for functional dyspepsia. [Not by prescription.]   ▶? ♀? ▶? $

ASTRAGALUS (*Astragalus membranaceus*, **huang qi, Jin Fu Kang, vetch**) Used in combination with other herbs in traditional Chinese medicine for CAD, CHF, chronic liver disease, kidney disease, viral infections, and upper respiratory tract infection. Possibly effective for improving survival and performance status with platinum-based chemotherapy for non-small-cell lung cancer. However, astragalus-based herbal formula (Jin Fu Kang) did not affect survival or pharmacokinetics of docetaxel in phase II study of patients with non-small-cell lung cancer. [Not by prescription.]   ▶? ♀? ▶? $

BUTTERBUR (*Petasites hybridus, Petadolex*) Migraine prophylaxis (effective): Petadolex 50 to 75 mg PO two times per day. Allergic rhinitis prophylaxis (possibly effective): Petadolex 50 mg PO two times per day. Efficacy unclear for asthma. [Not by prescription. Standardized pyrrolizidine-free extracts: Petadolex tabs 50, 75 mg.]   ▶? ♀− ▶− $$

CHAMOMILE (*Matricaria recutita*—**German** chamomile, *Anthemis nobilis*—**Roman** chamomile) Oral extract: Modest benefit in study for generalized anxiety disorder, but little to no benefit in study for primary chronic insomnia. Topical: Efficacy unclear for skin infections or inflammation. [Not by prescription.]   ▶? ♀− ▶? $

CHASTEBERRY (*Vitex agnus castus fruit extract, Femaprin*) Premenstrual syndrome (possibly effective): 20 mg PO daily of extract ZE 440. [Not by prescription.]   ▶? ♀− ▶− $

CHONDROITIN Does not appear effective for relief of OA pain overall. Chondroitin 400 mg PO three times per day + glucosamine may improve pain in subgroup of patients with moderate to severe knee OA. [Not by prescription.]   ▶K ♀? ▶? $

COENZYME Q10 (*CoQ-10*, **ubiquinone**) Heart failure: 100 mg/day PO divided two to three times per day (conflicting clinical trials; AHA does not recommend). Statin-induced myalgia: 100 to 200 mg PO daily (efficacy unclear; conflicting clinical trials). Parkinson's disease: 1200 mg/day PO divided four times per day ($$$$; efficacy unclear; might slow progression slightly, but the American Academy of Neurology does not recommend). Prevention of migraine (possibly effective): 100 mg PO three times per day. May be considered for migraine prevention per Am Academy Neurology and Am Headache Society. Efficacy unclear for hypertension and improving athletic performance. Appears ineffective for diabetes. [Not by prescription.] ▶Bile ♀– ▶– $

CRANBERRY (*Cranactin*, **Vaccinium macrocarpon**) Prevention of UTI (possibly effective): 300 mL/day PO cranberry juice cocktail. Usual dose of cranberry juice extract caps/tabs is 300 to 400 mg PO two times per day. Insufficient data to assess efficacy for treatment of UTI. Potential increase in INR with warfarin. [Not by prescription.] ▶? ♀+ in food, – in supplements ▶+ in food, – in supplements $

CREATINE Promoted to enhance athletic performance. No benefit for endurance exercise; modest benefit for intense anaerobic tasks lasting less than 30 sec. Usual loading dose of 20 g/day PO for 5 days, then 2 to 5 g/day divided two times per day. [Not by prescription.] ▶LK ♀– ▶– $

DEHYDROEPIANDROSTERONE (*DHEA*, *Aslera*, *Fidelin*, *Prasterone*) Does not improve cognition, quality of life, or sexual function in elderly. Not recommended as androgen replacement in late-onset male hypogonadism. To improve well being in women with adrenal insufficiency: 50 mg PO daily (possibly effective; conflicting clinical trials). [Not by prescription.] ▶Peripheral conversion to estrogens and androgens ♀– ▶– $

DEVIL'S CLAW (*Harpagophytum procumbens*, *Doloteffin*, *Harpadol*) OA, acute exacerbation of chronic low-back pain (possibly effective): 2400 mg extract/day (50 to 100 mg harpagoside/day) PO divided two to three times per day. [Not by prescription. Extracts standardized to harpagoside (iridoid glycoside) content.] ▶? ♀– ▶– $

ECHINACEA (*E. purpurea*, *E. angustifolia*, *E. pallida*, **cone flower**, *EchinaGuard*, *Echinacin Madaus*) Conflicting clinical trials for prevention or treatment of upper respiratory infections. Does not appear effective for treatment of common cold in adults. [Not by prescription.] ▶L ♀– ▶– $

ELDERBERRY (*Sambucus nigra*, *Rubini*, *Sambucol*, *Sinupret*) Efficacy unclear for influenza, sinusitis, and bronchitis. [Not by prescription.] ▶? ♀– ▶– $

FENUGREEK (*Trigonella foenum-graecum*) Efficacy unclear for diabetes or hyperlipidemia. [Not by prescription.] ▶? ♀– ▶? $$

FEVERFEW (*Chrysanthemum parthenium*, *MigraLief*, *Tanacetum parthenium L.*) Prevention of migraine (probably effective): 50 to 100 mg extract PO daily. May take 1 to 2 months to be effective. [Not by prescription.] ▶? ♀– ▶– $

FLAVOCOXID (*Limbrel*, *UP446*) OA (efficacy unclear): 250 to 500 mg PO two times per day. Hepatotoxicity reported. [Caps 250, 500 mg. Marketed as medical food by prescription only (not all medical foods require a prescription).] ▶L ♀– ▶– $$$

GARLIC SUPPLEMENTS (*Allium sativum, Kwai, Kyolic*) Ineffective for hyperlipidemia. Small reductions in BP, but efficacy in HTN unclear. Does not appear effective for diabetes. Significantly decreases saquinavir levels. May increase bleeding risk with warfarin with/without increase in INR. [Not by prescription.] ▶LK ♀− ▶− $

GINGER (*Zingiber officinale*) Acute chemotherapy-induced nausea (possibly effective adjunct to standard antiemetics): 250 to 500 mg PO two times per day for 6 days, starting 3 days before chemo. Possibly ineffective for prevention of motion sickness. Does not appear effective for postop N/V. American College of Obstetrics and Gynecology considers ginger 250 mg PO four times per day a nonpharmacologic option for N/V in pregnancy. Some experts advise pregnant women to limit dose to usual dietary amount (no more than 1 g/day). Some European countries advise pregnant women to avoid ginger supplements because it is cytotoxic in vitro. [Not by prescription.] ▶bile ♀? ▶? $

GINKGO BILOBA (*EGb 761, Ginkgold, Ginkoba*) Dementia (efficacy unclear): 40 mg PO three times per day of standardized extract containing 24% ginkgo flavone glycosides and 6% terpene lactones. The American Psychiatric Association and others find evidence too weak to recommend for Alzheimer's or other dementias. Does not prevent dementia in elderly or improve memory in people with normal cognitive function. Does not appear effective for intermittent claudication or prevention of acute altitude sickness. Possible risk of stroke. [Not by prescription.] ▶K ♀− ▶− $

GINSENG—AMERICAN (*Panax quinquefolius L., Cold-fX*) Reduction of postprandial glucose in type 2 diabetes (possibly effective): 3 g PO taken with or up to 2 h before meal. Cold-fX (1 cap PO two times per day) may modestly reduce the frequency of colds/flu; approved in Canada for adults and children 12 yo and older. [Not by prescription.] ▶K ♀− ▶− $

GINSENG—ASIAN (*Panax ginseng, Ginsana, G115, Korean red ginseng*) Promoted to improve vitality and well being: 200 mg PO daily. Ginsana: 2 caps PO daily or 1 cap PO two times per day. Preliminary evidence of efficacy for erectile dysfunction. Efficacy unclear for improving physical or psychomotor performance, diabetes, herpes simplex infections, cognitive, or immune function. American College of Obstetrics and Gynecologists and North American Menopause Society recommend against use for postmenopausal hot flashes. [Not by prescription.] ▶? ♀− ▶− $

GINSENG—SIBERIAN (*Eleutherococcus senticosus, Ci-wu-jia*) Does not appear effective for improving athletic endurance or chronic fatigue syndrome. May interfere with some digoxin assays. [Not by prescription.] ▶? ♀− ▶− $

GLUCOSAMINE (*Cosamin DS, Dona*) OA: Glucosamine HCl 500 mg PO three times per day or glucosamine sulfate (Dona $$) 1500 mg PO once daily. Appears ineffective overall for OA pain, but glucosamine plus chondroitin may improve pain in moderate to severe knee OA. [Not by prescription.] ▶LK ♀− ▶− $

GREEN TEA (*Camellia sinensis, Polyphenon E*) Efficacy unclear for cancer prevention, wt loss, hypercholesterolemia. Large doses might decrease

(cont.)

INR with warfarin due to vitamin K content. May contain caffeine. [Not by prescription. Green tea extract available in caps standardized to polyphenol content.] ▶LK ♀+ in moderate amount in food, – in supplements ▶+ in moderate amount in food, – in supplements $

HAWTHORN (*Crataegus laevigata, monogyna, oxyacantha, standardized extract WS 1442—Crataegutt novo, HeartCare*) Mild heart failure (possibly effective): 80 mg PO two times per day to 160 mg PO three times per day of standardized extract (19% oligomeric procyanidins; WS 1442; HeartCare 80 mg tabs). [Not by prescription.] ▶? ♀– ▶– $

HONEY (*Medihoney*) Topical for burn/wound (including diabetic foot, stasis leg ulcers, pressure ulcers, 1st- and 2nd-degree partial thickness burns): Apply Medihoney for 12 to 24 h/day. Oral for nocturnal cough due to upper respiratory tract infection in children (possibly effective): Give PO within 30 min before sleep. Dose is ½ tsp for 2 to 5 yo, 1 tsp for 6 to 11 yo, 2 tsp for 12 to 18 yo. Do not feed honey to children younger than 1 yo due to risk of infant botulism. [Mostly not by prescription. Medihoney is FDA approved.] ▶? ♀+ ▶+ $ for oral $$$ for Medihoney

HORSE CHESTNUT SEED EXTRACT (*Aesculus hippocastanum*, buckeye, *HCE50, Venastat*) Chronic venous insufficiency (effective): 1 cap Venastat (16% aescin standardized extract) PO two times per day with water before meals. American College of Cardiology found evidence insufficient to recommend for peripheral arterial disease. [Not by prescription.] ▶? ♀– ▶– $

LICORICE (*Cankermelt, Glycyrrhiza glabra, Glycyrrhiza uralensis*) Insufficient data to assess efficacy for postmenopausal vasomotor symptoms. Chronic high doses can cause pseudo-primary aldosteronism (with HTN, edema, hypokalemia). Cankermelt dissolving oral patch for aphthous ulcers (efficacy unclear): Apply patch to ulcer for 16 h/day until healed. [Not by prescription.] ▶Bile ♀– ▶– $

MELATONIN (*N-acetyl-5-methoxytryptamine*) To reduce jet lag after flights over more than 5 time zones (effective): 0.5 to 5 mg PO at bedtime for 3 to 6 nights starting on day of arrival. [Not by prescription.] ▶L ♀– ▶– $

MILK THISTLE (*Silybum marianum, Legalon*, silymarin, *Thisylin*) Hepatic cirrhosis (efficacy unclear): 100 to 200 mg PO three times per day of standardized extract with 70 to 80% silymarin. [Not by prescription.] ▶LK ♀– ▶– $

NONI (*Morinda citrifolia*) Promoted for many medical disorders; but insufficient data to assess efficacy. Potassium content comparable to orange juice; hyperkalemia reported in chronic renal failure. Case reports of hepatotoxicity. [Not by prescription.] ▶? ♀– ▶– $$$

PEPPERMINT OIL (*Mentha x piperita oil*) Irritable bowel syndrome (possibly effective): 0.2 to 0.4 mL enteric-coated caps PO three times per day. Peds, 8 yo or older: 0.1 to 0.2 mL enteric-coated caps PO three times per day. Take before meals. [Not by prescription.] ▶LK ♀+ in food, ? in supplements ▶+ in food, ? in supplements $

PROBIOTICS (*Acidophilus, Align, Bifantis, Bifidobacteria, Lactobacillus, Bacid, Culturelle, Florastor, Intestinex, Power-Dophilus, Primadophilus, Saccharomyces boulardii, VSL#3*) Prevention of antibiotic-associated

(cont.)

diarrhea (effective): Florastor (*Saccharomyces boulardii*) 2 caps PO two times per day for adults; 1 cap PO two times per day for peds. Culturelle (*Lactobacillus* GG) 1 cap PO once daily or two times per day for peds; give 2 h before/after antibiotic. IDSA recommends against probiotics to prevent *C. difficile*–associated diarrhea; safety and efficacy is unclear. Peds rotavirus gastroenteritis (effective): *Lactobacillus* GG at least 10 billion cells/day PO started early in illness. Ulcerative colitis or pouchitis: VSL#3 1 to 8 packets/day or 4 to 32 caps/day for adults; peds dose based on wt and number of bowel movements. Irritable bowel syndrome: VSL#3 either ½ to 1 packet PO daily or 2 to 4 caps PO daily to relieve gas/bloating. Align: 1 cap PO once daily to relieve abdominal pain/bloating. [Not by prescription. Culturelle contains *Lactobacillus* GG 10 billion cells/cap. Florastor contains *Saccharomyces boulardii* 5 billion cells/250 mg cap. VSL#3 (nonprescription medical food) contains 450 billion cells/packet, 225 billion cells/2 caps (*Bifidobacterium breve, longum, infantis; Lactobacillus acidophilus, plantarum, casei, bulgaricus; Streptococcus thermophilus*). Align contains *Bifidobacterium infantis* 35624, 1 billion cells/cap.] ▶? ♀+ ▶+ $

PYGEUM AFRICANUM (African plum tree) BPH (may have modest efficacy): 50 to 100 mg PO two times per day or 100 mg PO daily of standardized extract containing 14% triterpenes. [Not by prescription.] ▶? ♀– ▶– $

RED CLOVER (red clover isoflavone extract, *Trifolium pratense*, trefoil, *Promensil, Trinovin*) Postmenopausal vasomotor symptoms (conflicting evidence; does not appear effective overall, but may have modest benefit for severe symptoms): Promensil 1 tab PO daily to two times per day with meals. [Not by prescription. Isoflavone content (genistein, daidzein, biochanin, formononetin) is 40 mg/tab in Promensil and Trinovin.] ▶Gut, L, K ♀– ▶– $$

RED YEAST RICE (*Monascus purpureus, Xuezhikang, Zhibituo, Hypocol*) Hyperlipidemia: Usual dose is 1200 mg PO two times per day. Efficacy depends on whether formulation contains lovastatin or other statins. In the United States, red yeast rice should not contain more than trace amounts of statins, but some products contain up to 10 mg lovastatin per cap. Some clinicians consider red yeast rice an alternative for patients who develop myalgia with prescription statins. Can cause myopathy. Some formulations may contain citrinin, a potential nephrotoxin. [Not by prescription. Xuezhikang marketed in Asia, Norway (HypoCol).] ▶L ♀– ▶– $$

S-ADENOSYLMETHIONINE (*SAM-e*) Mild to moderate depression (effective): 800 to 1600 mg/day PO in divided doses with meals. Efficacy unclear for OA. [Not by prescription.] ▶L ♀? ▶? $$$

SAINT JOHN'S WORT (*Hypericum perforatum, Kira, LI-160*) Mild to moderate depression (effective): 300 mg PO three times per day of standardized extract (0.3% hypericin). Does not appear effective for ADHD. May decrease efficacy of other drugs (eg, ritonavir, oral contraceptives) by inducing liver metabolism. May cause serotonin syndrome with SSRIs, MAOIs. [Not by prescription.] ▶L ♀– ▶– $

SOY (*Genisoy, Healthy Woman, Novasoy, Phytosoya, Supro*) Soy protein or isoflavone supplements do not substantially reduce hyperlipidemia or

(cont.)

hypertension. Postmenopausal vasomotor symptoms (modest benefit): Per North Am Menopause Society, consider 50 mg/day or more of soy isoflavones for at least 12 weeks. Conflicting clinical trials for postmenopausal bone loss. [Not by prescription.] ▶Gut, L, K ♀+ for food, ? for supplements ▶+ for food, ? for supplements $

TEA TREE OIL (melaleuca oil, *Melaleuca alternifolia*) Not for oral use; CNS toxicity reported. Limited evidence for topical treatment of onychomycosis, tinea pedis, acne vulgaris, dandruff, pediculosis. [Not by prescription.] ▶? ♀− ▶− $

VALERIAN (*Valeriana officinalis, Alluna*) Insomnia (possibly modestly effective; conflicting clinical trials): 400 to 900 mg of standardized extract PO 30 min before bedtime. Alluna: 2 tabs PO 1 h before bedtime. [Not by prescription.] ▶? ♀− ▶− $

WILLOW BARK EXTRACT (*Salix alba, Salicis cortex*, salicin) OA, low-back pain (possibly effective): 60 to 240 mg/day salicin PO divided two to three times per day. [Not by prescription. Some products standardized to 15% salicin content.] ▶K ♀− ▶− $

IMMUNOLOGY

Immunizations

NOTE: *For vaccine info see CDC website (www.cdc.gov).*

BCG VACCINE (✦ *Oncotice, Immucyst*) 0.2 to 0.3 mL percutaneously. ▶Immune system ♀C ▶? $$$$ ■

COMVAX (*Haemophilus* B vaccine + hepatitis B vaccine) Infants born of HBsAg (negative) mothers: 0.5 mL IM for 3 doses, given at 2, 4, and 12 to 15 months. ▶Immune system ♀C ▶? $$$

DIPHTHERIA, TETANUS, AND ACELLULAR PERTUSSIS VACCINE (*DTaP, Tdap, Tripedia, Infanrix, Daptacel, Boostrix, Adacel, ✦ Tripacel*) 0.5 mL IM. Do not use Boostrix or Adacel for primary childhood vaccination series. ▶Immune system ♀C ▶− $$

DIPHTHERIA-TETANUS TOXOID (*Td, DT*) 0.5 mL IM. [Injection DT (pediatric: 6 weeks to 6 yo). Td (adult and children at least 7 yo).] ▶Immune system ♀C ▶? $

HAEMOPHILUS B VACCINE (*ActHIB, Hiberix, PedvaxHIB*) 0.5 mL IM. Dosing schedule varies depending on formulation used and age of child at 1st dose. ▶Immune system ♀C ▶? $$

HEPATITIS A VACCINE (*Havrix, Vaqta, ✦ Avaxim, Epaxal*) Adult formulation 1 mL IM, repeat in 6 to 12 months. Peds: 0.5 mL IM for age 1 yo or older, repeat 6 to 18 months later. [Single-dose vial (specify pediatric or adult).] ♀C ▶+ $$$

HEPATITIS B VACCINE (*Engerix-B, Recombivax HB*) Adults: 1 mL IM, repeat in 1 and 6 months later. Separate pediatric formulations and dosing. ♀C ▶+ $$$

HUMAN PAPILLOMAVIRUS RECOMBINANT VACCINE   (*Gardasil*) 0.5 mL IM at time 0, 2, and 6 months. ♀B ▶? $$$$$

INFLUENZA VACCINE—INACTIVATED INJECTION   (*Afluria, Fluarix, FluLaval, Fluzone, Fluvirin, ✦ Fluviral, Vaxigrip*) 0.5 mL IM or 0.1 mL intradermal (Fluzone Intradermal). FluLaval and Fluzone Intradermal not indicated for age younger than 18 yo, Fluvirin not indicated if age younger than 4 yo, Fluarix not indicated if age younger than 3 yo. ▶Immune system ♀C ▶+ $

INFLUENZA VACCINE—LIVE INTRANASAL   (*FluMist*) 1 dose (0.2 mL) intranasally. Use only if 2 to 49 yo. ▶Immune system ♀C ▶+ $

JAPANESE ENCEPHALITIS VACCINE   (*JE-Vax, ✦ Ixiaro*) 1 mL SC for 3 doses on days 0, 7, and 30. ♀C ▶? $$$$

MEASLES, MUMPS, & RUBELLA VACCINE   (*M-M-R II, ✦ Priorix*) 0.5 mL (1 vial) SC. ▶Immune system ♀C ▶+ $$$

MENINGOCOCCAL   VACCINE   (*Menomune-A/C/Y/W-135,   Menactra, ✦ Menjugate, Menveo*) 0.5 mL SC (Menomune) or IM (Menactra) at 11 to 12 yo. Repeat at 16 yo. ♀C ▶? $$$$

PEDIARIX   (diphtheria tetanus and acellular pertussis vaccine + hepatitis B vaccine + polio vaccine) 0.5 mL IM at 2, 4, 6 mo. ▶Immune system ♀C ▶? $$$

PLAGUE VACCINE   1 mL IM 1st dose, then 0.2 mL IM 1 to 3 months after the 1st injection, then 0.2 mL IM 5 to 6 months later for age 18 to 61 yo. ▶Immune system ♀C ▶+ $

PNEUMOCOCCAL 13-VALENT CONJUGATE VACCINE   (*Prevnar 13*) 0.5 mL IM for 3 doses at 2 mo, 4 mo, and 6 mo, followed by a 4th dose at 12 to 15 mo. ♀C ▶? $$$

PNEUMOCOCCAL 23-VALENT VACCINE   (*Pneumovax, ✦ Pneumo 23*) 0.5 mL IM or SC. ▶Immune system ♀C ▶+ $$

POLIO VACCINE   (*IPOL*) 0.5 mL IM or SC. ♀C ▶? $$

PROQUAD   (measles mumps & rubella vaccine + varicella vaccine, *MMRV*) 0.5 mL (1 vial) SC for age 12 mo to 12 yo. ▶Immune system ♀C ▶? $$$$

RABIES VACCINE   (*RabAvert, Imovax Rabies, BioRab, Rabies Vaccine Adsorbed*) 1 mL IM in deltoid region on days 0, 3, 7, 14, 28. ♀C ▶? $$$$$

ROTAVIRUS VACCINE   (*RotaTeq, Rotarix*) RotaTeq: First dose (2 mL PO) between 6 and 12 weeks of age, and then 2nd and 3rd doses at 4- to 10-week intervals thereafter (last dose no later than 32 weeks). Rotarix: First dose (1 mL) at 6 weeks of age, and 2nd dose (1 mL) at least 4 weeks later, and last dose prior to 24 weeks of age. [Trade only: Oral susp 2 mL (RotaTeq), 1 mL (Rotarix).] ▶? $$$$$

TETANUS TOXOID   0.5 mL IM or SC. ▶Immune system ♀C ▶+ $$

TRIHIBIT   (*Haemophilus* B vaccine + diphtheria tetanus and acellular pertussis vaccine) Use for 4th dose only, age 15 to 18 mo: 0.5 mL IM. ▶Immune system ♀C ▶– $$$

TWINRIX   (hepatitis A vaccine + hepatitis B vaccine) Adults: 1 mL IM in deltoid, repeat 1 and 6 months later. Accelerated dosing schedule: 0, 7, 21, and 30 days and booster dose at 12 months. ▶Immune system ♀C ▶? $$$$

TYPHOID VACCINE—INACTIVATED INJECTION (*Typhim Vi*, ✦ *Typherix*) 0.5 mL IM single dose. May revaccinate q 2 to 5 years if high risk. ▶Immune system ♀C ▶? $$

TYPHOID VACCINE—LIVE ORAL (*Vivotif Berna*) 1 cap every other day for 4 doses. May revaccinate q 2 to 5 years if high risk. [Trade only: Caps.] ▶Immune system ♀C ▶? $$

VARICELLA VACCINE (*Varivax*, ✦ *Varilrix*) Children 1 to 12 yo: 0.5 mL SC. Repeat dose at ages 4 to 6 yo. Age 13 yo or older: 0.5 mL SC, repeat 4 to 8 weeks later. ♀C ▶? $$$$

YELLOW FEVER VACCINE (*YF-Vax*) 0.5 mL SC. ♀C ▶+ $$$

ZOSTER VACCINE—LIVE (*Zostavax*) 0.65 mL SC single dose for age 50 yo or older. However, ACIP recommends immunizing those 60 yo and older. ▶Immune system ♀C ▶? $$$$

Immunoglobulins

ANTIVENIN—CROTALIDAE IMMUNE FAB OVINE POLYVALENT (*CroFab*) Rattlesnake envenomation: 4 to 6 vials IV infusion over 60 min, within 6 h of bite if possible. Administer 4 to 6 additional vials if no initial control of envenomation syndrome, then 2 vials q 6 h for up to 18 h (3 doses) after initial control has been established. ▶? ♀C ▶? $$$$$

BOTULISM IMMUNE GLOBULIN (*BabyBIG*) Infant botulism: Give 1 mL/kg (50 mg/kg) IV for age younger than 1 yo. ▶L ♀? ▶? $$$$$

HEPATITIS B IMMUNE GLOBULIN (*H-BIG, HyperHep B, HepaGam B, NABI-HB*) 0.06 mL/kg IM within 24 h of needlestick, ocular, or mucosal exposure to Hepatitis B, repeat in 1 month. ▶L ♀C ▶? $$$

IMMUNE GLOBULIN—INTRAMUSCULAR (*Baygam*, ✦ *Gamastan*) Hepatitis A prophylaxis: 0.02 to 0.06 mL/kg IM depending on length of travel to endemic area. Measles (within 6 days postexposure): 0.2 to 0.25 mL/kg IM. ▶L ♀C ▶? $$$$ ■

IMMUNE GLOBULIN—INTRAVENOUS (*Carimune, Flebogamma, Gammagard, Gammaplex, Gamunex, Octagam, Privigen*) IV dosage varies by indication and product. ▶L ♀C ▶? $$$$$ ■

IMMUNE GLOBULIN—SUBCUTANEOUS (*Vivaglobulin, Hizentra*) 100 to 200 mg/kg SC weekly. ▶L ♀C ▶? $$$$$ ■

LYMPHOCYTE IMMUNE GLOBULIN (*Atgam*) Specialized dosing. ▶L ♀C ▶? $$$$$

RABIES IMMUNE GLOBULIN HUMAN (*Imogam Rabies-HT, HyperRAB S/D*) 20 units/kg, as much as possible infiltrated around bite, the rest IM. ▶L ♀C ▶? $$$$$

RSV IMMUNE GLOBULIN (*RespiGam*) IV infusion for RSV. ▶Plasma ♀C ▶? $$$$$

TETANUS IMMUNE GLOBULIN (*BayTet*) Tetanus prophylaxis: 250 units IM. ▶L ♀C ▶? $$$$

VARICELLA-ZOSTER IMMUNE GLOBULIN (*VariZIG, VZIG*) Specialized dosing. ▶L ♀C ▶? $$$$$

CHILDHOOD IMMUNIZATION SCHEDULE*

	Months								Years		
Age	Birth	1	2	4	6	12	15	18	2	4–6	11–12
Hepatitis B	HB	HB				HB					
Rotavirus			Rota	Rota	Rota@						
DTP			DTaP	DTaP	DTaP		DTaP			DTaP	
H influenzae b			Hib	Hib	Hib	Hib^					
Pneumococci**			PCV	PCV	PCV	PCV					
Polio			IPV	IPV		IPV				IPV#	
Influenza†					Influenza (yearly)†						
MMR						MMR				MMR	
Varicella						Varicella				Vari cella	
Hepatitis A‡						Hep A × 2¶					
Papillomavirus §											HPV × 3¶
Meningococcal											MCV^

*2013 schedule from the CDC, ACIP, AAP, & AAFP, see CDC website (www.cdc.gov).
**Administer 1 dose Prevnar 13 to all healthy children 24 to 59 mo having an incomplete schedule.
***When immunizing adolescents 10 yo or older, consider DTaP if patient has never received a pertussis booster
(Boostrix if 10 yo or older, Adacel if 11 to 64 yo).
@If using Rotarix give at 2 and 4 mo (no earlier than 6 weeks). Give at 2, 4, and 6 mo if using Rotateq. Max age for final dose is 8 mo.
^Last IPV on or after 4th birthday, and at least 6 months since last dose.
^If using PedvaxHib or Comvax, dose at 6 mo not necessary, but booster at 12–15 mo indicated.
†For healthy patients age 2 yo or older can use intranasal form. If age younger than 9 yo and receiving for 1 time,
administer 2 doses 4 or more weeks apart for injected form and 6 or more weeks apart for intranasal form. FluLaval
not indicated for younger than 18 yo. Use Afluria only if 9 yo or older due to risk of febrile reaction.
†Two doses 6–18 months apart.
§Second and 3 doses 2 and 6 months after 1 dose. Also approved (Gardasil only) for males 9 to 18 yo to reduce risk of
genital warts.
^Vaccinate all children at 11 to 12 yo with Menactra, booster at 16 yo. Give one dose between 13 and 18 yo, if previously
unvaccinated. For children 9 months to 10 yo at high risk for meningococcal disease, vaccinate with meningococcal
vaccine. Refer to CDC for vaccine selection and booster recommendations.

Immunosuppression

BASILIXIMAB (**Simulect**) Specialized dosing for organ transplantation.
▶Plasma ♀B ▶? $$$$$
BELATACEPT (**Nulojix**) Specialized dosing for organ transplantation.
[injection.] ▶serum – ♀C ▶– $$$$$ ■
CYCLOSPORINE (**Sandimmune, Neoral, Gengraf**) Specialized dosing for organ
transplantation, RA, and psoriasis. [Generic/Trade: Microemulsion Caps 25, 100
mg. Generic/Trade: Caps (Sandimmune) 25, 100 mg. Soln (Sandimmune) 100 mg/
mL. Microemulsion soln (Neoral, Gengraf) 100 mg/mL.] ▶L ♀C ▶– $$$$$ ■
DACLIZUMAB (**Zenapax**) Specialized dosing for organ transplantation. ▶L
♀C ▶? $$$$$ ■
EVEROLIMUS (**Zortress**) Specialized dosing for organ transplantation.
[Trade: tab 0.25, 0,.5, 0.75 mg.] ▶L – ♀C ▶– $$$$$
MYCOPHENOLATE MOFETIL (**Cellcept, Myfortic**) Specialized dosing for
organ transplantation. [Generic/Trade: Caps 250 mg. Tabs 500 mg. Trade only
(cont.)

TETANUS WOUND CARE (www.cdc.gov)		
	Unknown or less than 3 prior tetanus immunizations	*3 or more prior tetanus immunizations*
Non-tetanus-prone wound (eg, clean and minor)	Td (DT age younger than 7 yo)	Td if more than 10 years since last dose
Tetanus-prone wound (eg, dirt, contamination, punctures, crush components)	Td (DT age younger than 7 yo), tetanus immune globulin 250 units IM at site other than Td	Td if more than 5 years since last dose

If patient age 10 yo or older has never received a pertussis booster consider DTaP (Boostrix if 10 yo or older, Adacel if 11–64 yo).

(CellCept): Susp 200 mg/mL (160 mL). Trade only (Myfortic): Tabs, Extended-release: 180, 360 mg.] ▶? ♀D ▶– $$ ■

SIROLIMUS (*Rapamune*) Specialized dosing for organ transplantation. [Trade only: Soln 1 mg/mL (60 mL). Tabs 1, 2 mg]. ▶L ♀C ▶– $$$$$

TACROLIMUS (*Prograf, FK 506, ✦ Advagraf*) Specialized dosing for organ transplantation. [Generic/Trade: Caps 0.5, 1, 5 mg]. ▶L ♀C ▶– $$$$$

Other

HYMENOPTERA VENOM Specialized desensitization dosing protocol. ▶Serum ♀C ▶? $$$$

TUBERCULIN PPD (*Aplisol, Tubersol, Mantoux, PPD*) 5 tuberculin units (0.1 mL) intradermally, read 48 to 72 h later. ▶L ♀C ▶+ $

NEUROLOGY

Alzheimer's Disease—Cholinesterase Inhibitors

DONEPEZIL (*Aricept*) Start 5 mg PO at bedtime. May increase to 10 mg PO at bedtime in 4 to 6 weeks. Max 10 mg/day for mild to moderate disease. For moderate to severe disease (MMSE 10 or less): may increase after 3 months to 23 mg/day. [Generic/Trade: Tabs 5, 10 mg, Orally disintegrating tabs 5, 10 mg. Trade only: Tab 23 mg.] ▶LK ♀C ▶? $$$$

GALANTAMINE (*Razadyne, Razadyne ER, ✦ Reminyl*) Extended-release: Start 8 mg PO q am with food; increase to 16 mg after 4 weeks. May increase to 24 mg after another 4 weeks. Immediate-release: Start 4 mg PO two times per day with food; increase to 8 mg two times per day after 4 weeks. May increase to 12 mg two times per day after another 4 weeks. [Generic/Trade: Tabs 4, 8, 12 mg. Extended-release caps 8, 16, 24 mg. Oral soln 4 mg/mL. Prior to April 2005 was called Reminyl in the US.] ▶LK ♀B ▶? $$$$

RIVASTIGMINE (*Exelon, Exelon Patch*) Alzheimer's disease: Start 1.5 mg PO two times per day with food. Increase to 3 mg two times per day after 2 weeks. Max 12 mg/day. Patch: Start 4.6 mg/24 h once daily; may increase after 1

(cont.)

month or more to recommended dose of 9.5 mg/24 h, max 13.3 mg/24 h. Rotate sites. Dementia in Parkinson's disease: Start 1.5 mg PO two times per day with food. Increase by 3 mg/day at intervals greater than 4 weeks to max 12 mg/day. Patch: Use dosing for Alzheimer's disease. [Generic/Trade: Caps 1.5, 3, 4.5, 6 mg. Trade only: Soln 2 mg/mL (120 mL). Transdermal patch: 4.6 mg/24h, 9.5 mg/24h, 13.3mg/24h] ▶K ♀B ▶? $$$$$

Alzheimer's Disease—NMDA Receptor Antagonists

MEMANTINE (*Namenda, Namenda XR, + Ebixa*) Start 5 mg PO daily. Increase by 5 mg/day at weekly intervals to max 20 mg/day. Doses greater than 5 mg/day should be divided two times per day. Extended-release: Start 7 mg once daily. Increase at weekly intervals to target dose of 28 mg/day. Reduce to 14 mg/day in renal impairment. [Generic/Trade: Tabs 5, 10 mg. Trade only: Oral soln 2 mg/mL. Extended-release caps 7, 14, 21, 28 mg.] ▶KL ♀B ▶? $$$$$

Anticonvulsants

CARBAMAZEPINE (*Tegretol, Tegretol XR, Carbatrol, Epitol, Equetro*) Epilepsy: 200 to 400 mg PO divided into two to four doses per day. Extended-release: 200 mg PO twice per day. Age younger than 6 yo: 10 to 20 mg/kg/day PO divided into two to four doses per day. Age 6 to 12 yo: 100 mg PO twice per day or 50 mg PO four times per day (susp); increase by 100 mg/day at weekly intervals divided three to four doses per day (immediate-release), twice per day (extended-release), or four times per day (susp). Bipolar disorder, acute manic/mixed episodes (Equetro): Start 200 mg PO two times per day; increase by 200 mg/day to max 1600 mg/day. Trigeminal neuralgia: Start 100 mg PO two times per day (regular and XR tabs) or 50 mg PO four times per day (susp). May increase by 200 mg/day to pain relief or max 1200 mg/day. Aplastic anemia, agranulocytosis, many drug interactions. [Generic/Trade: Tabs 200 mg, Chewable tabs 100 mg, Susp 100 mg/5 mL. Extended-release tabs (Tegretol XR) 100, 200, 400 mg. Extended-release caps (Carbatrol): 100, 200, 300 mg. Trade Only: Extended-Release Caps (Equetro): 100, 200, 300mg] ▶LK ♀D ▶+ $$ ■

CLOBAZAM (*ONFI, + FRISIUM*) US, adults and children 2 yo and older, weight greater than 30 kg: Start 5 mg PO twice daily. Increase to 10 mg PO twice daily after 1 week then to 20 mg PO twice daily after 2 weeks. Weight 30 kg or less: Start 5 mg PO daily. Increase to 5 mg PO twice daily after 1 week, then 10 mg PO twice daily after 2 weeks. Canada, adults: Start 5 to 15 mg PO daily. Increase prn to max 80 mg/day. Children younger than 2 yo: 0.5 to 1 mg/kg PO daily. Children age 2 to 16 yo: Start 5 mg PO daily. May increase prn to max 40 mg/day. [Trade only: Tabs 5,10, 20 mg. Oral susp 2.5 mg/mL] ▶L ♀X (1st trimester) D (2nd/3rd trimesters) ▶—©IV $$$$$

ETHOSUXIMIDE (*Zarontin*) Absence seizures, age 3 to 6 yo: Start 250 mg PO daily (or divided two times per day). Age older than 6 yo: Start 500 mg PO daily (or divided two times per day). Max 1.5 g/day. [Generic/Trade: Caps 250 mg. Syrup 250 mg/5 mL.] ▶LK ♀C ▶+ $$$$

EZOGABINE (*POTIGA*) Partial-onset seizures, adjunctive: Start 100 mg PO three times per day. Increase weekly by no more than 50 mg three times daily to usual maintenance dose of 200 to 400 mg PO three times daily or max of 250 mg three times daily if older than 65 yo. Reduce dose for moderate to severe renal or hepatic impairment. [Trade: Tabs 50, 200, 300, 400 mg.] ▶KL – ♀C ▶?

FELBAMATE (*Felbatol*) Start 400 mg PO three times per day. Max 3600 mg/day. Peds: Start 15 mg/kg/day PO divided three to four times per day. Max 45 mg/kg/day. Aplastic anemia, hepatotoxicity. Not first line. Requires written informed consent. [Generic/Trade: Tabs 400, 600 mg, Oral susp 600 mg/5 mL.] ▶KL ♀C ▶ – $$$$$ ■

FOSPHENYTOIN (*Cerebyx*) Load: 15 to 20 mg "phenytoin equivalents" (PE) per kg IM/IV no faster than 150 PE mg/min. Maintenance: 4 to 6 PE/kg/day. ▶L ♀D ▶+ $$$$$

GABAPENTIN (*Neurontin, Horizant, Gralise*) Partial seizures, adjunctive therapy: Start 300 mg PO at bedtime. Increase gradually to 300 to 600 mg PO three times per day. Max 3600 mg/day divided three times per day. Postherpetic neuralgia, immediate-release tabs: Start 300 mg PO on day 1; increase to 300 mg two times per day on day 2, and to 300 mg three times per day on day 3. Max 1800 mg/day divided three times per day. Postherpetic neuralgia (Gralise): Start 300 mg PO once daily with evening meal. Increase to 600 mg on day 2, 900 mg on days 3 to 6, 1200 mg on days 7 to 10, 1500 mg on days 11 to 14, and 1800 mg on day 15. Max 1800 mg/day. Postherpetic neuralgia (Horizant): Start 600 mg PO q am for 3 days, then increase to 600 mg PO twice per day. Max 1200 mg/day. Partial seizures, initial monotherapy: Titrate as above. Usual effective dose is 900 to 1800 mg/day. Restless legs syndrome (Horizant): 600 mg PO once daily around 5 pm taken with food. [Generic only: Tabs 100, 300, 400 mg. Generic/Trade: Caps 100, 300, 400 mg. Tabs, scored 600, 800 mg. Soln 50 mg/mL. Trade only: Tabs, extended-release 600 mg (gabapentin enacarbil, Horizant). Trade only (Gralise): Tabs 300, 600 mg.] ▶K ♀C ▶? $$$$

LACOSAMIDE (*Vimpat*) Partial-onset seizures, adjunctive (17 yo and older): Start 50 mg PO/IV two times per day. Increase by 50 mg twice per day to recommended dose of 100 to 200 mg twice per day. Max 600 mg/day (max 300 mg/day in mild/moderate hepatic or severe renal impairment. [Trade only: Tabs 50, 100, 150, 200 mg.] ▶KL ♀C ▶? $$$$$

LAMOTRIGINE (*Lamictal, Lamictal CD, Lamictal ODT, Lamictal XR*) Partial seizures, Lennox-Gastaut syndrome, or generalized tonic-clonic seizures adjunctive therapy with a single enzyme-inducing anticonvulsant. Age 2 to 12 yo: Dosing is based on wt and concomitant meds (see package insert). Age older than 12 yo: 50 mg PO daily for 2 weeks, then 50 mg two times per day for 2 weeks, then gradually increase to 150 to 250 mg PO two times per day. Extended-release: Start 50 mg PO daily for weeks 1 to 2, then increase to 100 mg PO daily for weeks 3 to 4. Then increase by 100 mg/day at weekly intervals to target dose of 400 to 600 mg/day. Partial seizures, Lennox-Gastaut syndrome, or generalized tonic-clonic seizures adjunctive therapy (NOT with

(cont.)

NEUROLOGY

valproate or enzyme-inducing anticonvulasant: Start 25 mg PO every day for weeks 1 to 2, then increase to 50 mg/day for weeks 3 to 4. Then increase by 50 mg/day every 1 to 2 weeks to target dose of 225 to 375 mg/day. Extended-release: Start 25 mg PO daily for weeks 1 to 2 then increase to 50 mg/day for weeks 3 to 4. Then increase weekly by 50 mg/day to target dose of 300 to 400 mg/day. Conversion to monotherapy (age 16 yo or older): See package insert. Drug interaction with valproate (see package insert for adjusted dosing guidelines). Potentially life-threatening rashes reported in 0.3% of adults and 0.8% of children; discontinue at first sign of rash. [Generic/Trade: Tabs, 25, 100, 150, 200 mg. Chewable dispersible tabs (Lamictal CD) 5, 25 mg. Extended-release Tabs (Lamictal XR) 25, 50,100, 200, 250, 300 mg. Trade only: Orally disintegrating tabs (Lamictal ODT) 25, 50, 100, 200 mg. Trade only: Chewable dispersible tabs 2 mg (Lamictal CD) may not be available in all pharmacies; obtain through manufacturer representative, or by calling 888-825-5249.] ▶LK ♀C (see notes) ▶– $$$$ ■

LEVETIRACETAM *(Keppra, Keppra XR)* Partial seizures, juvenile myoclonic epilepsy (JME), or primary generalized tonic-clonic seizures (GTC), adjunctive: Start 500 mg PO/IV twice per day (Keppra) or 1000 mg (Keppra XR, partial seizures only); increase by 1000 mg/day q 2 weeks prn to max 3000 mg/day (partial seizures) or to target dose of 3000 mg/day (JME or GTC). IV route not approved for GTC or if younger than 16 yo! [Generic/Trade: Tabs 250, 500, 750, 1000 mg, Oral soln 100 mg/mL, Tabs, extended-release 500, 750 mg.] ▶K ♀C ▶? $$$$$

OXCARBAZEPINE *(Trileptal, Oxtellar XR)* Immediate release: Start 300 mg PO two times per day. Titrate to 1200 mg/day (adjunctive) or 1200 to 2400 mg/day (monotherapy). Extended release (adjunctive): Start 600 mg PO daily. Increase by 600 mg/day weekly if needed, max 2400 mg/day. Peds 2 to 16 yo: Immediate release: Start 8 to 10 mg/kg/day divided two times per day. Extended release (adjunctive for 6 to 17 yo): Start 8 mg/kg to 10 mg/kg PO once daily not to exceed 600 mg/day. May increase weekly by 8 mg/kg to 10 mg/kg once daily if needed to max based on wt of 900 mg/day (20 to 29 kg), 1200 mg/day (29.1 to 39 kg), or 1800 mg/day (greater than 39 kg). Life-threatening rashes and hypersensitivity reactions. [Generic/Trade: Tabs (scored) 150, 300, 600 mg. Oral susp 300 mg/5 mL. Trade Only: Extended-release tabs (Oxtellar XR) 150, 300, 600 mg] ▶LK ♀C ▶– $$$$$

PHENOBARBITAL *(Luminal)* Load: 20 mg/kg IV at rate no faster than 60 mg/min. Maintenance: 100 to 300 mg/day PO given once daily or divided two times per day. Peds 3 to 5 mg/kg/day PO divided two to three times per day. Many drug interactions. [Generic only: Tabs 15, 16.2, 30, 32.4, 60, 100 mg. Elixir 20 mg/5 mL.] ▶L ♀D ▶–©IV $

PHENYTOIN *(Dilantin, Phenytek)* Status epilepticus: Load 15 to 20 mg/kg IV no faster than 50 mg/min, then 100 mg IV/PO q 6 to 8 h. Epilepsy: Oral load: 400 mg PO initially, then 300 mg in 2 h and 4 h. Maintenance: 5 mg/kg (or 300 mg PO) given once daily (extended-release) or divided three times per day (susp and chew tabs) and titrated to a therapeutic level. Limit dose increases to 10% or less due to saturable metabolism. [Generic/Trade: Extended-release

(cont.)

caps 100 mg (Dilantin). Susp 125 mg/5 mL. Extended-release caps 200, 300 mg (Phenytek). Chewable tabs 50 mg (Dilantin Infatabs). Trade only: Extended-release caps 30 mg (Dilantin).] ▶L ♀D ▶+ $$

PREGABALIN (**Lyrica**) Painful diabetic peripheral neuropathy: Start 50 mg PO three times per day; may increase within 1 week to max 100 mg PO three times per day. Postherpetic neuralgia: Start 150 mg/day PO divided two to three times per day. May increase within 1 week to 300 mg/day divided two to three times per day; max 600 mg/day. Partial seizures (adjunctive): Start 150 mg/day PO divided two to three times per day; may increase prn to max 600 mg/day divided two to three times per day. Fibromyalgia: Start 75 mg PO two times per day; may increase to 150 mg two times per day within 1 week; max 225 mg two times per day. Neuropathic pain associated with spinal cord injury: Start 75 mg PO two times per day; may increase to 150 mg two times per day within 1 week and then to 300 mg two times per day after 2 to 3 weeks if tolerated. [Trade only: Caps 25, 50, 75, 100, 150, 200, 225, 300 mg. Oral soln 20 mg/mL (480 mL).] ▶K ♀C ▶?©♥ $$$$$

PRIMIDONE (**Mysoline**) Start 100 to 125 mg PO at bedtime. Increase over 10 days to 250 mg three to four times per day. Max 2 g/day. Metabolized to phenobarbital. Essential tremor (unapproved): up to 750 mg/day. [Generic/Trade: Tabs 50, 250 mg.] ▶LK ♀D ▶– $$$$

RUFINAMIDE (**Banzel**) Start 400 to 800 mg/day PO divided two times per day. Increase by 400 to 800 mg/day q 2 days to max 3200 mg/day. [Trade only: Tabs 200, 400 mg. Susp 40 mg/mL.] ▶K ♀C ▶? $$$$$

TIAGABINE (**Gabitril**) Start 4 mg PO daily. Increase by 4 to 8 mg/day at weekly intervals prn to max 32 mg/day (age 12 to 18 yo) or max 56 mg/day (age older than 18 yo) divided two to four times per day. Avoid off-label use. [Trade only: Tabs 2, 4, 12, 16 mg.] ▶L ♀C ▶? $$$$$

TOPIRAMATE (**Topamax**) Partial seizures or primary generalized tonic-clonic seizures, monotherapy: Start 25 mg PO two times per day (week 1), 50 mg two times per day (week 2), 75 mg two times per day (week 3), 100 mg two times per day (week 4), 150 mg two times per day (week 5), then 200 mg two times per day as tolerated. Partial seizures, primary generalized tonic-clonic seizures or Lennox-Gastaut syndrome, adjunctive therapy: Start 25 to 50 mg PO at bedtime. Increase weekly by 25 to 50 mg per day to usual effective dose of 200 mg PO two times per day. Doses greater than 400 mg per day not shown to be more effective. Migraine prophylaxis: Start 25 mg PO at bedtime (week 1), then 25 mg two times per day (week 2), then 25 mg q am and 50 mg q pm (week 3), then 50 mg two times per day (week 4 and thereafter). Bipolar disorder (unapproved): Start 25 to 50 mg per day PO. Titrate prn to max 400 mg per day divided two times per day. [Generic/Trade: Tabs 25, 50, 100, 200 mg. Sprinkle Caps 15, 25 mg.] ▶K ♀D ▶? $$$$$

VALPROIC ACID—NEURO (**Depakene, Depakote, Depakote ER, Depacon, Stavzor,** divalproex, sodium valproate, ✦ **Epival**) Epilepsy: 10 to 15 mg/kg/day PO/IV divided two to four times per day (standard-release, delayed-release, or IV) or given once daily (Depakote ER). Titrate to max 60 mg/kg/day. Use rate no faster than 20 mg/min when given IV. Migraine prophylaxis:

(cont.)

Start 250 mg PO two times per day (Depakote or Stavzor) or 500 mg PO daily (Depakote ER) for 1 week, then increase to max 1000 mg/day PO divided two times per day (Depakote or Stavzor) or given once daily (Depakote ER). Hepatotoxicity, drug interactions, reduce dose in elderly. [Generic/Trade: Immediate-release caps 250 mg (Depakene), syrup (Depakene, valproic acid) 250 mg/5 mL. Delayed-release tabs (Depakote) 125, 250, 500 mg, Extended-release tabs (Depakote ER) 250, 500 mg, Delayed-release sprinkle caps (Depakote) 125 mg. Trade only (Stavzor): Delayed-release caps 125, 250, 500 mg.] ▶L ♀D ▶+ $$$$ ■

ZONISAMIDE (*Zonegran*) Start 100 mg PO daily. Titrate q 2 weeks to 200 to 400 mg/day given once daily or divided two times per day. Max 600 mg/day. Drug interactions. Contraindicated in sulfa allergy. [Generic/Trade: Caps 25, 50, 100 mg.] ▶LK ♀C ▶? $$$$

Migraine Therapy—Triptans (5-HT1 Receptor Agonists)

NOTE: *May cause vasospasm. Avoid in ischemic or vasospastic heart disease, cerebrovascular syndromes, peripheral arterial disease, uncontrolled HTN, and hemiplegic or basilar migraine. Do not use within 24 h of ergots or other triptans. Risk of serotonin syndrome if used with SSRIs or MAOIs.*

ALMOTRIPTAN (*Axert*) 6.25 to 12.5 mg PO. May repeat in 2 h prn. Max 25 mg/day. Avoid MAOIs. [Trade only: Tabs 6.25, 12.5 mg.] ▶LK ♀C ▶? $$

ELETRIPTAN (*Relpax*) 20 to 40 mg PO. May repeat in 2 h prn. Max 40 mg/ dose or 80 mg/day. Drug interactions. Avoid MAOIs. [Trade only: Tabs 20, 40 mg.] ▶LK ♀C ▶? $$$

FROVATRIPTAN (*Frova*) 2.5 mg PO. May repeat in 2 h prn. Max 7.5 mg/24 h. [Trade only: Tabs 2.5 mg.] ▶LK ♀C ▶? $

NARATRIPTAN (*Amerge*) 1 to 2.5 mg PO. May repeat in 4 h prn. Max 5 mg/ 24 h. [Generic/Trade: Tabs 1, 2.5 mg.] ▶KL ♀C ▶? $$$

RIZATRIPTAN (*Maxalt, Maxalt MLT*) 5 to 10 mg PO. May repeat in 2 h prn. Max 30 mg/24 h. MLT form dissolves on tongue without liquids. Avoid MAOIs. [Generic/ Trade: Tabs 5, 10 mg. Orally disintegrating tabs 5, 10 mg.] ▶LK ♀C ▶? $$$

SUMATRIPTAN (*Imitrex, Alsuma, Sumavel, Zecuity*) 4 to 6 mg SC. May repeat in 1 h prn. Max 12 mg/24 h. Tabs: 25 to 100 mg PO (50 mg most common). May repeat q 2 h prn with 25- to 100-mg doses. Max 200 mg/24 h. Intranasal spray: 5 to 20 mg q 2 h. Max 40 mg/24 h. Transdermal: one patch topically, max two patches/24 h with no less than 2 h before 2nd application. No evidence of increased benefit with 2nd patch. Avoid MAOIs. [Generic/Trade: Tabs 25, 50, 100 mg. Injection (STATdose System) 4-, 6-mg prefilled cartridges. Trade only: Nasal Spray (Imitrex Nasal) 5 mg and 20 mg (box of #6). Alsuma, Sumavel: Injection 6-mg prefilled cartridge. Zecuity Transdermal Patch: 6.5 mg/4 h. Generic only: Nasal Spray 5 mg and 20 mg (box of #6).] ▶LK ♀C ▶+ $

TREXIMET (**sumatriptan + naproxen**) 1 tab PO at onset of headache. Efficacy of more than one tablet not established. Max 2 tabs/24 h separated by at least 2 h. [Trade only: Tabs 85 mg sumatriptan + 500 mg naproxen sodium.] ▶LK ♀C ▶− $$

ZOLMITRIPTAN (*Zomig, Zomig ZMT*) 1.25 to 2.5 mg PO q 2 h. Max 10 mg/24 h. Orally disintegrating tabs (ZMT) 2.5 mg PO. May repeat in 2 h prn. Max 10 mg/24 h. Nasal spray: 5 mg (1 spray) in 1 nostril. May repeat in 2 h. Max 10 mg/24 h. [Generic/Trade: Tabs 2.5, 5 mg. Orally disintegrating tabs (ZMT) 2.5, 5 mg. Trade only: Nasal spray 5 mg/spray.] ▶L ♀C ▶? $$$$

Migraine Therapy—Other

CAFERGOT (*ergotamine + caffeine*) 2 tabs PO at onset, then 1 tab q 30 min prn. Max 6 tabs/attack or 10/week. Drug interactions. Fibrotic complications. [Trade only: Tabs 1/100 mg ergotamine/caffeine.] ▶L ♀X ▶– $ ■

DIHYDROERGOTAMINE (*D.H.E. 45, Migranal*) Soln (DHE 45) 1 mg IV/IM/SC. May repeat in 1 h prn. Max 2 mg (IV) or 3 mg (IM/SC) per day. Nasal spray (Migranal): 1 spray in each nostril. May repeat in 15 min prn. Max 6 sprays/24 h or 8 sprays/week. Drug interactions. Fibrotic complications. [Trade only: Nasal spray 0.5 mg/spray (Migranal). Self-injecting soln (D.H.E 45): 1 mg/mL.] ▶L ♀X ▶– $$ ■

FLUNARIZINE Canada only. 10 mg PO at bedtime. [Generic/Trade: Caps 5 mg.] ▶L ♀C ▶– $$

Multiple Sclerosis

DALFAMPRIDINE (*Ampyra, ✦ Fampyra*) 10 mg PO two times per day. Contraindicated in seizure disorders or moderate to severe renal impairment. [Trade: Extended-release tablets 10 mg.] ▶K– ♀C ▶? $$$$$

DIMETHYL FUMARATE (*Tecfidera*) Start 120 mg PO twice per day. Increase to maintenance dose after 7 days to 240 mg twice per day. [Delayed-release capsules: 120, 240 mg.] ▶esterases – ♀C ▶?

FINGOLIMOD (*Gilenya*) 0.5 mg PO once daily. Contraindicated in cerebral or cardiovascular disease. [Trade only: Caps 0.5 mg.] ▶L– ♀C ▶?

GLATIRAMER (*Copaxone*) 20 mg SC daily. [Trade only: Injection 20 mg single-dose vial.] ▶Serum ♀B ▶? $$$$$

INTERFERON BETA-1A (*Avonex, Rebif*) Avonex 30 mcg (6 million units) IM q week. Rebif: start 8.8 mcg SC 3 times a week; titrate over 4 weeks to maintenance dose of 44 mcg 3 times a week. Suicidality, hepatotoxicity, blood dyscrasias. Follow LFTs and CBC. [Trade only (Avonex): Injection 30 mcg single-dose vial with or without albumin. Prefilled syringe 30 mcg. Trade only (Rebif): Starter kit 20 mcg prefilled syringe. Prefilled syringe 22, 44 mcg.] ▶L ♀C ▶? $$$$$

INTERFERON BETA-1B (*Betaseron*) Start 0.0625 mg SC every other day; titrate over 6 weeks to 0.25 mg (8 million units) SC every other day. Suicidality, hepatotoxicity, blood dyscrasias. Follow LFTs. [Trade only: Injection 0.3 mg (9.6 million units) single-dose vial.] ▶L ♀C ▶? $$$$$

Myasthenia Gravis

EDROPHONIUM (*Tensilon, Enlon*) Evaluation for myasthenia gravis (diagnostic purposes only): 2 mg IV over 15 to 30 sec (test dose) while

(cont.)

on cardiac monitor, then 8 mg IV after 45 sec. Atropine should be readily available in case of cholinergic reaction. Duration of effect is 5 to 10 min. [10 mg/mL MDV vial.] ▶Plasma ♀C ▶? $

PYRIDOSTIGMINE (*Mestinon, Mestinon Timespan, Regonol*) 60 to 200 mg PO three times per day (standard-release) or 180 mg PO daily or divided two times per day (extended-release). [Generic/Trade: Tabs 60 mg. Trade only: Extended-release tabs 180 mg. Syrup 60 mg/ 5 mL.] ▶Plasma, K ♀C ▶+ $$

Parkinsonian Agents—Anticholinergics

BENZTROPINE MESYLATE (*Cogentin*) Parkinsonism: 0.5 to 2 mg IM/PO/IV given once daily or divided two times per day. Drug-induced extrapyramidal disorders: 1 to 4 mg PO/IM/IV given once daily or divided two times per day. [Generic only: Tabs 0.5, 1, 2 mg.] ▶LK ♀C ▶? $

BIPERIDEN (*Akineton*) 2 mg PO three to four times per day, max 16 mg/day. [Trade only: Tabs 2 mg.] ▶LK ♀C ▶? $$$

TRIHEXYPHENIDYL (*Artane*) Start 1 mg PO daily. Gradually increase to 6 to 10 mg/day divided three times per day. Max 15 mg/day. [Generic only: Tabs 2, 5 mg. Elixir 2 mg/5 mL.] ▶LK ♀C ▶? $

Parkinsonian Agents—COMT Inhibitors

ENTACAPONE (*Comtan*) Start 200 mg PO with each dose of carbidopa/levodopa. Max 8 tabs (1600 mg)/day. [Generic/Trade: Tabs 200 mg.] ▶L ♀C ▶? $$$$$

Parkinsonian Agents—Dopaminergic Agents and Combinations

APOMORPHINE (*Apokyn*) Start 0.2 mL SC prn. May increase in 0.1-mL increments every few days. Monitor for orthostatic hypotension after initial dose and with dose escalation. Max 0.6 mL/dose or 2 mL/day. Potent emetic, pretreat with trimethobenzamide 300 mg PO three times per day starting 3 days prior to use and continue for at least 6 weeks. Contains sulfites. [Trade only: Cartridges (for injector pen, 10 mg/mL) 3 mL. Ampules (10 mg/mL) 2 mL.] ▶L ♀C ▶? $$$$$

CARBIDOPA/LEVODOPA (*Sinemet, Sinemet CR, Parcopa, ✦ Duodopa*) Start 1 tab (25/100 mg) PO three times per day. Increase q 1 to 4 days prn. Controlled-release: Start 1 tab (50/200 mg) PO two times per day; increase q 3 days prn. [Generic/Trade: Tabs (carbidopa/levodopa) 10/100, 25/100, 25/250 mg. Tabs, sustained-release (Sinemet CR, carbidopa-levodopa ER) 25/100, 50/200 mg. Trade only: Orally disintegrating tabs (Parcopa) 10/100, 25/100, 25/250 mg.] ▶L ♀C ▶− $$$$

PRAMIPEXOLE (*Mirapex, Mirapex ER*) Parkinson's disease: Start 0.125 mg PO three times per day. Gradually increase to 0.5 to 1.5 mg PO three times per day. Extended-release: start 0.375 mg PO daily. May increase after 5 to 7 days to 0.75 mg daily, then by 0.75 mg/day increments q 5 to 7 days to max 4.5 mg/day. Restless legs syndrome: Start 0.125 mg PO 2 to 3 h before to bedtime. May increase q 4 to 7 days to max 0.5 mg/day given

(cont.)

Dermatomes

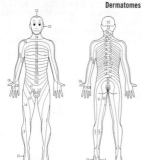

MOTOR FUNCTION BY NERVE ROOTS

Level	Motor Function
C3/C4/C5	Diaphragm
C5/C6	Deltoid/biceps
C7/C8	Triceps
C8/T1	Finger flexion/ intrinsics
T1–T12	Intercostal/ abd muscles
L2/L3	Hip flexion
L2/L3/L4	Hip adductor/quads
L4/L5	Ankle dorsiflexion
S1/S2	Ankle plantarflexion
S2/S3/S4	Rectal tone

LUMBOSACRAL NERVE ROOT COMPRESSIONS	Root	Motor	Sensory	Reflex
	L4	quadriceps	medial foot	knee-jerk
	L5	dorsiflexors	dorsum of foot	medial hamstring
	S1	plantarflexors	lateral foot	ankle-jerk

GLASGOW COMA SCALE

Eye Opening	Verbal Activity	Motor Activity
4. Spontaneous	5. Oriented	6. Obeys commands
3. To command	4. Confused	5. Localizes pain
2. To pain	3. Inappropriate	4. Withdraws to pain
1. None	2. Incomprehensible	3. Flexion to pain
	1. None	2. Extension to pain
		1. None

NEUROLOGY

2 to 3 h before bedtime. [Generic/Trade: Tabs 0.125, 0.25, 0.5, 0.75, 1, 1.5 mg. Trade only: Tabs, extended-release 0.375, 0.75, 1.5, 3, 4.5 mg.] ▶K ♀C ▶? $$$$$

ROPINIROLE (*Requip, Requip XL*) Parkinson's disease: Start 0.25 mg PO three times per day, then gradually increase over 4 weeks to 1 mg PO three times per day. Max 24 mg/day. Extended-release: Start 2 mg PO daily for 1 to 2 weeks, then gradually increase by 2 mg daily at weekly or longer intervals. Max 24 mg/day. Restless legs syndrome: Start 0.25 mg PO 1 to 3 h before bedtime for 2 days, then increase to 0.5 mg/day on days 3 to 7. Increase by 0.5 mg/day at weekly intervals prn to max 4 mg/day given 1 to 3 h before bedtime. [Generic/Trade: Tabs, immediate-release 0.25, 0.5, 1, 2, 3, 4, 5 mg. Tabs, extended-release 2, 4, 6, 8, 12 mg.] ▶L ♀C ▶? $$$

ROTIGOTINE (*Neupro*) Early stage Parkinson's disease: Start 2 mg/24 h patch daily; may increase by 2 mg/24 h at weekly intervals to max 6 mg/24 h. Advanced-stage Parkinson's disease: Start 4 mg/24 h patch daily; may increase by 2 mg/24 h at weekly intervals to max 8 mg/24 h. Restless legs syndrome: Start 1 mg/24 h patch daily; may be increased by 1 mg/24 h at weekly intervals to max 3 mg/24 h. [Trade: Transdermal patch 1, 2, 3, 4, 6 8 mg/24 h.] ▶L – ♀C ▶?

STALEVO (**carbidopa + levodopa + entacapone**) (conversion from carbidopa/levodopa with or without entacapone): Start Stalevo tab that contains the same amount of carbidopa/levodopa as the patient was previously taking, then titrate to desired response. May need to reduce levodopa dose if not already taking entacapone. [Trade only: Tabs (carbidopa/levodopa/entacapone): Stalevo 50 (12.5/50/200 mg), Stalevo 75 (18.75/75/200 mg), Stalevo 100 (25/100/200 mg), Stalevo 125 (31.25/125/200 mg), Stalevo 150 (37.5/150/200 mg), Stalevo 200 (50/200/200 mg).] ▶L ♀C ▶– $$$$$

Parkinsonian Agents—Monoamine Oxidase Inhibitors (MAOIs)

RASAGILINE (*Azilect*) Parkinson's disease, monotherapy: 1 mg PO q am. Parkinson's disease, adjunctive: 0.5 mg PO q am. Max 1 mg/day. Requires an MAOI diet recommended on PI, but not observed in clinical practice, and there is clinical research data to suggest that the diet is not needed. [Trade only: Tabs 0.5, 1 mg.] ▶L ♀C ▶? $$$$$

SELEGILINE (*Eldepryl, Zelapar*) Parkinson's disease: 5 mg PO q am and at noon, max 10 mg/day. Zelapar ODT: 1.25 to 2.5 mg q am, max 2.5 mg/day. [Generic/Trade: Caps 5 mg. Tabs 5 mg. Trade only: Oral disintegrating tabs (Zelapar ODT) 1.25 mg.] ▶LK ♀C ▶? $$$$

Other Agents

ABOBOTULINUMTOXIN A (*DYSPORT*) Cervical dystonia: 500 units IM total dose divided among affected muscles. May repeat q 12 weeks or longer. Max dose 1000 units per treatment. Glabellar lines (age youger than 65 yo): 50 units IM total dose divided into 10-unit injections at 5 sites (see prescribing information). May repeat q 12 weeks or longer. Risk of distant spread with symptoms of systemic botulism. Botulinum toxin products are not interchangeable. [Trade: vials 300, 500 units for reconstitution.] ♀C ▶? ■

DEXTROMETHORPHAN/QUINIDINE (*Nuedexta*) Start 1 cap PO daily for 7 days, then increase to maintenance dose of 1 cap PO twice daily. [Trade only: cap 10 mg dextromethorphan + 20 mg quinidine.] ▶LK – ♀C ▶?

INCOBOTULINUMTOXIN A (*Xeomin*) Cervical dystonia: Total 120 units IM divided among appropriate muscle groups. May repeat at intervals of at least 12 weeks. Blepharospasm in patients previously treated with Botox: Use same dose as Botox. If dose unknown, start 1.25 to 2.5 units per injection site. Do not exceed initial dose of 35 units/eye. May repeat at intervals of at least 12 weeks. [Trade only: 50 and 100 unit single use vials.] ▶not absorbed – ♀C ▶? ■

MANNITOL (*Osmitrol, Resectisol*) Intracranial HTN: 0.25 to 2 g/kg IV over 30 to 60 min. ▶K ♀C ▶? $$

MILNACIPRAN (*Savella*) Day 1: 12.5 mg PO once. Days 2 to 3: 12.5 mg two times per day. Days 4 to 7: 25 mg two times per day. After that: 50 mg two times per day. Max 200 mg/day. [Trade only: Tabs 12.5, 25, 50, 100 mg.] ▶KL ♀C ▶? $$$$

NIMODIPINE (*Nimotop, Nymalize*) Subarachnoid hemorrhage: 60 mg PO q 4 h for 21 days. [Generic only: Caps 30 mg. Trade only: 60 mg/20 mL oral solution (Nymalize)] ▶L ♀C ▶– $$$$$

ONABOTULINUM TOXIN TYPE A (*Botox, Botox Cosmetic*) Dose varies based on indication. Risk of distant spread with symptoms of systemic botulism. [Trade only: 100 unit single-use vials.] ▶Not absorbed ♀C ▶? $$$$$ ■

OXYBATE (*Xyrem, GHB, gamma hydroxybutyrate*) Cataplexy or excessive daytime sleepiness in narcolepsy: 2.25 g PO at bedtime. Repeat in 2.5 to 4 h. May increase by 1.5 g/day at 2-week intervals to max 9 g/day. From a centralized pharmacy. [Trade only: Soln 180 mL (500 mg/mL) supplied with measuring device and child-proof dosing cups.] ▶L ♀B ▶?©III $$$$$ ■

RILUZOLE (*Rilutek*) ALS: 50 mg PO q 12 h. Monitor LFTs. [Generic/Trade: Tabs 50 mg.] ▶LK ♀C ▶– $$$$$

TETRABENAZINE (*Xenazine, ✦Nitoman*) Chorea associated with Huntington's disease: Start 12.5 mg PO q am. Increase after 1 week to 12.5 mg PO two times per day. May increase by 12.5 mg/day weekly. Doses greater than 37.5 to 50 mg/day should be divided and given three times per day. For doses greater than 50 mg/day, genotype for CYP2D6, titrate by 12.5 mg/day weekly and divide in doses three times per day to max 37.5 mg/dose and 100 mg/day (extensive/intermediate metabolizers) or 25 mg/dose and 50 mg/day (poor metabolizers). Risk of depression, suicidality, and orthostatic hypotension. [Trade only: Tabs 12.5, 25 mg.] ▶L ♀C ▶? ? $$$$$ ■

OB/GYN

Contraceptives—Other

ETHINYLESTRADIOLVAGINALRING+ETONOGESTREL (*NuvaRing*) Contraception: 1 ring intravaginally for 3 weeks each month. [Trade only: Flexible intravaginal ring, 15 mcg ethinyl estradiol/0.120 mg etonogestrel/day in 1, 3 rings/box.] ▶L ♀X ▶– $$$

LEVONORGESTREL (*Plan B, Next Choice*) Emergency contraception: 1 tab PO ASAP but within 72 h of intercourse. 2nd tab 12 h later. [OTC Trade only: Kit contains 2 tabs 0.75 mg. Rx: Generic/Trade: Kit contains 2 tabs 0.75 mg.] ▶L ♀X ▶– $$

LEVONORGESTREL 1S (*Plan B One-Step, Next Choice One-Step*) Emergency contraception: 1 tab PO ASAP but within 72 h of intercourse. [OTC Trade only: Tabs 1.5 mg.] ▶L ♀X ▶– $$

NORELGESTROMIN + ETHINYL ESTRADIOL TRANSDERMAL (*Ortho Evra, ✦Evra*) Contraception: 1 patch q week for 3 weeks, then 1 week patch-free. [Trade only: Transdermal patch, 150 mcg norelgestromin/20 mcg ethinyl estradiol/day in 1, 3 patches/box.] ▶L ♀X ▶– $$$ ■

ULIPRISTAL ACETATE (*Ella*) Emergency contraception: 1 tab PO ASAP within 5 days of intercourse. [Trade only: Tabs 30 mg.] ▶L ♀X ▶?

Estrogens

NOTE: *See also Hormone Combinations.*

ESTERIFIED ESTROGENS (*Menest*) 0.3 to 1.25 mg PO daily. [Trade only: Tabs 0.3, 0.625, 1.25, 2.5 mg.] ▶L ♀X ▶– $$ ■

ESTRADIOL (*Estrace, Gynodiol*) 1 to 2 mg PO daily. [Generic/Trade: Tabs, micronized 0.5, 1, 2 mg, scored. Trade only: 1.5 mg (Gynodiol).] ▶L ♀X ▶– $ ■

ESTRADIOL ACETATE (*Femtrace*) 0.45 to 1.8 mg PO daily. [Trade only: Tabs, 0.45, 0.9, 1.8 mg.] ▶L ♀X ▶– $$ ■

ESTRADIOL ACETATE VAGINAL RING (*Femring*) Insert and replace after 90 days. [Trade only: 0.05 mg/day and 0.1 mg/day.] ▶L ♀X ▶– $$$ ■

ESTRADIOL CYPIONATE (*Depo-Estradiol*) 1 to 5 mg IM q 3 to 4 weeks. ▶L ♀X ▶– $ ■

ESTRADIOL GEL (*Divigel, Estrogel, Elestrin*) Thinly apply contents of 1 complete pump depression to one entire arm (Estrogel) or upper arm (Elestrin) or contents of 1 foil packet (Divigel) to one upper thigh. [Trade only: Gel 0.06% in nonaerosol, metered-dose pump with #64 or #32 1.25 g doses (Estrogel), #100 0.87 g doses (Elestrin). Gel 0.1% in single-dose foil packets of 0.25, 0.5, 1.0 g, carton of 30 (Divigel).] ▶L ♀X ▶– $$$ ■

ESTRADIOL TOPICAL EMULSION (*Estrasorb*) Rub in contents of 1 pouch each to left and right legs (spread over thighs and calves) q am. Daily dose is equivalent to two 1.74 g pouches. [Trade only: Topical emulsion, 56 pouches/carton.] ▶L ♀X ▶– $$ ■

ESTRADIOL TRANSDERMAL PATCH (*Alora, Climara, Menostar, Vivelle Dot, Minivelle, ✦ Estradot, Oesclim*) Apply 1 patch weekly (Climara, Estradiol, Menostar) or two times per week (Minivelle, Vivelle Dot, Alora). [Generic/Trade: Transdermal patches doses in mg/day: Climara (once a week) 0.025, 0.0375, 0.05, 0.06, 0.075, 0.1. Trade only: Vivelle Dot (two times per week) 0.025, 0.0375, 0.05, 0.075, 0.1. Alora (twice per week) 0.025, 0.05, 0.075, 0.1. Minivelle (twice per week) 0.0375, 0.05, 0.075, 0.1mg/day. Menostar (once a week) 0.014mg] ▶L ♀X ▶– $$$ ■

ESTRADIOL TRANSDERMAL SPRAY (*Evamist*) 1 to 3 sprays daily to forearm. [Trade only: Spray: 1.53 mg estradiol per 90 mcL spray, 56 sprays per metered-dose pump.] ▶L ♀X ▶– $$$ ■

ESTRADIOL VAGINAL RING (*Estring*) Insert and replace after 90 days. [Trade only: 2 mg ring single pack.] ▶L ♀X ▶– $$$ ■

ESTRADIOL VAGINAL TAB (*Vagifem*) 1 tab vaginally daily for 2 weeks, then 1 tab vaginally two times per week. [Trade only: Vaginal tab: 10 mcg or 25 mcg in disposable single-use applicators, 8, 18/pack.] ▶L ♀X ▶– $$$ ■

ESTRADIOL VALERATE (*Delestrogen*) 10 to 20 mg IM q 4 weeks. ▶L ♀X ▶– $$ ■

ESTROGEN VAGINAL CREAM (*Premarin, Estrace*) Menopausal atrophic vaginitis: Premarin: 0.5 to 2 g daily. Estrace: 2 to 4 g daily for 2 weeks,
(cont.)

EMERGENCY CONTRACEPTION

Emergency contraception within 72 h of unprotected sex.

<u>Progestin-only methods (causes less nausea and may be more effective):</u> Plan B One-Step (OTC) (levonorgestrel 1.5 mg): Take 1 pill. Next Choice or Plan B (levonorgestrel 0.75 mg): Take 1 pill ASAP and 2nd dose 12 h later.

<u>Progestin and estrogen method:</u> Dose is defined as 2 pills of Ogestrel, 4 pills of Cryselle, Enpresse*, Levora, Lo/Ovral, Low-Ogestrel, Nordette, Portia, Quasense, Seasonale, Seasonique, or Trivora*, or 5 pills of Aviane, Lessina, LoSeasonique, Lutera, or Sronyx. Take first dose ASAP and 2nd dose 12 h later. If vomiting occurs within 1 h of taking dose, consider repeating that dose with an antiemetic 1 h prior.

Emergency contraception within 120 h of unprotected sex.
Ella (ulipristal 30mg): Take 1 pill.
More info at: www.not-2-late.com

*Use 0.125 mg levonorgestrel/30 mcg ethinyl estradiol tabs.

then reduce. Moderate to severe menopausal dyspareunia: Premarin: 0.5 g daily, then reduce to two times per week. [Trade only: Premarin: 0.625 mg conjugated estrogens/g in 42.5 g with or without calibrated applicator. Estrace: 0.1 mg estradiol/g in 42.5 g with calibrated applicator. Generic only: Cream 0.625 mg synthetic conjugated estrogens/g in 30 g with calibrated applicator.] ▶L ♀X ▶? $$$$ ■

ESTROGENS CONJUGATED (*Premarin, C.E.S., Congest*) 0.3 to 1.25 mg PO daily. Abnormal uterine bleeding: 25 mg IV/IM. Repeat in 6 to 12 h if needed. [Trade only: Tabs 0.3, 0.45, 0.625, 0.9, 1.25 mg.] ▶L ♀X ▶− $$$ ■

ESTROGENS SYNTHETIC CONJUGATED A (*Cenestin*) 0.3 to 1.25 mg PO daily. [Trade only: Tabs 0.3, 0.45, 0.625, 0.9, 1.25 mg.] ▶L ♀X ▶− $$$ ■

ESTROGENS SYNTHETIC CONJUGATED B (*Enjuvia*) 0.3 to 1.25 mg PO daily. [Trade only: Tabs 0.3, 0.45, 0.625, 0.9, 1.25 mg.] ▶L ♀X ▶− $$ ■

ESTROPIPATE (*Ogen, Ortho-Est*) 0.75 to 6 mg PO daily. [Generic/Trade: Tabs 0.75, 1.5, 3, 6 mg of estropipate.] ▶L ♀X ▶− $ ■

Hormone Combinations

NOTE: *See also Estrogens.*

ACTIVELLA (estradiol + norethindrone) 1 tab PO daily. [Trade only: Tabs 1/0.5 mg and 0.5/0.1 mg estradiol/norethindrone acetate in calendar dial pack dispenser.] ▶L ♀X ▶− $$$ ■

ANGELIQ (estradiol + drospirenone) 1 tab PO daily. [Trade only: Tabs 1 mg estradiol/0.5 mg drospirenone.] ▶L ♀X ▶− $$$ ■

CLIMARA PRO (estradiol + levonorgestrel) 1 patch weekly. [Trade only: Transdermal 0.045/0.015 estradiol/levonorgestrel in mg/day, 4 patches/box.] ▶L ♀X ▶− $$$ ■

COMBIPATCH (estradiol + norethindrone, ✦Estalis) 1 patch two times per week. [Trade only: Transdermal patch 0.05 estradiol/0.14 norethindrone and 0.05 estradiol/0.25 norethindrone in mg/day, 8 patches/box.] ▶L ♀X ▶− $$$ ■

EEMT (esterified estrogens + methyltestosterone) 1 tab PO daily. [Generic only: Tabs 1.25 mg esterified estrogens/2.5 mg methyltestosterone.] ▶L ♀X ▶− $$$$ ■

ORAL CONTRACEPTIVES* ▶L CX	Estrogen (mcg)	Progestin (mg)
Monophasic		
Lo Loestrin Fe, Lo Minastrin Fe	10 ethinyl estradiol	1 norethindrone
Beyaz, Loryna, *Yaz*	20 ethinyl estradiol	3 drospirenone
Aviane, Falmina, Lessina, Lutera, Orsythia, Sronyx		0.1 levonorgestrel
Gildess Fe 1/20, Junel 1/20, Junel Fe 1/20, *Loestrin-21 1/20, Loestrin Fe 1/20,* Loestrin-24 Fe, Microgestin 1/20, Microgestin Fe 1/20, Minastrin 24 Fe		1 norethindrone
Generess Fe chewable	25 ethinyl estradiol	0.8 norethindrone
Desogen, Emoquette, *Ortho-Cept*	30 ethinyl estradiol	0.15 desogestrel
Safyral, Syeda, *Yasmin*		3 drospirenone
Altavera, Kurvelo, Levora, Marlissa, *Nordette,* Portia		0.15 levonorgestrel
Gildess Fe 1.5/30, 1.5/30, Junel 1.5/30, Junel 1.5/30 Fe, *Loestrin 1.5/30, Loestrin Fe 1.5/30,* Microgestin 1.5/30, Microgestin Fe 1.5/30		1.5 norethindrone
Cryselle, Elinest, Lo/Ovral, *Low-Ogestrel*		0.3 norgestrel
Kelnor 1/35, *Zovia 1/35E*	35 ethinyl estradiol	1 ethynodiol
Balziva, Briellyn, Femcon Fe, Gildagia, *Ovcon-35,* Philith		0.4 norethindrone
Brevicon, *Modicon,* Necon 0.5/35, Nortrel 0.5/35, Wera		0.5 norethindrone
Alyacen 1/35, Cyclafem 1/35, Dasetta 1/35, Necon 1/35, Norinyl 1+35, Nortrel 1/35, **Norethin** 1/35, *Ortho-Novum 1/35,* Pirmella 1/35		1 norethindrone
Mono-Linyah, *Ortho-Cyclen,* Previfem, Sprintec-28		0.25 norgestimate
Zovia 1/50E	50 ethinyl estradiol	1 ethynodiol
Ovcon-50		1 norethindrone
Ogestrel		0.5 norgestrel
Necon 1/50, *Norinyl 1+50*	50 mestranol	1 norethindrone
Progestin only		
Camila, Errin, Heather, Jencycla, Jolivette, *Micronor,* Nor-Q.D., Nora-BE	None	0.35 norethindrone
Biphasic (estrogen and progestin contents vary)		
Azurette, Kariva, *Mircette,* Viorele	20/10 ethinyl estradiol	0.15 desogestrel

(cont.)

Necon 10/11	35 ethinyl estradiol	0.5/1 norethindrone
Triphasic (estrogen and progestin contents vary)		
Estrostep Fe, Tri-Legest, Tri-Legest Fe	20/30/35 ethinyl estradiol	1 norethindrone
Caziant, *Cyclessa*, Velivet	25 ethinyl estradiol	0.1/0.125/0.150 desogestrel
Ortho Tri-Cyclen Lo		0.18/0.215/0.25 norgestimate
Enpresse, Levonest, Myzilra, *Trivora-28*	30/40/30 ethinyl estradiol	0.5/0.75/0.125 levonorgestrel
Alyacen 7/7/7, Cyclafem 7/7/7, Dasetta 7/7/7, Necon 7/7/7, Nortrel 7/7/7, *Ortho-Novum 7/7/7*, Primella 7/7/7	35 ethinyl estradiol	0.5/0.75/1 norethindrone
Aranelle, *Tri-Norinyl*		0.5/1/0.5 norethindrone
Ortho Tri-Cyclen, Tri-Estarylla, Tri-Linyah, Tri-Previfem, Tri-Sprintec		0.18/0.215/0.25 norgestimate
Quadphasic		
Natazia	3 mg/2 mg estradiol valerate	2/3/1 dienogest
Extended Cycle		
Lybrel†	20 ethinyl estradiol	0.09 levonorgestrel
LoSeasonique††	20/10 ethinyl estradiol	0.1 levonorgestrel
Quartette††	20/25/30/10 ethinyl estradiol	0.15 levonorgestrel
Introvale, Quasense, *Seasonale*	30 ethinyl estradiol	
Daysee, *Seasonique*††	30/10 ethinyl estradiol	

*All: Not recommended in smokers. Increases risk of thromboembolism, CVA, MI, hepatic neoplasia, and gallbladder disease. Nausea, breast tenderness, headache and breakthrough bleeding are common transient side effects. Effectiveness reduced by hepatic enzyme-inducing drugs such as certain anticonvulsants and barbiturates, rifampin, rifabutin, griseofulvin, and protease inhibitors. Coadministration with St. John's wort may decrease efficacy. Vomiting or diarrhea may also increase the risk of contraceptive failure. Consider an additional form of birth control in above circumstances. See product insert for instructions on missing doses.

Progestin only: Must be taken at the same time every day. Because much of the literature regarding OC adverse effects pertains mainly to estrogen/progestin combinations, the extent to which progestin-only contraceptives cause these effects is unclear. No significant interaction has been found with broad-spectrum antibiotics. The effect of St. John's wort is unclear. No placebo days, start new pack immediately after finishing current one. Available in 28-day packs. Readers may find the following website useful: www.managingcontraception.com.
† Approved for continuous use without a "pill-free" period.
†† 84 active pills and 7 ethinyl estradiol only pills.

EEMT H.S. (esterified estrogens + methyltestosterone) 1 tab PO daily. [Generic only: Tabs 0.625 mg esterified estrogens/1.25 mg methyltestosterone.] ▶L ♀X ▶– $$$ ■

FEMHRT (ethinyl estradiol + norethindrone) 1 tab PO daily. [Trade only: Tabs 5/1, 2.5/0.5 mcg ethinyl estradiol/mg norethindrone, 28/blister card.] ▶L ♀X ▶– $$$ ■

PREFEST (estradiol + norgestimate) 1 pink tab PO daily for 3 days followed by 1 white tab PO daily for 3 days, sequentially throughout the month. [Trade only: Tabs in 30-day blister packs 1 mg estradiol (15 pink), 1 mg estradiol/0.09 mg norgestimate (15 white).] ▶L ♀X ▶– $$$ ■

PREMPHASE (estrogens conjugated + medroxyprogesterone) 1 tab PO daily. [Trade only: Tabs in 28-day EZ-Dial dispensers: 0.625 mg conjugated estrogens (14), 0.625 mg/5 mg conjugated estrogens/medroxyprogesterone (14).] ▶L ♀X ▶– $$$ ■

PREMPRO (estrogens conjugated + medroxyprogesterone, ✦ Premplus) 1 tab PO daily. [Trade only: Tabs in 28-day EZ-Dial dispensers: 0.625 mg/5 mg, 0.625 mg/2.5 mg, 0.45 mg/1.5 mg (Prempro low dose), or 0.3 mg/1.5 mg conjugated estrogens/medroxyprogesterone.] ▶L ♀X ▶– $$$ ■

Labor Induction / Cervical Ripening

DINOPROSTONE (*PGE2, Prepidil, Cervidil, Prostin E2*) Cervical ripening: 1 syringe of gel placed directly into the cervical os for cervical ripening or 1 insert in the posterior fornix of the vagina. [Trade only: Gel (Prepidil) 0.5 mg/3 g syringe. Vaginal insert (Cervidil) 10 mg. Vaginal supps (Prostin E2) 20 mg.] ▶Lung ♀C ▶? $$$$$

MISOPROSTOL—OB (*PGE1, Cytotec*) Cervical ripening: 25 mcg intravaginally q 3 to 6 h (or 50 mcg q 6 h). First trimester pregnancy failure: 800 mcg intravaginally, repeat on day 3 if expulsion incomplete. Postpartum hemorrhage: 800 mcg PR. [Generic/Trade: Oral tabs 100, 200 mcg.] ▶LK ♀X ▶– $$ ■

OXYTOCIN (*Pitocin*) Labor induction: 10 units in 1000 mL NS (10 milliunits/mL), start at 6 to 12 mL/h (1 to 2 milliunits/min). Postpartum bleeding: 10 units IM or 10 to 40 units in 1000 mL NS IV, infuse 20 to 40 milliunits/min. ▶LK ♀? ▶– $

Ovulation Stimulants

NOTE: *Potentially serious adverse effects include DVT/PE, ovarian hyperstimulation syndrome, adnexal torsion, ovarian enlargement and cysts, and febrile reactions.*

CLOMIPHENE (*Clomid, Serophene*) Specialized dosing for ovulation induction. [Generic/Trade: Tabs 50 mg, scored.] ▶L ♀D ▶? $$$$$

Progestins

MEDROXYPROGESTERONE (*Provera*) 10 mg PO daily for last 10 to 12 days of month, or 2.5 to 5 mg PO daily. Secondary amenorrhea, abnormal uterine bleeding: 5 to 10 mg PO daily for 5 to 10 days. Endometrial hyperplasia: 10 to 30 mg PO daily. [Generic/Trade: Tabs 2.5, 5, 10 mg, scored.] ▶L ♀X ▶+ $

MEDROXYPROGESTERONE—INJECTABLE (*Depo-Provera, depo-subQ provera 104*) Contraception/endometriosis: 150 mg IM in deltoid or gluteus maximus or 104 mg SC in anterior thigh or abdomen q 13 weeks. ▶L ♀X ▶+ $ ■

MEGESTROL (*Megace, Megace ES*) Endometrial hyperplasia: 40 to 160 mg PO daily for 3 to 4 months. AIDS anorexia: 800 mg (20 mL) susp PO daily or 625 mg (5 mL) ES daily. [Generic/Trade: Tabs 20, 40 mg. Susp 40 mg/mL in 240 mL. Trade only: Megace ES susp 125 mg/mL (150 mL).] ▶L ♀D ▶? $$$$$

NORETHINDRONE (*Aygestin, Micronor, Nor-Q.D., Camila, Errin, Heather, Jolivette, Nora-BE*) Amenorrhea, abnormal uterine bleeding: 2.5 to 10 mg PO daily for 5 to 10 days during the 2nd half of the menstrual cycle. Endometriosis: 5 mg PO daily for 2 weeks. Increase by 2.5 mg q 2 weeks to 15 mg. [Generic/Trade: Tabs 0.35 mg and scored 5 mg.] ▶L ♀D/X ▶See notes $$ ■

PROGESTERONE GEL (*Crinone, Prochieve*) Secondary amenorrhea: 45 mg (4%) intravaginally every other day up to 6 doses. If no response, use 90 mg (8%) every other day up to 6 doses. Infertility: Special dosing. [Trade only: 4%, 8% single-use, prefilled applicators.] ▶Plasma ♀– ▶? $$$

PROGESTERONE MICRONIZED (*Prometrium*) 200 mg PO at bedtime 10 to 12 days per month or 100 mg at bedtime daily. Secondary amenorrhea: 400 mg PO at bedtime for 10 days. Contraindicated in peanut allergy. [Generic/Trade: Caps 100, 200 mg.] ▶L ♀B ▶+ $$

PROGESTERONE VAGINAL INSERT (*Endometrin*) Infertility: Special dosing. [Trade only: 100 mg vaginal insert.] ▶Plasma ♀– ▶? $$$$

Selective Estrogen Receptor Modulators

OSPEMIFENE (*Osphena*) Dyspareunia: 1 tab PO daily with food. [Trade only: Tabs 60 mg.] ▶L – ♀X ▶– $$$$ ■

RALOXIFENE (*Evista*) Osteoporosis prevention/treatment, breast cancer prevention: 60 mg PO daily. [Trade only: Tabs 60 mg.] ▶L ♀X ▶– $$$$ ■

TAMOXIFEN (*Nolvadex, Soltamox, Tamone*) Breast cancer prevention: 20 mg PO daily for 5 years. Breast cancer: 10 to 20 mg PO two times per day. [Generic/Trade: Tabs 10, 20 mg. Trade only (Soltamox): Sugar-free soln 10 mg/5 mL (150 mL).] ▶L ♀D ▶– $$ ■

Uterotonics

CARBOPROST (*Hemabate, 15-methyl-prostaglandin F2 alpha*) Refractory postpartum uterine bleeding: 250 mcg deep IM. ▶LK ♀C ▶? $$$

METHYLERGONOVINE (*Methergine*) Refractory postpartum uterine bleeding: 0.2 mg IM/PO three to four times per day prn. [Trade only: Tabs 0.2 mg.] ▶LK ♀C ▶– $$

Vaginitis Preparations

NOTE: See also STD/vaginitis table in antimicrobial section.

BORIC ACID   Resistant vulvovaginal candidiasis: 1 vaginal suppository at bedtime for 2 weeks. [No commercial preparation; must be compounded by pharmacist. Vaginal supps 600 mg in gelatin caps.]   ▶Not absorbed ♀? ▶– $

BUTOCONAZOLE   (*Gynazole, Mycelex-3*)   Vulvovaginal candidiasis: Mycelex-3: 1 applicatorful at bedtime for 3 to 6 days. Gynazole-1: 1 applicatorful intravaginally once at bedtime. [OTC: Trade only (Mycelex-3): 2% vaginal cream in 5 g prefilled applicators (3s), 20 g tube with applicators. Rx: Trade only (Gynazole-1): 2% vaginal cream in 5 g prefilled applicator.]   ▶LK ♀C ▶? $(OTC), $$$(Rx)

CLINDAMYCIN—VAGINAL   (*Cleocin, Clindesse,   ✦ Dalacin*)   Bacterial vaginosis: Cleocin: 1 applicatorful cream at bedtime for 7 days or 1 vaginal suppository at bedtime for 3 days. Clindesse: 1 applicatorful once. [Generic/ Trade: 2% vaginal cream in 40 g tube with 7 disposable applicators (Cleocin). Vaginal supp (Cleocin Ovules) 100 mg (3) with applicator. 2% vaginal cream in a single-dose prefilled applicator (Clindesse).]   ▶L ♀– ▶+ $$

CLOTRIMAZOLE—VAGINAL   (*Mycelex 7, Gyne-Lotrimin,   ✦ Canesten, Clotrimaderm*)   Vulvovaginal candidiasis: 1 applicatorful 1% cream at bedtime for 7 days. 1 applicatorful 2% cream at bedtime for 3 days. 1 vaginal suppository 100 mg at bedtime for 7 days. 200 mg suppository at bedtime for 3 days. [OTC Generic/Trade: 1% vaginal cream with applicator (some prefilled). 2% vaginal cream with applicator and 1% topical cream in some combination packs. OTC Trade only (Gyne-Lotrimin): Vaginal supp 100 mg (7), 200 mg (3) with applicators.]   ▶LK ♀B ▶? $

METRONIDAZOLE—VAGINAL   (*MetroGel-Vaginal, Vandazole*)   Bacterial vaginosis: 1 applicatorful at bedtime or two times per day for 5 days. [Generic/ Trade: 0.75% gel in 70 g tube with applicator.]   ▶LK ♀B ▶? $$

MICONAZOLE   (*Monistat, Femizol-M, M-Zole, Micozole, Monazole*)   Vulvovaginal candidiasis: 1 applicatorful at bedtime for 3 (4%) or 7 (2%) days. 100 mg vaginal suppository at bedtime for 7 days. 400 mg vaginal suppository at bedtime for 3 days. 1200 mg vaginal suppository once. [OTC Generic/Trade: 2% vaginal cream in 45 g with 1 applicator or 7 disposable applicators. Vaginal supp 100 mg (7). OTC Trade only: 400 mg (3), 1200 mg (1) with applicator. Generic/Trade: 4% vaginal cream in 25 g tubes or 3 prefilled applicators. Some in combination packs with 2% miconazole cream for external use.]   ▶LK ♀+ ▶? $

NYSTATIN—VAGINAL   (*Mycostatin,   ✦ Nyaderm*)   Vulvovaginal candidiasis: 1 vaginal tab at bedtime for 14 days. [Generic only: Vaginal tabs 100,000 units in 15s with applicator.]   ▶Not metabolized ♀A ▶? $$

TERCONAZOLE   (*Terazol*)   Vulvovaginal candidiasis: 1 applicatorful of 0.4% cream at bedtime for 7 days, or 1 applicatorful of 0.8% cream at bedtime for 3 days, or 80 mg vaginal suppository at bedtime for 3 days. [All forms supplied with applicators: Generic/Trade: Vaginal cream 0.4% (Terazol 7) in 45 g tube, 0.8% (Terazol 3) in 20 g tube. Vaginal supp (Terazol 3) 80 mg (#3).]   ▶LK ♀C ▶– $$

TIOCONAZOLE   (*Monistat 1-Day, Vagistat-1*)   Vulvovaginal candidiasis: 1 applicatorful of 6.5% ointment intravaginally at bedtime single-dose. [OTC Trade only: Vaginal ointment: 6.5% (300 mg) in 4.6 g prefilled single-dose applicator.]   ▶Not absorbed ♀C ▶– $

Other OB/GYN Agents

DANAZOL (*Danocrine*, ✦*Cyclomen*) Endometriosis: Start 400 mg PO two times per day, then titrate downward to maintain amenorrhea for 3 to 6 months. Fibrocystic breast disease: 100 to 200 mg PO two times per day for 4 to 6 months. [Generic only: Caps 50, 100, 200 mg.] ▶L ♀X▶– $$$$$

HYDROXYPROGESTERONE CAPROATE (*Makena*) Specialized dosing (1 mL IM weekly) to reduce risk of preterm birth. [Trade only. 5 mL MDV (250 mg/mL) hydroxyprogesterone caproate in castor oil soln.] ▶L + glucuronidation ♀B ▶? $$$$$

MIFEPRISTONE (*Mifeprex*, *RU-486*) Termination of pregnancy, up to 49 days: 600 mg PO followed by 400 mcg misoprostol on day 3, if abortion not confirmed. [Trade only: Tabs 200 mg.] ▶L ♀X ▶? $$$$$ ■

PREMESIS-RX (pyridoxine + folic acid + cyanocobalamin + calcium carbonate) Pregnancy-induced nausea: 1 tab PO daily. [Trade only: Tabs 75 mg vitamin B6 (pyridoxine), sustained-release, 12 mcg vitamin B12 (cyanocobalamin), 1 mg folic acid, and 200 mg calcium carbonate.] ▶L ♀A ▶+ $$

RHO IMMUNE GLOBULIN (*HyperRHO S/D*, *MICRhoGAM*, *RhoGAM*, *Rhophylac*, *WinRho SDF*) Prevention of hemolytic disease of the newborn if mother Rh– and baby is or might be Rh+: 300 mcg vial IM to mother at 28 weeks' gestation followed by a 2nd dose within 72 h of delivery. Microdose (50 mcg, MICRhoGAM) is appropriate if spontaneous abortion less than 12 weeks' gestation. ▶L ♀C ▶? $$$$$

DRUGS GENERALLY ACCEPTED AS SAFE IN PREGNANCY (selected)

Analgesics	acetaminophen, codeine*, meperidine*, methadone*, oxycodone*
Antimicrobials	azithromycin, cephalosporins, clotrimazole, erythromycins (not estolate), metronidazole, penicillins, permethrin, nitrofurantoin***, nystatin
Antivirals	acyclovir, famciclovir, valacyclovir
CV	hydralazine*, labetalol, methyldopa, nifedipine
Derm	benzoyl peroxide, clindamycin, erythromycin
Endo	insulin, levothyroxine, liothyronine
ENT	chlorpheniramine, diphenhydramine, dextromethorphan, guaifenesin, nasal steroids, nasal cromolyn
GI	antacids*, bisacodyl, cimetidine, docusate, doxylamine, famotidine, lactulose, loperamide, meclizine, metoclopramide, nizatidine, ondansetron, psyllium, ranitidine, simethicone, trimethobenzamide
Heme	heparin, low molecular wt heparins
Psych	bupropion, buspirone, desipramine, doxepin
Pulmonary	beclomethasone, budesonide, cromolyn, montelukast, nedocromil, prednisone**, short-acting inhaled beta-2 agonists, theophylline

*Except if used long-term or in high dose at term.
**Except 1st trimester.
***Contraindicated at term and during labor and delivery.

ONCOLOGY

ALKYLATING AGENTS altretamine (*Hexalen*), bendamustine (*Treanda*), busulfan (*Myleran, Busulfex*), carmustine (*BCNU, BiCNU, Gliadel*), chlorambucil (*Leukeran*), cyclophosphamide (*Cytoxan, Neosar*), dacarbazine (*DTIC-Dome*), ifosfamide (*Ifex*), lomustine (*CeeNu, CCNU*), mechlorethamine (*Mustargen*), melphalan (*Alkeran*), procarbazine (*Matulane*), streptozocin (*Zanosar*), temozolomide (*Temodar, ◆Temodal*), thiotepa (*Thioplex*). **ANTIBIOTICS:** bleomycin (*Blenoxane*), dactinomycin (*Cosmegen*), daunorubicin (*Cerubidine*), doxorubicin liposomal (*Doxil, ◆Caelyx, Myocet*), doxorubicin non-liposomal (*Adriamycin, Rubex*), epirubicin (*Ellence, ◆Pharmorubicin*), idarubicin (*Idamycin*), mitomycin (*Mutamycin, Mitomycin-C*), mitoxantrone (*Novantrone*), valrubicin (*Valstar, ◆Valtaxin*). **ANTIMETABOLITES:** azacitidine (*Vidaza*), capecitabine (*Xeloda*), cladribine (*Leustatin, chlorodeoxyadenosine*), clofarabine (*Clolar*), cytarabine (*Cytosar, AraC*), cytarabine liposomal (*Depo-Cyt*),decitabine (*Dacogen*), floxuridine (*FUDR*), fludarabine (*Fludara*), fluorouracil (*Adrucil, 5-FU*), gemcitabine (*Gemzar*), hydroxyurea (*Hydrea, Droxia*), mercaptopurine (*6-MP, Purinethol*), methotrexate (*Rheumatrex, Trexall*), nelarabine (*Arranon*), pemetrexed (*Alimta*), pentostatin (*Nipent*), pralatrexate (*Folotyn*), thioguanine (*Tabloid, ◆Lanvis*). **CYTOPROTECTIVE AGENTS:** amifostine (*Ethyol*), dexrazoxane (*Zinecard, Totect*), leucovorin (folinic acid), levoleucovorin (*Fusilev*), mesna (*Mesnex, ◆Uromitexan*), palifermin (*Kepivance*). **HORMONES:** anastrozole (*Arimidex*), bicalutamide (*Casodex*), cyproterone, (*Androcur, Androcur Depot*), degarelix (*Firmagon*), estramustine (*Emcyt*), exemestane (*Aromasin*), flutamide (*Eulexin, ◆Euflex*), fulvestrant (*Faslodex*), goserelin (*Zoladex*), histrelin (*Vantas, Supprelin LA*), letrozole (*Femara*), leuprolide (*Eligard, Lupron, Lupron Depot, Lupron Depot-Ped*), nilutamide (*Nilandron*), raloxifene (*Evista*), tamoxifen (*Nolvadex*), toremifene (*Fareston*), triptorelin (*Trelstar Depot*). **IMMUNOMODULATORS:** aldesleukin (*Proleukin, interleukin-2*), alemtuzumab (*Campath, ◆MabCampath*), BCG (*Bacillus of Calmette & Guerin, Pacis, TheraCys, Tice BCG, ◆OncoTICE, ◆Immucyst*), bevacizumab (*Avastin*), cetuximab (*Erbitux*), denileukin (*Ontak*), everolimus (*Afinitor*), ibritumomab (*Zevalin*), interferon alfa-2b (*Intron-A*), lenalidomide (*Revlimid*), ofatumumab (*Arzerra*), panitumumab (*Vectibix*), rituximab (*Rituxan*), temsirolimus (*Torisel*), thalidomide (*Thalomid*) tositumomab (*Bexxar*), trastuzumab (*Herceptin*). **MITOTIC INHIBITORS:** Cabazitaxel (*Jevtana*), Docetaxel (*Taxotere*), eribulin (*Halaven*), ixabepilone (*Ixempra*), paclitaxel (*Taxol, Abraxane, Onxol*), vinblastine (*Velban, VLB*), vincristine (*Oncovin, Vincasar, VCR*), vinorelbine (*Navelbine*). **PLATINUM-CONTAINING AGENTS:** carboplatin (*Paraplatin*), cisplatin (*Platinol-AQ*), oxaliplatin (*Eloxatin*). **RADIOPHARMACEUTICALS:** samarium 153 (*Quadramet*), strontium-89 (*Metastron*). **TOPOISOMERASE INHIBITORS:** etoposide (*VP-16, Etopophos, Toposar, VePesid*), irinotecan (*Camptosar*), teniposide (*Vumon, VM-26*), topotecan (*Hycamtin*). **MISCELLANEOUS:** arsenic trioxide (*Trisenox*), asparaginase (*Elspar, ◆Kidrolase*), bexarotene (*Targretin*), bortezomib (*Velcade*), dasatinib (*Sprycel*), erlotinib (*Tarceva*) gefitinib (*Iressa*), imatinib (*Gleevec*), lapatinib (*Tykerb*), mitotane (*Lysodren*), nilotinib (*Tasigna*), pazopanib (*Votrient*), pegaspargase (*Oncaspar*), porfimer (*Photofrin*), rasburicase (*Elitek*), romidepsin (*Istodax*), sorafenib (*Nexavar*), sunitinib (*Sutent*), tretinoin (*Vesanoid*), vorinostat (*Zolinza*).

OPHTHALMOLOGY

NOTE: *Most eye medications can be administered 1 gtt at a time despite common manufacturer recommendations of 1 to 2 gtts concurrently. Even a single gtt is typically more than the eye can hold, and thus a 2nd gtt is wasteful and increases the possibility of systemic toxicity. If 2 gtts of the medication are desired, separate each gtt by at least 5 min.*

Antiallergy—Decongestants & Combinations

NAPHAZOLINE (*Albalon, All Clear, AK-Con, Naphcon, Clear Eyes*) 1 to 2 gtts in each affected eye four times per day for up to 3 days. [OTC Generic/Trade: Soln 0.012, 0.025% (15, 30 mL). Rx Generic/Trade: 0.1% (15 mL).] ▶? ♀C ▶? $

NAPHCON-A (*naphazoline + pheniramine, Visine-A*) 1 gtt in each affected eye four times per day prn for up to 3 days. [OTC Trade only: Soln 0.025% + 0.3% (15 mL).] ▶L ♀C ▶? $

VASOCON-A (*naphazoline + antazoline*) 1 gtt in each affected eye four times per day prn for up to 3 days. [OTC Trade only: Soln 0.05% + 0.5% (15 mL).] ▶L ♀C ▶? $

Antiallergy—Dual Antihistamine & Mast Cell Stabilizer

ALCAFTADINE (*Lastacaft*) 1 gtt in each eye daily. [Soln 0.25%, 3 mL.] ▶not absorbed – ♀B ▶? $$$

AZELASTINE—OPHTHALMIC (*Optivar*) 1 gtt in each affected eye two times per day. [Trade/Generic: Soln 0.05% (6 mL).] ▶L ♀C ▶? $$$

EPINASTINE (*Elestat*) 1 gtt in each affected eye two times per day. [Trade only: Soln 0.05% (5 mL).] ▶K ♀C ▶? $$$$

KETOTIFEN—OPHTHALMIC (*Alaway, Zaditor*) 1 gtt in each affected eye q 8 to 12 h. [OTC Generic/Trade: Soln 0.025% (5 mL, 10 mL).] ▶Minimal absorption ♀C ▶? $

OLOPATADINE (*Pataday, Patanol*) 1 gtt of 0.1% soln in each affected eye two times per day (Patanol) or 1 gtt of 0.2% soln in each affected eye daily (Pataday). [Trade only: Soln 0.1% (5 mL, Patanol), 0.2% (2.5 mL, Pataday).] ▶K ♀C ▶? $$$$

Antiallergy—Pure Antihistamines

BEPOTASTINE (*Bepreve*) 1 gtt in each affected eye two times per day. [Trade only: Soln 1.5% (2.5, 5, 10 mL)] ▶L (but minimal absorption) – ♀C ▶? $$$

EMEDASTINE (*Emadine*) 1 gtt in each affected eye daily to four times per day. [Trade only: Soln 0.05% (5 mL).] ▶L ♀B ▶? $$$

LEVOCABASTINE—OPHTHALMIC (*Livostin*) 1 gtt in each affected eye two to four times per day for 2 weeks. [Trade only: Susp 0.05% (5, 10 mL).] ▶Minimal absorption ♀C ▶? $$$

Antiallergy—Pure Mast Cell Stabilizers

CROMOLYN—OPHTHALMIC (*Crolom, Opticrom*) 1 to 2 gtts in each affected eye four to six times per day. [Generic/Trade: Soln 4% (10 mL).] ▶LK ♀B ▶? $$

LODOXAMIDE (*Alomide*) 1 to 2 gtts in each affected eye four times per day. [Trade only: Soln 0.1% (10 mL).] ▶K ♀B ▶? $$$

NEDOCROMIL—OPHTHALMIC (*Alocril*) 1 to 2 gtts in each affected eye two times per day. [Trade only: Soln 2% (5 mL).] ▶L ♀B ▶? $$$

PEMIROLAST (*Alamast*) 1 to 2 gtts in each affected eye four times per day. [Trade only: Soln 0.1% (10 mL).] ▶? ♀C ▶? $$$

Antibacterials—Aminoglycosides

GENTAMICIN—OPHTHALMIC (*Garamycin, Genoptic, Gentak, ✦ Diogent*) 1 to 2 gtts in each affected eye q 2 to 4 h; ½ inch ribbon of ointment two to three times per day. [Generic/Trade: Soln 0.3% (5, 15 mL). Ointment 0.3% (3.5 g tube).] ▶K ♀C ▶? $

TOBRAMYCIN—OPHTHALMIC (*Tobrex*) 1 to 2 gtts in each affected eye q 1 to 4 h or ½ inch ribbon of ointment q 3 to 4 h or two or three times per day. [Generic/Trade: Soln 0.3% (5 mL). Trade only: Ointment 0.3% (3.5 g tube).] ▶K ♀B ▶– $

Antibacterials—Fluoroquinolones

BESIFLOXACIN (*Besivance*) 1 gtt in each affected eye three times per day for 7 days. [Trade: Soln 0.6% (5 mL).] ▶LK ♀C ▶? $$$

CIPROFLOXACIN—OPHTHALMIC (*Ciloxan*) 1 to 2 gtts in each affected eye q 1 to 6 h or ½ inch ribbon ointment two to three times per day. [Generic/Trade: Soln 0.3% (2.5, 5, 10 mL). Trade only: Ointment 0.3% (3.5 g tube).] ▶LK ♀C ▶? $$

GATIFLOXACIN—OPHTHALMIC (*Zymaxid, ✦ Zymar*) 1 to 2 gtts in each affected eye q 2 h while awake (up to 8 times per day) on days 1 and 2, then 1 to 2 gtts four times per day on days 3 to 7. [Trade only: Soln 0.5% (5 mL).] ▶K ♀C ▶? $$$

LEVOFLOXACIN—OPHTHALMIC (*Iquix, Quixin*) Quixin: 1 to 2 gtts in each affected eye q 2 h while awake (up to 8 times per day) on days 1 and 2, then 1 to 2 gtts q 4 h (up to four times per day) on days 3 to 7. Iquix: 1 to 2 gtts q 30 min to 2 h while awake and q 4 to 6 h overnight on days 1 to 3, then 1 to 2 gtts q 1 to 4 h while awake on day 4 to completion of therapy. [Generic only: Soln 0.5% (5 mL)] ▶KL ♀C ▶? $$$

MOXIFLOXACIN—OPHTHALMIC (*Vigamox, Moxeza*) 1 gtt in each affected eye three times per day for 7 days (Vigamox) or 1 gtt in each affected eye two times per day for 7 days (Moxeza). [Trade only: Soln 0.5% (3 mL, Vigamox and Moxeza).] ▶LK ♀C ▶? $$$

OFLOXACIN—OPHTHALMIC (*Ocuflox*) 1 to 2 gtts in each affected eye q 1 to 6 h for 7 to 10 days. [Generic/Trade: Soln 0.3% (5, 10 mL).] ▶LK ♀C ▶? $$

Antibacterials—Other

AZITHROMYCIN—OPHTHALMIC (***Azasite***) 1 gtt in each affected eye two times per day for 2 days, then 1 gtt once daily for 5 more days. [Trade only: Soln 1% (2.5 mL).] ▶L ♀B ▶? $$$

BACITRACIN—OPHTHALMIC (***AK Tracin***) Apply ¼ to ½ inch ribbon of ointment in each affected eye q 3 to 4 h or two to four times per day for 7 to 10 days. [Generic/Trade: Ointment 500 units/g (3.5 g tube).] ▶Minimal absorption ♀C ▶? $

ERYTHROMYCIN—OPHTHALMIC (***Ilotycin, AK-Mycin***) ½ inch ribbon of ointment in each affected eye q 3 to 4 h or two to six times per day. [Generic only: Ointment 0.5% (1, 3.5 g tube).] ▶L ♀B ▶+ $

NEOSPORIN OINTMENT—OPHTHALMIC (neomycin + bacitracin + polymyxin) ½ inch ribbon of ointment in each affected eye q 3 to 4 h for 7 to 10 days or ½ inch ribbon 2 to 3 times per day for mild to moderate infection. [Generic only: Ointment. (3.5 g tube).] ▶K ♀C ▶? $

NEOSPORIN SOLUTION—OPHTHALMIC (neomycin + polymyxin + gramicidin) 1 to 2 gtts in each affected eye q 4 to 6 h for 7 to 10 days. [Generic/Trade: Soln (10 mL).] ▶KL ♀C ▶? $$

POLYSPORIN—OPHTHALMIC (polymyxin + bacitracin) ½ inch ribbon of ointment in each affected eye q 3 to 4 h for 7 to 10 days or ½ inch ribbon two to three times per day for mild to moderate infection. [Generic only: Ointment (3.5 g tube).] ▶K ♀C ▶? $$

POLYTRIM—OPHTHALMIC (polymyxin + trimethoprim) 1 to 2 gtts in each affected eye q 4 to 6 h (up to 6 gtts per day) for 7 to 10 days. [Generic/Trade: Soln (10 mL).] ▶KL ♀C ▶? $$

SULFACETAMIDE—OPHTHALMIC (***Bleph-10, Sulf-10***) 1 to 2 gtts in each affected eye q 2 to 6 h for 7 to 10 days or ½ inch ribbon of ointment q 3 to 8 h for 7 to 10 days. [Generic/Trade: Soln 10% (15 mL), Ointment 10% (3.5 g tube). Generic only: Soln 30% (15 mL).] ▶K ♀C ▶– $

Antiviral Agents

GANCICLOVIR (***Zirgan***) Herpetic keratitis: 1 gtt five times per day (approximately q 3 h) until ulcer heals, then 1 gtt 3 times/day for 7 days. [Trade only: Gel 0.15% (5g).] ▶Minimal absorption ♀C ▶? $$$$

TRIFLURIDINE (***Viroptic***) Herpetic keratitis: 1 gtt q 2 to 4 h for 7 to 14 days, max 9 gtts per day and max of 21 days of therapy. [Generic/Trade Soln 1% (7.5 mL).] ▶Minimal absorption ♀C ▶– $$$

Corticosteroid & Antibacterial Combinations

NOTE: *Recommend that only ophthalmologists or optometrists prescribe due to infection, cataract, corneal/scleral perforation, and glaucoma risk from prolonged use. Monitor intraocular pressure.*

BLEPHAMIDE (prednisolone—ophthalmic + sulfacetamide) 2 gtts in each affected eye q 4 h and at bedtime or ½ inch ribbon to lower conjunctival sac 3

(cont.)

to 4 times per day and at bedtime. [Generic/Trade: Soln/Susp (5, 10 mL), Trade only: Ointment (3.5 g tube).] ▶KL ♀C ▶? $

CORTISPORIN—OPHTHALMIC (neomycin + polymyxin + hydrocortisone—ophthalmic) 1 to 2 gtts or ½ inch ribbon of ointment in each affected eye q 3 to 4 h or more frequently prn. [Generic only: Susp (7.5 mL), Ointment (3.5 g tube).] ▶LK ♀C ▶? $

FML-S LIQUIFILM (prednisolone—ophthalmic + sulfacetamide) 1 to 2 gtts in each affected eye q 1 to 8 h. [Trade only: Susp (10 mL).] ▶KL ♀C ▶? $$

MAXITROL (dexamethasone—ophthalmic + neomycin + polymyxin) Small amount (about ½ inch) ointment in affected eye 3 to 4 times per day or at bedtime as an adjunct with gtts. 1 to 2 gtts susp into affected eye 4 to 6 times daily; in severe disease, gtts may be used hourly and tapered to discontinuation. [Generic/Trade: Susp (5 mL), Ointment (3.5 g tube).] ▶KL ♀C ▶? $

PRED G (prednisolone—ophthalmic + gentamicin) 1 to 2 gtts in each affected eye two to four times per day or ½ inch ribbon of ointment one to three times per day. [Trade only: Susp (2, 5, 10 mL), Ointment (3.5 g tube).] ▶KL ♀C ▶? $$

TOBRADEX (tobramycin + dexamethasone—ophthalmic) 1 to 2 gtts in each affected eye q 2 to 6 h or ½ inch ribbon of ointment three to four times per day. [Trade/generic: Susp (tobramycin 0.3%/dexamethasone 0.1%, 2.5, 5, 10 mL) Trade: Ointment (tobramycin 0.3%/dexamethasone 0.1%, 3.5 g tube).] ▶L ♀C ▶? $$$

TOBRADEX ST (tobramycin + dexamethasone—ophthalmic) 1 gtt in each affected eye q 2 to 6 h. [Trade only: Tobramycin 0.3%/dexamethasone 0.05%: Susp (2.5, 5, 10 mL).] ▶L ♀C ▶? $$$

VASOCIDIN (prednisolone—ophthalmic + sulfacetamide) 1 to 2 gtts in each affected eye q 1 to 8 h or ½ inch ribbon of ointment one to four times per day. [Generic only: Soln (5, 10 mL).] ▶KL ♀C ▶? $$

ZYLET (loteprednol + tobramycin) 1 to 2 gtts in each affected eye q 1 to 2 h for 1 to 2 days then 1 to 2 gtts q 4 to 6 h. [Trade only: Susp 0.5% loteprednol + 0.3% tobramycin (2.5, 5, 10 mL).] ▶LK ♀C ▶? $$$

Corticosteroids

NOTE: *Recommend that only ophthalmologists or optometrists prescribe due to increased risk of infection, cataract, corneal/scleral perforation, and glaucoma risk from prolonged use. Monitor intraocular pressure.*

DIFLUPREDNATE (*Durezol*) Inflammation and pain associated with ocular surgery: 1 gtt into affected eye four times per day, beginning 24 h after surgery for 2 weeks, then 1 gtt into affected eye two times per day for 1 week, then taper based on response. Endogenous anterior uveitis: 1 gtt into affected eye 4 times daily for 14 days followed by tapering as indicated. [Trade only: Ophthalmic emulsion 0.05% (2.5, 5 mL).] ▶Not absorbed ♀C ▶? $$$$

FLUOROMETHOLONE (*FML, FML Forte, Flarex*) 1 to 2 gtts in each affected eye q 1 to 12 h or ½ inch ribbon of ointment q 4 to 24 h. [Trade only: Susp 0.1% (5, 10, 15 mL), 0.25% (2, 5, 10, 15 mL), Ointment 0.1% (3.5 g tube).] ▶L ♀C ▶? $$

LOTEPREDNOL (*Alrex, Lotemax*) 1 to 2 gtts in each affected eye four times per day or ½ inch ointment four times daily beginning 24 h after surgery. [Trade only: Susp 0.2% (Alrex 5, 10 mL), 0.5% (Lotemax 2.5, 5, 10, 15 mL). Ointment 0.5% 3.5 g, Gel drop 0.5% (Lotemax 10 mL).] ▶L ♀C ▶? $$$

PREDNISOLONE—OPHTHALMIC (*Pred Forte, Pred Mild, Inflamase Forte, Econopred Plus, ✦ Diopred*) Soln: 1 to 2 gtts in each affected eye (up to q 1 h during day and q 2 h at night); when response observed, then 1 gtt in each affected eye q 4 h, then 1 gtt three to four times per day. Susp: 1 to 2 gtts in each affected eye two to four times per day. [Generic/Trade: Soln, Susp 1% (5, 10, 15 mL). Trade only (Pred Mild): Susp 0.12% (5, 10 mL), Susp (Pred Forte) 1% (1 mL).] ▶L ♀C ▶? $

RIMEXOLONE (*Vexol*) 1 to 2 gtts in each affected eye q 1 to 6 h. [Trade only: Susp 1% (5, 10 mL).] ▶L ♀C ▶? $$

Glaucoma Agents—Beta-Blockers

NOTE: *Use caution in cardiac conditions and asthma.*

BETAXOLOL—OPHTHALMIC (*Betoptic, Betoptic S*) 1 to 2 gtts in each affected eye two times per day. [Trade only: Susp 0.25% (10, 15 mL). Generic only: Soln 0.5% (5, 10, 15 mL).] ▶LK ♀C ▶? $$

CARTEOLOL—OPHTHALMIC (*Ocupress*) 1 gtt in each affected eye two times per day. [Generic only: Soln 1% (5, 10, 15 mL).] ▶KL ♀C ▶? $

LEVOBUNOLOL (*Betagan*) 1 to 2 gtts in each affected eye one to two times per day. [Generic/Trade: Soln 0.25% (5, 10 mL), 0.5% (5, 10 mL).] ▶? ♀C ▶– $$

METIPRANOLOL (*Optipranolol*) 1 gtt in each affected eye two times per day. [Generic/Trade: Soln 0.3% (5, 10 mL).] ▶? ♀C ▶? $$

TIMOLOL—OPHTHALMIC (*Betimol, Timoptic, Timoptic XE, Istalol, Timoptic Ocudose*) 1 gtt in each affected eye two times per day. Timoptic XE, Istalol: 1 gtt in each affected eye daily. [Generic/Trade: Soln 0.25, 0.5% (5, 10, 15 mL), Preservative-free soln (Timoptic Ocudose) 0.25% (0.2 mL), Gel-forming soln (Timoptic XE) 0.25, 0.5% (5 mL).] ▶LK ♀C ▶+ $$

Glaucoma Agents—Carbonic Anhydrase Inhibitors

NOTE: *Sulfonamide derivatives; verify absence of sulfa allergy before prescribing.*

BRINZOLAMIDE (*Azopt*) 1 gtt in each affected eye three times per day. [Trade only: Susp 1% (10, 15 mL).] ▶LK ♀C ▶? $$$

DORZOLAMIDE (*Trusopt*) 1 gtt in each affected eye three times per day. [Generic/Trade: Soln 2% (10 mL).] ▶KL ♀C ▶– $$$

METHAZOLAMIDE 25 to 50 mg PO daily (up to three times per day). [Generic only: Tabs 25, 50 mg.] ▶LK ♀C ▶? $$

Glaucoma Agents—Combinations and Other

COMBIGAN (brimonidine + timolol) 1 gtt in each affected eye two times per day. Contraindicated in children younger than 2 yo. [Trade only: Soln brimonidine 0.2% + timolol 0.5% (5, 10 mL).] ▶LK ♀C ▶– $$$

COSOPT (dorzolamide + timolol) 1 gtt in each affected eye two times per day. [Generic/Trade: Soln dorzolamide 2% + timolol 0.5% (5, 10 mL). Trade only: Soln preservative free dorzolamide 2% + timolol 0.5% (30 single use containers).] ▶LK ♀D ▶– $$$

SIMBRINZA (brinzolamide + brimonidine) 1 gtt in each affected eye three times per day. [Trade: brinzolamide 1% and brimonidine 0.2% 8 mL.] ▶LK – ♀C ▶? $$$$

UNOPROSTONE (Rescula) 1 gtt in each affect eye two times a day. [Trade: 0.15% (5 mL).] ▶esterases – ♀C ▶? $$$

Glaucoma Agents—Miotics

PILOCARPINE—OPHTHALMIC (Pilopine HS, Isopto Carpine, ✦ Diocarpine, Akarpine) 1 gtt in each affected eye up to four times per day or ½ inch ribbon of gel at bedtime. [Generic/Trade: Soln 0.5% (15 mL), 1% (2 mL, 15 mL), 2% (2 mL, 15 mL), 4% (2 mL, 15 mL), 6% (15 mL). Trade only (Pilopine HS): Gel 4% (4 g tube).] ▶Plasma ♀C ▶? $

Glaucoma Agents—Prostaglandin Analogs

BIMATOPROST (Lumigan, Latisse) Glaucoma (Lumigan): 1 gtt to affected eye(s) at bedtime. Hypotrichosis of the eyelashes (Latisse): 1 gtt to eyelashes at bedtime. [Trade only: Soln 0.01%, 0.03% (Lumigan, 2.5, 5, 7.5 mL), (Latisse, 3 mL with 60 sterile, disposable applicators).] ▶LK ♀C ▶? $$$

LATANOPROST (Xalatan) 1 gtt in each affected eye at bedtime. [Generic/Trade: Soln 0.005% (2.5 mL).] ▶LK ♀C ▶? $$$

TAFLUPROST (Zioptan) 1 gtt in each affect eye q pm. [Trade: Soln 0.0015%] ▶L – ♀C ▶? $$$

TRAVOPROST (Travatan Z) 1 gtt in each affected eye at bedtime. [Trade only: benzalkonium chloride-free (Travatan Z) 0.004% (2.5, 5 mL). Generic only: travoprost 0.004% (2.5 mL, 5 mL)] ▶L ♀C ▶? $$$$

Glaucoma Agents—Sympathomimetics

BRIMONIDINE (Alphagan P, ✦ Alphagan) 1 gtt in each affected eye three times per day. [Trade only: Soln 0.1% (5, 10, 15 mL). Generic/Trade: Soln 0.15% (5, 10, 15 mL). Generic only: Soln 0.2% (5, 10, 15 mL).] ▶LK ♀B ▶? $$

Mydriatics & Cycloplegics

ATROPINE—OPHTHALMIC (Isopto Atropine, Atropine Care) 1 to 2 gtts in each affected eye before procedure or daily to four times per day or ⅛ to ¼

(cont.)

inch ointment before procedure or one to three times per day. Cycloplegia may last up to 5 to 10 days and mydriasis may last up to 7 to 14 days. [Generic/Trade: Soln 1% (2, 5, 15 mL). Generic only: Ointment 1% (3.5 g tube).] ▶L ♀C ▶+ $

CYCLOPENTOLATE (*AK-Pentolate, Cyclogyl, Pentolair*) 1 to 2 gtts in each affected eye for 1 to 2 doses before procedure. Cycloplegia may last 6 to 24 h; mydriasis may last 1 day. [Generic/Trade: Soln 1% (2, 15 mL). Trade only (Cyclogyl): 0.5% (15 mL), 1% (5 mL), 2% (2, 5, 15 mL).] ▶? ♀C ▶? $

HOMATROPINE (*Isopto Homatropine*) 1 to 2 gtts in each affected eye before procedure or two to three times per day. Cycloplegia and mydriasis last 1 to 3 days. [Trade only: Soln 2% (5 mL), 5% (15 mL). Generic/Trade: Soln 5% (5 mL).] ▶? ♀C ▶? $

PHENYLEPHRINE—OPHTHALMIC (*AK-Dilate, Altafrin, Mydfrin, Refresh*) 1 to 2 gtts in each affected eye before procedure or three to four times per day. No cycloplegia; mydriasis may last up to 5 h. Red eyes: 1 or 2 gtts (0.12%) in affected eyes up to four times daily. [Rx Generic/Trade: Soln 2.5% (2, 3, 5, 15 mL), 10% (5 mL). OTC Trade only (Altafrin and Refresh): Soln 0.12% (15 mL).] ▶Plasma, L ♀C ▶? $

TROPICAMIDE (*Mydriacyl, Tropicacyl*) 1 to 2 gtts in each affected eye before procedure. Mydriasis may last 6 h. [Generic/Trade: Soln 0.5% (15 mL), 1% (3, 15 mL). Generic only: Soln 1% (2 mL).] ▶? ♀C ▶? $

Non-Steroidal Anti-Inflammatories

BROMFENAC—OPHTHALMIC (*Bromday, Prolensa*) 1 gtt in each affected eye once daily beginning 1 day prior to surgery and continuing for 14 days after surgery (Bromday, Prolensa) or twice daily (generic). [Trade only: Soln 0.09% (Bromday) 1.7 mL, 3.4 mL (two 1.7 mL twin pack), Soln 0.07% (Prolensa) 1.6, 3 mL. Generic only: Soln 0.09% (twice-daily soln 2.5, 5 mL).] ▶Minimal absorption ♀C, D (3rd trimester) ▶? $$$$$

DICLOFENAC—OPHTHALMIC (*Voltaren*, ✦ *Voltaren Ophtha*) 1 gtt in each affected eye one to four times per day. [Generic/Trade: Soln 0.1% (2.5, 5 mL).] ▶L ♀C ▶? $$$

KETOROLAC—OPHTHALMIC (*Acular, Acular LS, Acuvail*) Acular, Acular LS: 1 gtt in each affected eye four times per day. Acuvail: 1 gtt in each affected eye twice daily. [Generic/Trade: Soln (Acular LS) 0.4% (5 mL). Trade only: Acular 0.5% (3, 5, 10 mL), preservative-free Acuvail 0.45% unit dose (0.4 mL).] ▶L ♀C ▶? $$$$

NEPAFENAC (*Nevanac, Ilevro*) 1 gtt in each affected eye three times per day for 2 weeks. [Trade only: Susp 0.1% (Nevanac-3 mL). Susp 0.3% (Ilevro 1.7ml)] ▶Minimal absorption ♀C, D in 3rd trimester ▶? $$$$

Other Ophthalmologic Agents

AFLIBERCEPT (*Eylea*) 2 mg (0.05 mL) intravitreal injection q 4 weeks for 3 months, then 2 mg (0.05 mL) intravitreal injection q 8 weeks. [Sterile powder for reconstitution.] ▶minimal absorption − ♀C ▶− $$$$$

ARTIFICIAL TEARS (*Tears Naturale, Hypotears, Refresh Tears, GenTeal, Systane*) 1 to 2 gtts prn. [OTC Generic/Trade: Soln (15, 30 mL, among others).] ▶Minimal absorption ♀A ▶+ $

CYCLOSPORINE—OPHTHALMIC (*Restasis*) 1 gtt in each eye q 12 h. [Trade only: Emulsion 0.05% (0.4 mL single-use vials).] ▶Minimal absorption ♀C ▶? $$$$

CYSTEAMINE (*Cystaran*) Corneal cysteine crystal accumulation: 1 gtt in each eye q waking h. [Trade: 0.44% soln, 15 mL.] ▶minimal absorption – ♀C ▶? $$$$$

HYDROXYPROPYL CELLULOSE (*Lacrisert*) Moderate to severe dry eyes: 1 insert in each eye daily. Some patients may require twice daily use. [Trade only: Ocular insert 5 mg.] ▶Minimal absorption ♀+ ▶+ $$$

LIDOCAINE—OPHTHALMIC (*Akten*) Do not prescribe for unsupervised or prolonged use. Corneal toxicity and ocular infections may occur with repeated use. 2 gtts before procedure, repeat prn. [Generic only: Gel 3.5% (5 mL).] ▶L ♀B ▶? ?

OCRIPLASMIN (*Jetrea*) 0.125 mg (0.1 mL) intravitreal injection as a single dose. [Sterile soln of 0.5 mg in 0.2 mL. Dilution required with 0.2 mL of normal saline (0.5 mg/0.4 mL). Final concentration 0.125 mg/0.1 mL.] ▶minimal absorption – ♀C ▶? $$$$$

PETROLATUM (*Lacrilube, Dry Eyes, Refresh PM, ✦ Duolube*) Apply ¼ to ½ inch ointment to inside of lower lid prn. [OTC Trade only: Ointment (3.5, 7 g) tube.] ▶Minimal absorption ♀A ▶+ $

PROPARACAINE (*Ophthaine, Ophthetic, ✦ Alcaine*) Do not prescribe for unsupervised or prolonged use. Corneal toxicity and ocular infections may occur with repeated use. 1 to 2 gtts into affected eye before procedure. [Generic/Trade: Soln 0.5% (15 mL).] ▶L ♀C ▶? $

TETRACAINE—OPHTHALMIC (*Pontocaine*) Do not prescribe for unsupervised or prolonged use. Corneal toxicity and ocular infections may occur with repeated use. 1 to 2 gtts or ½ to 1 inch ribbon of ointment in each affected eye before procedure. [Generic only: Soln 0.5% (15 mL), unit-dose vials (0.7, 2 mL).] ▶Plasma ♀C ▶? $

PSYCHIATRY

Antidepressants—Heterocyclic Compounds

AMITRIPTYLINE (*Elavil*) Depression: Start 25 to 100 mg PO at bedtime; gradually increase to usual effective dose of 50 to 300 mg/day. Primarily inhibits serotonin reuptake. Demethylated to nortriptyline, which primarily inhibits norepinephrine reuptake. Suicidality. [Generic: Tabs 10, 25, 50, 75, 100, 150 mg. Elavil brand name no longer available; has been retained in this entry for name recognition purposes only.] ▶L ♀D ▶– $$ ■

CLOMIPRAMINE (*Anafranil*) OCD: Start 25 mg PO at bedtime; gradually increase to usual effective dose of 150 to 250 mg/day. Max 250 mg/day. Primarily inhibits serotonin reuptake. Suicidality. [Generic/Trade: Caps 25, 50, 75 mg.] ▶L ♀C ▶+ $$$ ■

DESIPRAMINE (*Norpramin*) Depression: Start 25 to 100 mg PO given once daily or in divided doses. Gradually increase to usual effective dose of 100 to 200 mg/day, max 300 mg/day. Primarily inhibits norepinephrine reuptake. Suicidality. [Generic/Trade: Tabs 10, 25, 50, 75, 100, 150 mg.] ▶L ♀C ▶+ $$ ■

DOXEPIN (*Sinequan, Silenor*) Depression: Start 75 mg PO at bedtime. Gradually increase to usual effective dose of 75 to 150 mg/day, max 300 mg/day. Primarily inhibits norepinephrine reuptake. Insomnia (Silenor): 6 mg PO 30 min before bedtime, 3 mg in age 65 yo or older. Suicidality. [Generic only: Caps 10, 25, 50, 75, 100, 150 mg. Oral concentrate 10 mg/mL. Trade only: Tabs 3, 6 mg (Silenor)] ▶L ♀C ▶– $$ ■

IMIPRAMINE (*Tofranil, Tofranil PM*) Depression: Start 75 to 100 mg PO at bedtime or in divided doses; gradually increase to max 300 mg/day. Enuresis: 25 to 75 mg PO at bedtime. Suicidality. [Generic/Trade: Tabs 10, 25, 50 mg. Caps 75, 100, 125, 150 mg (as pamoate salt).] ▶L ♀D ▶– $$$ ■

NORTRIPTYLINE (*Aventyl, Pamelor*) Depression: Start 25 mg PO given once daily or divided two to four times per day. Usual effective dose is 75 to 100 mg/day, max 150 mg/day. Primarily inhibits norepinephrine reuptake. Suicidality. [Generic/Trade: Caps 10, 25, 50, 75 mg. Oral soln 10 mg/5 mL.] ▶L ♀D ▶+ $$$ ■

PROTRIPTYLINE (*Vivactil*) Depression: 15 to 40 mg/day PO divided three to four times per day. Max 60 mg/day. Suicidality. [Generic/Trade: Tabs 5, 10 mg.] ▶L ♀C ▶+ $$$$ ■

VILAZODONE (*Viibryd*) Depression: Start 10 mg PO once daily. Max 40 mg/day. [Trade only: Tabs 10, 20, 40 mg.] Give this medication with food. ▶L – ♀C ▶? ■

Antidepressants—Monoamine Oxidase Inhibitors (MAOIs)

NOTE: Must be on tyramine-free diet throughout treatment and for 2 weeks after discontinuation. Numerous drug interactions; risk of hypertensive crisis and serotonin syndrome with many medications, including OTC. Allow at least 2 weeks wash-out when converting from an MAOI to an SSRI (6 weeks after fluoxetine), TCA, or other antidepressant.

ISOCARBOXAZID (*Marplan*) Depression: Start 10 mg PO two times per day; increase by 10 mg q 2 to 4 days. Usual effective dose is 20 to 40 mg/day. MAOI diet. Suicidality. [Trade only: Tabs 10 mg.] ▶L ♀C ▶? $$$ ■

PHENELZINE (*Nardil*) Depression: Start 15 mg PO three times per day. Usual effective dose is 60 to 90 mg/day in divided doses. MAOI diet. Suicidality. [Trade only: Tabs 15 mg.] ▶L ♀C ▶? $$$ ■

SELEGILINE—TRANSDERMAL (*Emsam*) Depression: Start 6 mg/24 h patch, change daily. Max 12 mg/24 h. MAOI diet for doses 9 mg/day or higher. Suicidality. [Trade only: Transdermal patch 6 mg/day, 9 mg/24 h, 12 mg/24 h.] ▶L ♀C ▶? $$$$$ ■

TRANYLCYPROMINE (*Parnate*) Depression: Start 10 mg PO q am; increase by 10 mg/day at 1- to 3-week intervals to usual effective dose of 10 to 40 mg/day divided two times per day. MAOI diet. Suicidality. [Generic/Trade: Tabs 10 mg.] ▶L ♀C ▶– $$ ■

Antidepressants—Selective Serotonin Reuptake Inhibitors (SSRIs)

CITALOPRAM (*Celexa*) Depression: Start 20 mg PO daily. May increase after 1 or more weeks to max 40 mg PO daily or 20 mg daily if older than 60 yo. Suicidality. [Generic/Trade: Tabs 10, 20, 40 mg. Oral soln 10 mg/5 mL. Generic only: Orally disintegrating tab 10, 20, 40 mg.] ▶LK ♀C but – in 3rd trimester ▶– $$$ ■

ESCITALOPRAM (*Lexapro*, ✦*Cipralex*) Depression, generalized anxiety disorder, adults and age 12 yo or older: Start 10 mg PO daily; max 20 mg/day. Suicidality. [Generic/Trade: Tabs 5, 10, 20 mg. Oral soln 1 mg/mL.] ▶LK ♀C but – in 3rd trimester ▶– $$$$ ■

FLUOXETINE (*Prozac, Prozac Weekly, Sarafem*) Depression, OCD: Start 20 mg PO q am; usual effective dose is 20 to 40 mg/day, max 80 mg/day. Depression, maintenance: 20 to 40 mg/day (standard-release) or 90 mg PO once a week (Prozac Weekly) starting 7 days after last standard-release dose. Bulimia: 60 mg PO daily; may need to titrate slowly, over several days. Panic disorder: Start 10 mg PO q am; titrate to 20 mg/day after 1 week, max 60 mg/day. Premenstrual dysphoric disorder (Sarafem): 20 mg PO daily, given either throughout the menstrual cycle or for 14 days prior to menses; max 80 mg/day. Doses greater than 20 mg/day can be divided two times per day (in morning and at noon). Bipolar depression, olanzapine + fluoxetine: Start 5 mg olanzapine + 20 mg fluoxetine in the evening. Increase to usual range of 5 to 12.5 mg olanzapine plus 20 to 50 mg fluoxetine as tolerated. Treatment-resistant depression, olanzapine + fluoxetine: Start 5 mg olanzapine + 20 mg fluoxetine daily in the evening. Increase to usual range of 5 to 20 mg olanzapine plus 20 to 50 mg fluoxetine as tolerated. Suicidality, many drug interactions. [Generic/Trade: Tabs 10 mg. Caps 10, 20, 40 mg. Oral soln 20 mg/5 mL. Caps (Sarafem) 10, 20 mg. Trade only: Tabs (Sarafem) 10, 15, 20 mg. Caps, delayed-release (Prozac Weekly) 90 mg. Generic only: Tabs 20, 40 mg.] ▶L ♀C but – in 3rd trimester ▶– $$$ ■

FLUVOXAMINE (*Luvox, Luvox CR*) OCD: Start 50 mg PO at bedtime; usual effective dose is 100 to 300 mg/day divided two times per day, max 300 mg/day. OCD (children age 8 yo or older): Start 25 mg PO at bedtime; usual effective dose is 50 to 200 mg/day divided two times per day, max 200 mg/day. Do not use with thioridazine, pimozide, alosetron, cisapride, tizanidine, tryptophan, or MAOIs; use caution with benzodiazepines, TCAs, theophylline, and warfarin. Suicidality. [Generic/Trade: Tabs 25, 50, 100 mg. Caps, extended-release 100, 150 mg.] ▶L ♀C but – in 3rd trimester ▶– $$$$ ■

PAROXETINE (*Paxil, Paxil CR, Pexeva*) Depression: Start 20 mg PO q am, max 50 mg/day. Depression, controlled-release: Start 25 mg PO q am, max 62.5 mg/day. OCD: Start 10 to 20 mg PO q am, max 60 mg/day. Social anxiety disorder: Start 10 to 20 mg PO q am, max 60 mg/day. Social anxiety disorder, controlled-release: Start 12.5 mg PO q am, max 37.5 mg/day. Generalized anxiety disorder: Start 20 mg PO q am, max 50 mg/day. Panic disorder: Start 10 mg PO q am, increase by 10 mg/day at intervals of 1 week or more to usual effective dose of 10 to 60 mg/day; max 60 mg/day. Panic disorder, controlled-release: Start

(cont.)

12.5 mg PO q am, max 75 mg/day. Post-traumatic stress disorder: Start 20 mg PO q am, max 50 mg/day. Premenstrual dysphoric disorder (PMDD), continuous dosing: Start 12.5 mg PO q am (controlled-release); may increase dose after 1 week to max 25 mg q am. PMDD, intermittent dosing (given for 2 weeks prior to menses): 12.5 mg PO q am (controlled-release), max 25 mg/day. Suicidality, many drug interactions. [Generic/Trade: Tabs 10, 20, 30, 40 mg. Oral susp 10 mg/5 mL. Controlled-release tabs 12.5, 25 mg. Trade only: (Paxil CR) 37.5 mg.] ▶LK ♀D ▶? $$$ ■

SERTRALINE   (Zoloft) Depression, OCD: Start 50 mg PO daily; usual effective dose is 50 to 200 mg/day, max 200 mg/day. Panic disorder, post-traumatic stress disorder, social anxiety disorder: Start 25 mg PO daily, max 200 mg/day. PMDD, continuous dosing: Start 50 mg PO daily, max 150 mg/day. PMDD, intermittent dosing (given for 14 days prior to menses): Start 50 mg PO daily for 3 days, then increase to 100 mg/day. Suicidality. [Generic/Trade: Tabs 25, 50, 100 mg. Oral concentrate 20 mg/mL (60 mL).] ▶LK ♀C but – in 3rd trimester ▶+ $$$ ■

Antidepressants—Serotonin-Norepinephrine Reuptake Inhibitors (SNRIs)

DESVENLAFAXINE   (Pristiq) 50 mg PO daily. Max 400 mg/day. [Trade only: Tabs (Pristiq), extended-release 50, 100 mg. Generic only: Extended-release tabs 50, 100 mg.] ▶LK ♀C ▶? $$$$ ■

DULOXETINE   (Cymbalta) Depression: 20 mg PO two times per day; max 60 mg/day given once daily or divided two times per day. Generalized anxiety disorder: Start 30 to 60 mg PO daily, max 120 mg/day. Diabetic peripheral neuropathic pain: 60 mg PO daily. Fibromyalgia: Start 30 to 60 mg PO daily, max 60 mg/day. Suicidality, hepatotoxicity, many drug interactions. [Trade only: Caps 20, 30, 60 mg.] ▶L ♀C ▶? $$$$ ■

VENLAFAXINE   (Effexor, Effexor XR) Depression/anxiety: Start 37.5 to 75 mg PO daily (Effexor XR) or 75 mg/day divided two to three times per day (Effexor). Usual effective dose is 150 to 225 mg/day, max 225 mg/day (Effexor XR) or 375 mg/day (Effexor). Generalized anxiety disorder: Start 37.5 to 75 mg PO daily (Effexor XR), max 225 mg/day. Social anxiety disorder: 75 mg PO daily (Effexor XR). Panic disorder: Start 37.5 mg PO daily (Effexor XR), may titrate by 75 mg/day at weekly intervals to max 225 mg/day. Suicidality, seizures, HTN. [Generic/Trade: Caps, extended-release 37.5, 75, 150 mg. Tabs 25, 37.5, 50, 75, 100 mg. Generic only: Tabs, extended-release 37.5, 75, 150, 225 mg.] ▶LK ♀C but – in 3rd trimester ▶? $$$$ ■

Antidepressants—Other

BUPROPION   (Wellbutrin, Wellbutrin SR, Wellbutrin XL, Aplenzin, Zyban, Buproban, Forfivo XL) Depression: Start 100 mg PO two times per day (immediate-release tabs); can increase to 100 mg three times per day after 4 to 7 days. Usual effective dose is 300 to 450 mg/day, max 150 mg/dose and 450 mg/day. Sustained-release: Start 150 mg PO q am; may increase

(cont.)

to 150 mg two times per day after 4 to 7 days, max 400 mg/day. Give last dose no later than 5 pm. Extended-release: Start 150 mg PO q am; may increase to 300 mg q am after 4 days, max 450 mg q morning. Extended-release (Aplenzin): Start 174 mg PO q am; increase to target dose of 348 mg/day after 4 days or more. May increase to max dose of 522 mg/day after 4 weeks or more. Extended-release (Forfivo XL): Do not use to initiate therapy. If standard tabs tolerated and pateint requires more than 300 mg/day may use 450 mg PO daily, max 450 mg/day. Seasonal affective disorder: Start 150 mg of extended-release PO q am in autumn; can increase to 300 mg q am after 1 week, max 300 mg/day. In the spring, decrease to 150 mg/day for 2 weeks and then discontinue. Extended-release (Aplenzin): Start 174 mg PO each morning. Increase to 348 mg/day after 7 days. Smoking cessation: Start 150 mg PO q am for 3 days, then increase to 150 mg PO two times per day for 7 to 12 weeks. Max 150 mg PO two times per day. Give last dose no later than 5 pm. Seizures, suicidality. [Generic/Trade (for depression, bupropion HCl): Tabs 75, 100 mg. Sustained-release tabs 100, 150, 200 mg. Extended-release tabs 150, 300 mg (Wellbutrin XL). Generic/Trade (Smoking cessation): Sustained-release tabs 150 mg (Zyban, Buproban). Trade only: Extended-release (Aplenzin, bupropion hydrobromide) tabs 174, 348, 522 mg. Extended-release (Forfivo XL) tabs 450 mg.] ▶LK ♀C ▶– $$ ■

MIRTAZAPINE (*Remeron, Remeron SolTab*) Start 15 mg PO at bedtime. Usual effective dose is 15 to 45 mg/day. Agranulocytosis in 0.1% of patients. Suicidality. [Generic/Trade: Tabs 15, 30, 45 mg. Tabs, orally disintegrating (SolTab) 15, 30, 45 mg. Generic only: Tabs 7.5 mg.] ▶LK ♀C ▶? $$ ■

TRAZODONE (*Desyrel, Oleptro*) Depression: Start 50 to 150 mg/day PO in divided doses; usual effective dose is 400 to 600 mg/day. Extended-release: Start 150 mg PO at bedtime. May increase by 75 mg/day q 3 days to max 375 mg/day. Insomnia: 50 to 150 mg PO at bedtime. [Trade only: Extended-release tabs (Oleptro) 150, 300 mg. Generic only: Tabs 50, 100, 150, 300 mg.] ▶L ♀C ▶– $ ■

Antimanic (Bipolar) Agents

LAMOTRIGINE (*Lamictal, Lamictal CD, Lamictal ODT, Lamictal XR*) bipolar disorder (maintenance): Start 25 mg PO daily, 50 mg PO daily if on enzyme-inducing drugs, or 25 mg PO every other day if on valproate; titrate to 200 mg/day, 400 mg/day divided two times per day if on enzyme-inducing drugs, or 100 mg/day if on valproate. Potentially life-threatening rashes in 0.3% of adults and 0.8% of children; discontinue at first sign of rash. Drug interaction with valproic acid; see prescribing information for adjusted dosing guidelines. [Generic/Trade: Chewable dispersible tabs (Lamictal CD) 5, 25 mg. Tabs 25, 100, 150, 200 mg. Extended-release tabs (XR) 25, 50, 100, 200, 250, 300 mg. Trade only: Orally disintegrating tabs (ODT) 25, 50, 100, 200 mg. Chewable dispersible tabs 2 mg.] ▶LK ♀C (see notes) ▶– $$$$ ■

LITHIUM (*Eskalith, Eskalith CR, Lithobid, ✦ Lithane*) Acute mania: Start 300 to 600 mg PO two to three times per day; usual effective dose is 900 to

(cont.)

1800 mg/day. Steady state is achieved in 5 days. Bipolar maintenance usually 900 to 1200 mg/day titrated to therapeutic trough level of 0.6 to 1.2 mEq/L. [Generic/Trade: Caps 150, Extended-release tabs 300, 450 mg. Generic only: Caps 150, 600 mg, Tabs 300 mg, Syrup 300 mg/5 mL.] ▶K ♀D ▶– $ ■

TOPIRAMATE (*Topamax*) Bipolar disorder (unapproved): Start 25 to 50 mg/day PO. Titrate prn to max 400 mg/day divided two times per day. [Generic/Trade: Tabs 25, 50, 100, 200 mg. Sprinkle Caps 15, 25 mg.] ▶K ♀D ▶? $$$$$

VALPROIC ACID—PSYCH (*Depakote, Depakote ER, Stavzor, divalproex, ✦ Epival*) Mania: 250 mg PO three times per day (Depakote) or 25 mg/kg once daily (Depakote ER); max 60 mg/kg/day. Hepatotoxicity, drug interactions, reduce dose in the elderly. [Generic only: Syrup (Valproic acid) 250 mg/5 mL. Generic/Trade: Delayed-release tabs (Depakote) 125, 250, 500 mg. Extended-release tabs (Depakote ER) 250, 500 mg. Delayed-release sprinkle caps (Depakote) 125 mg. Trade only (Stavzor): Delayed-release caps 125, 250, 500 mg.] ▶L ♀D ▶+ $$$$ ■

Antipsychotics—First Generation (Typical)

CHLORPROMAZINE (*Thorazine*) Start 10 to 50 mg PO/IM two to three times per day, usual dose 300 to 800 mg/day. [Generic only: Tabs 10, 25, 50, 100, 200 mg. Generic/Trade: Oral concentrate 30 mg/mL, 100 mg/mL. Trade only: Syrup 10 mg/5 mL, Supps 25, 100 mg.] ▶LK ♀C ▶– $$$ ■

FLUPHENAZINE (*Prolixin, ✦ Modecate*) 1.25 to 10 mg/day IM divided q 6 to 8 h. Start 0.5 to 10 mg/day PO divided q 6 to 8 h. Usual effective dose 1 to 20 mg/day. Depot (fluphenazine decanoate/enanthate): 12.5 to 25 mg IM/SC q 3 weeks is equivalent to 10 to 20 mg/day PO fluphenazine. [Generic/Trade: Tabs 1, 2.5, 5, 10 mg. Elixir 2.5 mg/5 mL. Oral concentrate 5 mg/mL.] ▶LK ♀C ▶? $$$ ■

HALOPERIDOL (*Haldol*) 2 to 5 mg IM. Start 0.5 to 5 mg PO two to three times per day, usual effective dose 6 to 20 mg/day. Therapeutic range 2 to 15 ng/mL. Depot haloperidol (haloperidol decanoate): 100 to 200 mg IM q 4 weeks is equivalent to 10 mg/day oral haloperidol. [Generic only: Tabs 0.5, 1, 2, 5, 10, 20 mg. Oral concentrate 2 mg/mL.] ▶LK ♀C ▶– $$ ■

PERPHENAZINE Start 4 to 8 mg PO three times per day or 8 to 16 mg PO two to four times per day (hospitalized patients), maximum 64 mg/day PO. Can give 5 to 10 mg IM q 6 h, maximum 30 mg/day IM. [Generic only: Tabs 2, 4, 8, 16 mg. Oral concentrate 16 mg/5 mL.] ▶LK ♀C ▶? $$$ ■

PIMOZIDE (*Orap*) Tourette syndrome: Start 1 to 2 mg/day PO in divided doses, increase q 2 days to usual effective dose of 1 to 10 mg/day. [Trade only: Tabs 1, 2 mg.] ▶L ♀C ▶– $$$ ■

THIORIDAZINE (*Mellaril*) Start 50 to 100 mg PO three times per day, usual dose 200 to 800 mg/day. Not 1st-line therapy. Causes QTc prolongation, torsades de pointes, and sudden death. Contraindicated with SSRIs, propranolol, pindolol. Monitor baseline ECG and potassium. Pigmentary retinopathy with doses greater than 800 mg/day. [Generic only: Tabs 10, 15, 25, 50, 100, 150, 200 mg. Oral concentrate 30, 100 mg/mL.] ▶LK ♀C ▶? $$ ■

THIOTHIXENE   (*Navane*) Start 2 mg PO three times per day. Usual effective dose is 20 to 30 mg/day, maximum 60 mg/day PO. [Generic/Trade: Caps 1, 2, 5, 10. Oral concentrate 5 mg/mL. Trade only: Caps 20 mg.] ▶LK ♀C ▶? $$$ ■

TRIFLUOPERAZINE   (*Stelazine*) Start 2 to 5 mg PO two times per day. Usual effective dose is 15 to 20 mg/day. [Generic/Trade: Tabs 1, 2, 5, 10 mg. Trade only: Oral concentrate 10 mg/mL.] ▶LK ♀C ▶ − $$$ ■

Antipsychotics—Second Generation (Atypical)

ARIPIPRAZOLE   (*Abilify, Abilify Discmelt, Abilify Maintena*) Schizophrenia: Start 10 to 15 mg PO daily. Max 30 mg daily. Schizophrenia, maintenance (Maintena): 400 mg IM monthly. May reduce to 300 mg IM monthly if adverse reactions to higher dose. Bipolar disorder: Start 15 mg PO daily. Max 30 mg/day. Agitation associated with schizophrenia or bipolar disorder: 9.75 mg IM recommended. May consider 5.25 to 15 mg if indicated. May repeat in 2 h up to max 30 mg/day. Depression, adjunctive therapy: Start 2 to 5 mg PO daily. Max 15 mg/day. [Trade only: Tabs 2, 5, 10, 15, 20, 30 mg. Oral soln 1 mg/mL (150 mL). Orally disintegrating tabs (Discmelt) 10 and 15 mg. Soln for injection 9.75 mg/1.3 mL, Susp Extended-release for Injection (Abilify Maintena) 300 mg and 400 mg/vial.] ▶L ♀C ▶? $$$$$ ■

ASENAPINE   (*Saphris*) Schizophrenia: Acute and maintenance: 5 mg SL twice per day. Max 10 mg twice per day. Bipolar disorder, acute manic or mixed episodes, monotherapy: Start 5 mg SL two times per day (adjunctive) or 10 mg SL two times per day (monotherapy). Max 20 mg/day. [Trade: Sublingual tabs 5, 10 mg] ▶L ♀C ▶− ■

CLOZAPINE   (*Clozaril, FazaClo ODT*) Start 12.5 mg PO one to two times per day. Usual effective dose is 300 to 450 mg/day divided two times per day, max 900 mg/day. Agranulocytosis 1 to 2%; check WBC and ANC weekly for 6 months, then q 2 weeks. Seizures, myocarditis, cardiopulmonary arrest. [Generic/Trade: Tabs 25, 100 mg. Generic only: Tabs 12.5, 50, 200 mg. Orally disintegrating tabs 12.5, 25, 100 mg. Trade only: Orally disintegrating tabs (Fazaclo ODT) 12.5, 25, 100, 150, 200 mg (scored).] ▶L ♀B ▶− $$$$$ ■

ILOPERIDONE   (*Fanapt*) Start 1 mg PO two times per day. Increase to 2 mg PO two times per day on day 2, then by 2 mg per dose each day to usual effective range of 6 to 12 mg PO two times per day. Max 24 mg/day. [Trade: Tabs 1, 2, 4, 6, 8, 10, 12 mg.] ▶L ♀C ▶−? ■

LURASIDONE   (*Latuda*) Start 40 mg PO daily. Effective dose range is 40 to 160 mg/day, max 160 mg/day. Take with food. Reduce starting dose to 20 mg PO daily if moderate to severe renal or hepatic insufficiency or use with moderate CYP3A4 inhibitors, max 80 mg/day unless severe hepatic insufficiency which is 40 mg/day. [Trade only: Tabs 20, 40, 80, 120 mg.] ▶K − ♀B ▶? ■

OLANZAPINE   (*Zyprexa, Zyprexa Zydis, Zyprexa Relprevv*) Agitation in acute bipolar mania or schizophrenia: Start 10 mg IM (2.5 to 5 mg in elderly or debilitated patients); may repeat in 2 h to max 30 mg/day. Schizophrenia,

(cont.)

ANTIPSYCHOTIC RELATIVE ADVERSE EFFECTS[a]

Gener-ation	Antipsychotic	Anti-choli nergic	Sedation	Hypo-tension	EPS	Weight Gain	Diabetes/ Hyper-gly cemia	Dyslipid-emia
1st	chlorpromazine	+++	+++	++	++	++	?	?
1st	fluphenazine	++	+	+	++++	++	?	?
1st	haloperidol	+	+	+	++++	++	0	?
1st	loxapine	++	+	+	++	+	?	?
1st	molindone	++	++	+	++	+	?	?
1st	perphenazine	++	++	+	++	+	+/?	?
1st	pimozide	+	+	+	+++	?	?	?
1st	thioridazine	++++	+++	+++	+	+++	+/?	?
1st	thiothixene	+	++	++	+++	++	?	/
1st	trifluoperazine	++	+	+	+++	++	?	?
2nd	aripiprazole	++	+	0	0	0/+	0	0
2nd	asenapine	+	+	++	++	+	?	?
2nd	clozapine	++++	+++	+++	0	+++	+	+
2nd	iloperidone	++	+	+++	+	++	?	?
2nd	olanzapine	+++	++	+	0[b]	+++	+	+
2nd	paliperidone	+	+	++	++	++	?	?
2nd	risperidone	+	++	+	+[b]	++	?	?
2nd	quetiapine	+	+++	++	0	++	?	?
2nd	ziprasidone	+	+	0	0	0/+	0	0

[a]Risk of specific adverse effects is graded from 0 (absent) to ++++ (high). ? = Limited or inconsistent comparative data.

[b]Extrapyramidal symptoms (EPS) are dose-related and are more likely for risperidone greater than 6 to 8 mg/day, olanzapine greater than 20 mg/day. Akathisia risk remains unclear and may not be reflected in these ratings. There are limited comparative data for aripiprazole iloperidone, paliperidone, and asenapine relative to other 2nd-generation antipsychotics.

References: Goodman & Gilman 11e p461-500, Applied Therapeutics 8e p78, APA schizophrenia practice guideline, Psychiatry Q 2002; 73:297, Diabetes Care 2004;27:596, Pharmacotherapy. A Pathophysiologic Approach, 8. pg 1158, 2011.

oral therapy: Start 5 to 10 mg PO daily; usual effective dose is 10 to 15 mg/day. Schizophrenia, long-acting injection: dose based on prior oral dose and ranges from 150 mg to 300 mg deep IM (gluteal) q 2 weeks or 300 mg to 405 mg q 4 weeks. See prescribing information. Bipolar disorder, maintenance treatment, or monotherapy for acute manic or mixed episodes: Start 10 to 15 mg PO daily. Increase by 5 mg/day at intervals of 24 h to usual effective dose of 5 to 20 mg/day, max 20 mg/day. Bipolar disorder, adjunctive for acute manic or mixed episodes: Start 10 mg PO daily; usual effective dose is 5 to 20 mg/day, max 20 mg/day. Bipolar depression, olanzapine + fluoxetine: Start 5 mg olanzapine + 20 mg fluoxetine daily in the evening. Increase to usual range of 5 to 12.5 mg olanzapine plus 20 to 50 mg fluoxetine as tolerated. Treatment-resistant depression, olanzapine + fluoxetine: Start 5 mg olanzapine + 20 mg fluoxetine daily in the evening. Increase to usual range of 5 to 20 mg olanzapine plus 20 to 50 mg fluoxetine as tolerated. [Generic/

(cont.)

Trade: Tabs 2.5, 5, 7.5, 10, 15, 20 mg. Tabs, orally disintegrating (Zyprexa Zydis) 5, 10, 15, 20 mg. Trade only: Long-acting injection (Zyprexa Relprevv) 210, 300, 405 mg/vial.] ▶L ♀C ▶– $$$$$ ■

PALIPERIDONE (*Invega, Invega Sustenna*) Schizophrenia and schizoaffective disorder (adjunctive and monotherapy): Start 6 mg PO q am. 3 mg/day may be sufficient in some. Max 12 mg/day. Extended-release injection: Start 234 mg IM (deltoid) and then 156 mg IM 1 week later. Recommended monthly dose 117 mg IM (deltoid or gluteal) or within range of 39 to 234 mg, based on response. [Trade only: Extended-release tabs 1.5, 3, 6, 9 mg.] ▶KL ♀C ▶– $$$$$ ■

QUETIAPINE (*Seroquel, Seroquel XR*) Schizophrenia: Start 25 mg two times per day (regular tabs); increase by 25 to 50 mg two to three times per day on days 2 and 3, and then to target dose of 300 to 400 mg/day divided two to three times per day on day 4. Usual effective dose is 150 to 750 mg/day, max 800 mg/day. Schizophrenia, extended-release tabs: Start 300 mg PO daily in evening, increase by up to 300 mg/day at intervals of more than 1 day to usual effective range of 400 to 800 mg/day. Acute bipolar mania, monotherapy, or adjunctive: Start 50 mg PO two times per day on day 1, then increase to no higher than 100 mg two times per day on day 2, 150 mg two times per day on day 3, and 200 mg two times per day on day 4. May increase prn to 300 mg two times per day on day 5 and 400 mg two times per day thereafter. Usual effective dose is 400 to 800 mg/day. Acute bipolar mania, monotherapy or adjunctive, extended-release: Start 300 mg PO evening of day 1, 600 mg day 2, and 400 to 800 mg/day thereafter. Bipolar depression, regular and extended-release: 50 mg PO at bedtime on day 1, 100 mg at bedtime day 2, 200 mg at bedtime day 3, and 300 mg at bedtime day 4. May increase prn to 400 mg at bedtime on day 5 and 600 mg at bedtime on day 8. Bipolar maintenance: Continue dose required to maintain remission. Major depressive disorder, adjunctive to antidepressants, extended-release: Start 50 mg evening of day 1, may increase to 150 mg on day 3. Max 300 mg/day. Eye exam for cataracts recommended q 6 months. [Generic/Trade: Tabs 25, 50, 100, 200, 300, 400 mg. Trade only: Extended-release tabs 50, 150, 200, 300, 400 mg.] ▶LK ♀C ▶– $$$$ ■

RISPERIDONE (*Risperdal, Risperdal Consta, Risperdal M-Tab*) Schizophrenia (adults): Start 2 mg/day PO given once daily or divided two times per day (0.5 mg two times per day in the elderly, debilitated, or with hypotension, severe renal or hepatic disease); increase by 1 to 2 mg/day (no more than 0.5 mg two times per day in elderly and debilitated) at intervals of 24 h or more to usual effective dose of 4 to 8 mg/day given once daily or divided two times per day, max 16 mg/day. Long-acting injection (Consta): Schizophrenia, Bipolar type 1 maintenance: Start 25 mg IM q 2 weeks while continuing oral dose for 3 weeks. May increase at 4-week intervals to max 50 mg q 2 weeks. Schizophrenia (13 to 17 yo): Start 0.5 mg PO daily; increase by 0.5 to 1 mg/day at intervals of 24 h or more to target dose of 3 mg daily. Max 6 mg/day. Bipolar mania (adults): Start 2 to 3 mg PO daily; may increase by 1 mg/day at 24-h intervals to max 6 mg/day. Bipolar mania (10 to 17 yo): Start 0.5 mg PO daily; increase by 0.5 to 1 mg/day at intervals of 24 h to recommended dose of 2.5 mg/day. Max 6 mg/day. Autistic

(cont.)

disorder irritability (age 5 to 16 yo): Start 0.25 mg (for wt less than 20 kg) or 0.5 mg (wt 20 kg or greater) PO daily. May increase after 4 days to 0.5 mg/day (for wt less than 20 kg) or 1.0 mg/day (wt 20 kg or greater). Maintain at least 14 days. May then increase at 14-day intervals or more by increments of 0.25 mg/day (for wt less than 20 kg) or 0.5 mg/day (wt 20 kg or greater) to max 1.0 mg/day (for wt less than 20 kg), 2.5 mg/day (20 to 44 kg) or 3.0 mg/day (wt more than 45 kg). [Generic/Trade: Tabs 0.25, 0.5, 1, 2, 3, 4 mg. Oral soln 1 mg/mL (30 mL). Orally disintegrating tabs 0.5, 1, 2, 3, 4 mg. Generic only: Orally disintegrating tabs 0.25 mg. Trade Only: IM Injection (Risperdal Consta) 12.5, 25, 37.5, 50mg] ▶LK ♀C ▶– $$$$ ■

ZIPRASIDONE (*Geodon*, ✦ *Zeldox*) Schizophrenia: Start 20 mg PO two times per day with food; may adjust at more than 2-day intervals to max 80 mg PO two times per day. Acute agitation: 10 to 20 mg IM, max 40 mg IM. Bipolar mania: Start 40 mg PO two times per day with food; may increase to 60 to 80 mg two times per day on day 2. Usual effective dose is 40 to 80 mg two times per day. [Trade/Generic: Caps 20, 40, 60, 80 mg. Trade only: 20 mg/mL Injection.] ▶L ♀C ▶– $$$$$

Anxiolytics/Hypnotics—Benzodiazepines—Long Half-Life (25 to 100 h)

BROMAZEPAM (✦ *Lectopam*) Canada only. 6 to 18 mg/day PO in divided doses. [Generic/Trade: Tabs 1.5, 3, 6 mg.] ▶L ♀D ▶– $

CHLORDIAZEPOXIDE (*Librium*) Anxiety: 5 to 25 mg PO or 25 to 50 mg IM/IV three to four times per day. Acute alcohol withdrawal: 50 to 100 mg PO/IM/IV, repeat q 3 to 4 h prn up to 300 mg/day. Half-life 5 to 30 h. [Generic/Trade: Caps 5, 10, 25 mg.] ▶LK ♀D ▶–©IV $$

CLONAZEPAM (*Klonopin, Klonopin Wafer*, ✦ *Rivotril, Clonapam*) Panic disorder: Start 0.25 to 0.5 mg PO two to three times per day, max 4 mg/day. Half-life 18 to 50 h. Epilepsy: Start 0.5 mg PO three times per day. Max 20 mg/day. [Generic/Trade: Tabs 0.5, 1, 2 mg. Orally disintegrating tabs (approved for panic disorder only) 0.125, 0.25, 0.5, 1, 2 mg.] ▶LK ♀D ▶–©IV $$

CLORAZEPATE (*Tranxene*) Start 7.5 to 15 mg PO at bedtime or two to three times per day, usual effective dose is 15 to 60 mg/day. Acute alcohol withdrawal: 60 to 90 mg/day on 1st day divided two to three times per day, reduce dose to 7.5 to 15 mg/day over 5 days. [Generic/Trade: Tabs 3.75, 7.5, 15 mg.] ▶LK ♀D ▶–©IV $$$$

DIAZEPAM (*Valium, Diastat, Diastat AcuDial, Diazemuls*) Active seizures: 5 to 10 mg IV q 10 to 15 min to max 30 mg, or 0.2 to 0.5 mg/kg rectal gel PR. Skeletal muscle spasm, spasticity related to cerebral palsy, paraplegia, athetosis, "stiff man syndrome": 2 to 10 mg PO/PR three to four times per day. Anxiety: 2 to 10 mg PO two to four times per day. Half-life 20 to 80 h. Alcohol withdrawal: 10 mg PO three to four times per day for 24 h then 5 mg PO three to four times per day prn. [Generic/Trade: Tabs 2, 5, 10 mg. Generic only: Oral soln 5 mg/5 mL. Oral concentrate (Intensol) 5 mg/mL. Trade only: Rectal gel (Diastat) 2.5, 5, 10, 15, 20 mg. Rectal gel (Diastat AcuDial) 10, 20 mg.] ▶LK ♀D ▶–©IV $

FLURAZEPAM (*Dalmane*) 15 to 30 mg PO at bedtime. Half-life 70 to 90 h. [Generic/Trade: Caps 15, 30 mg.] ▶LK ♀X ▶–©IV $

Anxiolytics/Hypnotics—Benzodiazepines—Medium Half-Life (10 to 15 h)

NOTE: *To avoid withdrawal, gradually taper when discontinuing after prolonged use. Sedative-hypnotics have been associated with severe allergic reactions and complex sleep behaviors including sleep driving. Use caution and discuss with patients.*

ESTAZOLAM (*ProSom*) 1 to 2 mg PO at bedtime. [Generic/Trade: Tabs 1, 2 mg.] ▶LK ♀X ▶–©IV $$

LORAZEPAM (*Ativan*) Anxiety: 0.5 to 2 mg IV/IM/PO q 6 to 8 h, max 10 mg/day. Half-life 10 to 20 h. Status epilepticus: Adult: 4 mg IV over 2 min; may repeat in 10 to 15 min. Status epilepticus: Peds: 0.05 to 0.1 mg/kg (max 4 mg) IV over 2 to 5 min; may repeat 0.05 mg/kg once in 10 to 15 min. [Generic/Trade: Tabs 0.5, 1, 2 mg. Generic only: Oral concentrate 2 mg/mL.] ▶LK ♀D ▶–©IV $

TEMAZEPAM (*Restoril*) 7.5 to 30 mg PO at bedtime. Half-life 8 to 25 h. [Generic/Trade: Caps 7.5, 15, 22.5, 30 mg]. ▶LK ♀X ▶–©IV $

Anxiolytics/Hypnotics—Benzodiazepines—Short Half-Life (< 12 h)

NOTE: *To avoid withdrawal, gradually taper when discontinuing after prolonged use. Sedative-hypnotics have been associated with severe allergic reactions and complex sleep behaviors including sleep driving. Use caution and discuss with patients.*

ALPRAZOLAM (*Xanax, Xanax XR, Niravam*) 0.25 to 0.5 mg PO two to three times per day. Half-life 12 h. Multiple drug interactions. [Generic/Trade: Tabs 0.25, 0.5, 1, 2 mg. Tabs, extended-release 0.5, 1, 2, 3 mg. Orally disintegrating tabs (Niravam) 0.25, 0.5, 1, 2 mg. Generic only: Oral concentrate (Intensol) 1 mg/mL.] ▶LK ♀D ▶–©IV $

OXAZEPAM (*Serax*) 10 to 30 mg PO three to four times per day. Half-life 8 h. [Generic/Trade: Caps 10, 15, 30 mg. Trade only: Tabs 15 mg.] ▶LK ♀D ▶–©IV $$$

TRIAZOLAM (*Halcion*) 0.125 to 0.5 mg PO at bedtime. 0.125 mg/day in elderly. Half-life 2 to 3 h. [Generic/Trade: Tabs 0.25 mg. Generic only: Tabs 0.125 mg] ▶LK ♀X ▶–©IV $

Anxiolytics/Hypnotics—Other

BUSPIRONE (*BuSpar, Vanspar*) Anxiety: Start 15 mg "dividose" daily (7.5 mg PO two times per day), usual effective dose 30 mg/day. Max 60 mg/day. [Generic/Trade: Tabs 5, 10, Dividose Tabs 15, 30 mg (scored to be easily bisected or trisected). Generic only: Tabs 7.5 mg.] ▶K ♀B ▶– $$$

ESZOPICLONE (*Lunesta*) Insomina: 2 mg PO at bedtime prn. Max 3 mg. Elderly: 1 mg PO at bedtime prn, max 2 mg. [Trade only: Tabs 1, 2, 3 mg.] ▶L ♀C ▶?©IV $$$$

RAMELTEON (*Rozerem*) Insomnia: 8 mg PO at bedtime. [Trade only: Tabs 8 mg.] ▶L ♀C ▶? $$$$

ZALEPLON (*Sonata*) 5 to 10 mg PO at bedtime prn, max 20 mg. Do not use for benzodiazepine or alcohol withdrawal. [Generic/Trade: Caps 5, 10 mg.] ▶L ♀C ▶–©IV $$$$

ZOLPIDEM (*Ambien, Ambien CR, Zolpimist, Intermezzo, Edluar, ♣ Sublinox*) Adult: Insomnia: Standard tabs: women 5 mg and men 5 to 10 mg PO at bedtime. The 5 mg dose may be increased to 10 mg if needed. For age older than 65 yo or debilitated: 5 mg PO at bedtime. Oral spray: women 5 mg and men 5 to 10 mg PO at bedtime. May increase the 5 mg dose to 10 mg if needed. For age older than 65 yo or debilitated: 5 mg PO at bedtime. Controlled-release tabs: women 6.25 mg and men 6.25 to 12.5 mg PO at bedtime. May increase the 6.25 mg dose to 12.5 mg if needed. For age older than 65 yo or debilitated: Give 6.25 mg PO at bedtime. Sublingual tabs (Edluar): women 5 mg and men 5 to 10 mg SL at bedtime. May increase the 5 mg dose to 10 mg if needed. Sublingual tabs (Intermezzo) for middle of the night awakening: women 1.75 mg SL and men 3.5 mg once nightly with at least 4 h of sleep remaining. Do not use for benzodiazepine or alcohol withdrawal. [Generic/Trade: Tabs 5, 10 mg. Controlled-release tabs 6.25, 12.5 mg. Trade only: Oral spray 5 mg/ actuation (Zolpimist), Sublingual tab 5, 10 mg (Edluar), Sublingual tab 1.75, 3.5 mg (Intermezzo).] ▶L ♀C ▶+©IV $$$$

ZOPICLONE (♣ *Imovane*) Canada only. Adults: Insomina: 5 to 7.5 mg PO at bedtime. Reduce dose in elderly. [Generic/Trade: Tabs 5, 7.5 mg. Generic only: Tabs 3.75 mg.] ▶L ♀D ▶– $

Combination Drugs

SYMBYAX (olanzapine + fluoxetine) Bipolar type 1 with depression and treatment-resistant depression: Start 6/25 mg PO at bedtime. Max 18/75 mg/day. [Generic/Trade: Caps (olanzapine/fluoxetine) 3/25, 6/25, 6/50, 12/25, 12/50 mg.] ▶LK ♀C ▶– $$$$$ ■

Drug Dependence Therapy

ACAMPROSATE (*Campral*) Maintenance of abstinence from alcohol: 666 mg (2 tabs) PO three times per day. Start after alcohol withdrawal and when patient is abstinent. [Trade only: Tabs, delayed-release 333 mg.] ▶K ♀C ▶? $$$$

DISULFIRAM (*Antabuse*) Sobriety: 125 to 500 mg PO daily. Patient must abstain from any alcohol for at least 12 h before using. Metronidazole and alcohol in any form (cough syrups, tonics, etc.) contraindicated. [Generic/Trade: Tabs 250, 500 mg.] ▶L ♀C ▶? $$

NALTREXONE (*ReVia, Depade, Vivitrol*) Alcohol/opioid dependence: 25 to 50 mg PO daily. Extened-release injectable susp: 380 mg IM q 4 weeks or monthly. Avoid if recent ingestion of opioids (past 7 to 10 days). Hepatotoxicity with higher than approved doses. [Generic/Trade: Tabs 50 mg. Trade only (Vivitrol): Extended-release injectable susp kits 380 mg.] ▶LK ♀C ▶? $$$$$ ■

PSYCHIATRY

NICOTINE GUM (*Nicorette, Nicorette DS*) Smoking cessation: Gradually taper: 1 piece q 1 to 2 h for 6 weeks, 1 piece q 2 to 4 h for 3 weeks, then 1 piece q 4 to 8 h for 3 weeks, max 30 pieces/day of 2 mg or 24 pieces/day of 4 mg. Use Nicorette DS 4 mg/piece in high cigarette use (more than 24 cigarettes/day). [OTC/Generic/Trade: Gum 2, 4 mg.] ▶LK ♀C ▶– $$$$

NICOTINE INHALATION SYSTEM (*Nicotrol Inhaler, ✦Nicorette inhaler*) 6 to 16 cartridges/day for 12 weeks. [Trade only: Oral inhaler 10 mg/cartridge (4 mg nicotine delivered), 42 cartridges/box.] ▶LK ♀D ▶– $$$$$

NICOTINE LOZENGE (*Commit, Nicorette*) Smoking cessation: In those who smoke within 30 min of waking use 4 mg lozenge; others use 2 mg. Take 1 to 2 lozenges q 1 to 2 h for 6 weeks, then q 2 to 4 h in weeks 7 to 9, then q 4 to 8 h weeks 10 to 12. Length of therapy 12 weeks. [OTC Generic/Trade: Lozenge 2, 4 mg in 48, 72, 168 count packages.] ▶LK ♀D ▶– $$$$$

NICOTINE NASAL SPRAY (*Nicotrol NS*) Smoking cessation: 1 to 2 doses q 1 h, each dose is 2 sprays, 1 in each nostril (1 spray contains 0.5 mg nicotine). Minimum recommended: 8 doses/day, max 40 doses/day. [Trade only: Nasal soln 10 mg/mL (0.5 mg/inhalation); 10 mL bottles.] ▶LK ♀D ▶– $$$$$

NICOTINE PATCHES (*Habitrol, NicoDerm CQ, Nicotrol*) Smoking cessation: Start 1 patch (14 to 22 mg) daily, taper after 6 weeks. Ensure patient has stopped smoking. [OTC/Rx/Generic/Trade: Patches 11, 22 mg/24 h, 7, 14, 21 mg/24 h (Habitrol and NicoDerm). OTC/Trade: 15 mg/16 h (Nicotrol).] ▶LK ♀D ▶– $$$$

SUBOXONE (buprenorphine + naloxone) Treatment of opioid dependence: Maintenance: 16 mg SL daily. Can individualize to range of 4 to 24 mg SL daily. [Generic only: SL tabs 2/0.5 mg and 8/2 mg buprenorphine/naloxone. Trade only: SL film 2/0.5 mg, 4/1 mg, 8/2 mg, and 12/3 mg buprenorphine/naloxone.] ▶L ♀C ▶–©III $$$$$

VARENICLINE (*Chantix, ✦Champix*) Smoking cessation: Start 0.5 mg PO daily for 1 to 3, then 0.5 mg two times per day on days 4 to 7, then 1 mg two times per day thereafter. Take after meals with full glass of water. Start 1 week prior to cessation and continue for 12 weeks or patient may start the drug and stop smoking between days 8 and 35 of treatment. [Trade only: Tabs 0.5, 1 mg.] ▶K ♀C ▶? $$$$ ■

Stimulants/ADHD/Anorexiants

ADDERALL (dextroamphetamine + amphetamine, *Adderall XR*) ADHD, standard-release tabs: Start 2.5 mg (3 to 5 yo) or 5 mg (age 6 yo or older) PO one to two times per day, increase by 2.5 to 5 mg q week, max 40 mg/day. ADHD, extended-release caps (Adderall XR): If age 6 to 12 yo, then start 5 to 10 mg PO daily to a max of 30 mg/day. If 13 to 17 yo, then start 10 mg PO daily to a max of 20 mg/day. If adult, then 20 mg PO daily. Narcolepsy, standard-release: Start 5 to 10 mg PO q am, increase by 5 to 10 mg q week, max 60 mg/day. Avoid evening doses. Monitor growth and use drug holidays when appropriate. [Generic/Trade: Tabs 5, 7.5, 10, 12.5, 15, 20, 30 mg. Caps, extended-release (Adderall XR) 5, 10, 15, 20, 25, 30 mg.] ▶L ♀C ▶–©II $$$$ ■

ARMODAFINIL (*Nuvigil*) Obstructive sleep apnea/hypopnea syndrome and narcolepsy: 150 to 250 mg PO q am. Inconsistent evidence for improved efficacy of 250 mg/day dose. Shift work sleep disorder: 150 mg PO 1 h prior to start of shift. [Trade only: Tabs 50, 100, 150, 200, 250 mg.] ▶L ♀C ▶?☺IV $$$$$

ATOMOXETINE (*Strattera*) ADHD: All ages wt greater than 70 kg: Start 40 mg PO daily, then increase after more than 3 days to target of 80 mg/day divided one to two times per day. Max 100 mg/day. [Trade only: Caps 10, 18, 25, 40, 60, 80, 100 mg.] ▶L ♀C ▶? $$$$$ ■

CAFFEINE (*NoDoz, Vivarin, Caffedrine, Stay Awake, Quick-Pep, Cafcit*) 100 to 200 mg PO q 3 to 4 h prn. [OTC Generic/Trade: Tabs/Caps 200 mg. Oral soln caffeine citrate (Cafcit) 20 mg/mL. OTC Trade only: Tabs, extended-release 200 mg. Lozenges 75 mg.] ▶L ♀B/C ▶? $

DEXMETHYLPHENIDATE (*Focalin, Focalin XR*) ADHD, extended-release, not already on stimulants: Start 5 mg (children) or 10 mg (adults) PO q am. Max 30 mg/day (children) or 40 mg/day (Adults). Immediate-release, not already on stimulants: 2.5 mg PO two times per day. Max 20 mg/day. If taking racemic methylphenidate, use conversion of 2.5 mg for each 5 mg of methylphenidate. [Generic/Trade: Tabs, immediate-release 2.5, 5, 10 mg. Trade only: Extended-release caps (Focalin XR) 5, 10, 15, 20, 30 mg.] ▶LK ♀C ▶?☺II $$$

DEXTROAMPHETAMINE (*Dexedrine, Procentra, Zenzedi*) Narcolepsy: Age 6 to 12 yo: Start 5 mg PO q am, increase by 5 mg/day q week. Age older than 12 yo: Start 10 mg PO q am, increase by 10 mg/day q week. Usual dose range 5 to 60 mg/day in divided doses (tabs) or daily (extended-release). ADHD: 2.5 to 5 mg PO q am, usual max 40 mg/day. Avoid evening doses. Monitor growth and use drug holidays when appropriate. [Generic/Trade: Caps, extended-release 5, 10, 15 mg. Tabs 5, 10 mg. Oral soln 5 mg/5 mL. Trade only: Tabs 2.5, 7.5mg (Zenzedi)] ▶L ♀C ▶–☺II $$$$$ ■

GUANFACINE (*Intuniv*) Start 1 mg PO q am. Increase by 1 mg/week to max 4 mg/day. [Trade only: Tabs 1, 2, 3, 4 mg.] ▶LK – ♀B ▶?

LISDEXAMFETAMINE (*Vyvanse*) ADHD, adults and adolescents, and children age 6 yo and older: Start 30 mg PO q am. May increase weekly by 10 to 20 mg/day to max 70 mg/day. Avoid evening doses. Monitor growth and use drug holidays when appropriate. [Trade: Caps 20, 30, 40, 50, 60, 70 mg.] ▶L ♀C ▶–☺II $$$$$ ■

BODY MASS INDEX* (Heights are in feet and inches; weights are in pounds)

BMI	Class	4' 10"	5' 0"	5' 4"	5' 8"	6' 0"	6' 4"
<19	Underweight	<91	<97	<110	<125	<140	<156
19–24	Healthy weight	91–119	97–127	110–144	125–163	140–183	156–204
25–29	Overweight	120–143	128–152	145–173	164–196	184–220	205–245
30–40	Obese	144–191	153–204	174–233	197–262	221–293	246–328
>40	Very Obese	>191	>204	>233	>262	>293	>328

*BMI = kg/m^2 = (wt in pounds)(703)/(height in inches)^2. Anorectants appropriate if BMI ≥30 (with comorbidities ≥27); surgery an option if BMI >40 (with comorbidities 35–40). www.nhlbi.nih.gov

METHYLPHENIDATE (*Ritalin, Ritalin LA, Ritalin SR, Methylin, Methylin ER, Metadate ER, Metadate CD, Concerta, Daytrana, Quillivant XR, ♦ Biphentin*) ADHD/narcolepsy: 5 to 10 mg PO two to three times per day or 20 mg PO q am (sustained- and extended-release), max 60 mg/day. Or 18 to 36 mg PO q am (Concerta), max 72 mg/day. ADHD: Sustained-release suspension (6 yo and older): Start 20 mg PO in the morning. May increase weekly by 10 to 20 mg daily to max 60 mg/day. Avoid evening doses. Monitor growth and use drug holidays when appropriate. [Trade only: Tabs, chewable 2.5, 5, 10 mg (Methylin). Tabs, extended-release 10, 20 mg (Methylin ER, Metadate ER). Tabs, sustained-release 20 mg (Ritalin SR). Transdermal patch (Daytrana) 10 mg/9 h, 15 mg/9 h, 20 mg/9 h, 30 mg/9 h. Susp, extended-release 5 mg/mL (Quillivant XR). Generic/Trade: Tabs 5, 10, 20 mg (Ritalin). Tabs, extended-release 18, 27, 36, 54 mg (Concerta). Caps, extended-release 10, 20, 30, 40, 50, 60 mg (Metadate CD), may be sprinkled on food. Caps, extended-release 10, 20, 30, 40 mg (Ritalin LA). Oral soln 5 mg/5 mL, 10 mg/5 mL. Generic only: Tabs 5, 10, 20 mg; tabs, extended-release 10, 20 mg; tabs, sustained-release 20 mg.]   ▶LK ♀C ▶?©II $$

MODAFINIL (*Provigil, ♦ Alertec*) Narcolepsy and sleep apnea/hypopnea: 200 mg PO q am. Shift work sleep disorder: 200 mg PO 1 h before shift. [Generic/Trade: Tabs 100, 200 mg.]   ▶L ♀C ▶?©IV $$$$$

PHENTERMINE (*Adipex-P, Ionamin, Suprenza*) 8 mg PO three times per day or 15 to 37.5 mg/day q am or 10 to 14 h before retiring. For short-term use. [Generic/Trade: Caps 15, 30, 37.5 mg. Tabs 37.5 mg. Trade only: Orally disintegrating tables (Suprenza) 15, 30 mg. Generic only: Caps extended-release 15, 30 mg (Ionamin).]   ▶KL ♀C ▶–©IV $

PULMONARY

Beta Agonists—Long-Acting

ARFORMOTEROL (*Brovana*) COPD: 15 mcg nebulized two times per day. [Trade only: Soln for inhalation 15 mcg in 2 mL vial.]   ▶L ♀C ▶? $$$$$ ■

FORMOTEROL (*Foradil, Perforomist, ♦ Oxeze Turbuhaler*) 1 puff two times per day. Nebulized: 20 mcg q 12 h. Not for acute bronchospasm. For asthma, use only in combination with corticosteroids. [Trade only: DPI 12 mcg, 12, 60 blisters/pack (Foradil). To be used only with Aerolizer device. Soln for inhalation: 20 mcg in 2 mL vial (Perforomist). Canada only (Oxeze): DPI 6, 12 mcg 60 blisters/pack.]   ▶L ♀C ▶? $$$ ■

INDACATEROL (*Arcapta, ♦ Onbrez*) COPD: DPI: 75 mcg inhaled once daily. [Trade only: DPI: 75 mcg caps for inhalation, 30 blisters. To be used with Neohaler device.]   ▶L– ♀C ▶? ■

SALMETEROL (*Serevent Diskus*) 1 puff two times per day. Not for acute bronchospasm. For asthma, use only in combination with corticosteroids. [Trade only: DPI (Diskus): 50 mcg, 60 blisters.]   ▶L ♀C ▶? $$$$ ■

Beta Agonists—Short-Acting

ALBUTEROL (*AccuNeb, Ventolin HFA, Proventil HFA, ProAir HFA, VoSpire ER, ♦Airomir, salbutamol*) MDI: 2 puffs q 4 to 6 h prn. Soln: 0.5 mL of 0.5% soln (2.5 mg) nebulized three to four times per day. One 3 mL unit dose (0.083%) nebulized three to four times per day. Caps for inhalation: 200 to 400 mcg q 4 to 6 h. Tabs: 2 to 4 mg PO three times per day to four times per day or extended-release 4 to 8 mg PO q 12 h up to 16 mg PO q 12 h. Peds: 0.1 to 0.2 mg/kg/dose PO three times per day up to 4 mg three times per day for age 2 to 5 yo, 2 to 4 mg or extended-release 4 mg PO q 12 h for age 6 to 12 yo. Prevention of exercise-induced bronchospasm: MDI: 2 puffs 10 to 30 min before exercise. [Trade only: MDI 90 mcg/actuation, 200 metered doses/canister. "HFA" inhalers use hydrofluoroalkane propellant instead of CFCs but are otherwise equivalent. Generic/Trade: Soln for inhalation 0.021% (AccuNeb), 0.042% (AccuNeb), and 0.083% in 3 mL vials, 0.5% (5 mg/mL) in 20 mL with dropper. Tabs, extended-release 4, 8 mg (VoSpire ER). Generic only: Syrup 2 mg/5 mL. Tabs, immediate-release 2, 4 mg.] ▶L ♀C ▶? $$

LEVALBUTEROL (*Xopenex, Xopenex HFA*) MDI 2 puffs q 4 to 6 h prn. Nebulizer 0.63 to 1.25 mg q 6 to 8 h. Peds: 0.31 mg nebulized three times per day for age 6 to 11 yo. [Generic/Trade: Soln for inhalation 0.31, 0.63, 1.25 mg in 3 mL and 1.25 mg in 0.5 mL unit-dose vials. Trade only: HFA MDI 45 mcg/actuation, 15 g 200/canister. "HFA" inhalers use hydrofluoroalkane propellant.] ▶L ♀C ▶? $$$

METAPROTERENOL (*Alupent*) MDI: 2 to 3 puffs q 3 to 4 h. Soln: 0.2 to 0.3 mL 5% soln nebulized q 4 h. Peds: Tabs: 20 mg PO three to four times per day age older than 9 yo, 10 mg PO three to four times per day if age 6 to 9 yo, 1.3 to 2.6 mg/kg/day divided three to four times per day if age 2 to 5 yo. [Trade only: MDI 0.65 mg/actuation, 14 g 200/canister. Generic/Trade: Soln for inhalation 0.4%, 0.6% in 2.5 mL unit-dose vials. Generic only: Syrup 10 mg/5 mL, Tabs 10, 20 mg.] ▶L ♀C ▶? $$

PIRBUTEROL (*Maxair Autohaler*) MDI: 1 to 2 puffs q 4 to 6 h. [Trade only: MDI 200 mcg/actuation, 14 g 400/canister.] ▶L ♀C ▶? $$$$

PREDICTED PEAK EXPIRATORY FLOW (liters/min) *Am Rev Resp Dis* 1963;88:644.

Age (yo)	Women (height in inches)					Men (height in inches)					Child (height in inches)	
	55"	60"	65"	70"	75"	60"	65"	70"	75"	80"		
20	390	423	460	496	529	554	602	649	693	740	44"	160
30	380	413	448	483	516	532	577	622	664	710	46"	187
40	370	402	436	470	502	509	552	596	636	680	48"	214
50	360	391	424	457	488	486	527	569	607	649	50"	240
60	350	380	412	445	475	463	502	542	578	618	52"	267
70	340	369	400	432	461	440	477	515	550	587	54"	293

PULMONARY

INHALED STEROIDS: ESTIMATED COMPARATIVE DAILY DOSES*

Adults and Children older than 12 yo				
Drug	Form	Low Dose	Medium Dose	High Dose
beclomethasone HFA MDI	40 mcg/puff	2–6 puffs/day	6–12 puffs/day	>12 puffs/day
	80 mcg/puff	1–3 puffs/day	3–6 puffs/day	>6 puffs/day
budesonide DPI	90 mcg/dose	2–6 inhalations/day	6–13 inhalations/day	>13 inhalations/day
	180 mcg/dose	1–3 inhalations/day	3–7 inhalations/day	>7 inhalations/day
budesonide	soln for nebs	—	—	—
flunisolide HFA MDI	80 mcg/puff	4puffs/day	5–8 puffs/day	>8 puffs/day
fluticasone HFA MDI	44 mcg/puff	2–6 puffs/day	6–10 puffs/day	>10 puffs/day
	110 mcg/puff	1–2 puffs/day	2–4 puffs/day	>4 puffs/day
	220 mcg/puff	1 puff/day	1–2 puffs/day	>2 puffs/day
fluticasone DPI	50 mcg/dose	2–6 inhalations/day	6–10 inhalations/day	>10 inhalations/day
	100 mcg/dose	1–3 inhalations/day	3–5 inhalations/day	>5 inhalations/day
	250 mcg/dose	1 inhalation/day	2 inhalations/day	>2 inhalations/day
mometasone DPI	220 mcg/dose	1 inhalations/day	2 inhalations/day	>2 inhalations/day
Children (age 5 to 11 yo)				
Drug	Form	Low Dose	Medium Dose	High Dose
beclomethasone HFA MDI	40 mcg/puff	2–4 puffs/day	4–8 puffs/day	>8 puffs/day
	80 mcg/puff	1–2 puffs/day	2–4 puffs/day	>4 puffs/day
budesonide DPI	90 mcg/dose	2–4 inhalations/day	4–9 inhalations/day	>9 inhalations/day
	180 mcg/dose	1–2 inhalations/day	2–4 inhalations/day	>4 inhalations/day
budesonide	soln for nebs	0.5 mg 0.25–0.5 mg (0–4 yo)	1 mg >0.5–1 mg (0–4 yo)	2 mg >1 mg (0–4 yo)
flunisolide HFA MDI	80 mcg/puff	2 puffs/day	4 puffs/day	≥8 puffs/day
fluticasone HFA MDI (0–11 yo)	44 mcg/puff	2–4 puffs/day	4–8 puffs/day	>8 puffs/day
	110 mcg/puff	1–2 puff/day	2–3 puffs/day	>4 puffs/day
	220 mcg/puff	n/a	1–2 puffs/day	>2 puffs/day
fluticasone	50 mcg/dose	2–4 inhalations/day	4–8 inhalations/day	>8 inhalations/day
	100 mcg/dose	1–2 inhalations/day	2–4 inhalations/day	>4 inhalations/day
	250 mcg/dose	n/a	1 inhalation/day	>1 inhalation/day
mometasone DPI	220 mcg/dose	n/a	n/a	n/a

*HFA = Hydrofluoroalkane (propellant). MDI = metered dose inhaler. DPI = dry powder inhaler.
Reference: http://www.nhlbi.nih.gov/guidelines/asthma/asthsumm.pdf

Combinations

ADVAIR (fluticasone—inhaled + salmeterol, *Advair HFA*) Asthma: DPI: 1 puff two times per day (all strengths). MDI: 2 puffs two times per day (all strengths). COPD: DPI: 1 puff two times per day (250/50 only). [Trade only: DPI: 100/50, 250/50, 500/50 mcg fluticasone/salmeterol per actuation; 60 doses/ DPI. Trade only (Advair HFA): MDI 45/21, 115/21, 230/21 mcg fluticasone/ salmeterol per actuation; 120 doses/canister.] ▶L ♀C ▶? $$$$$ ■

BREO ELLIPTA (fluticasone—inhaled + vilanterol) COPD: 1 inhalation once daily. [Trade only: DPI: 100/25 mcg fluticasone/vilanterol per actuation; 30 doses/DPI.] ▶L – ♀C ▶? ■

COMBIVENT, COMBIVENT RESPIMAT (albuterol + ipratropium) MDI: 2 puffs four times per day, max 12 puffs/day. Contraindicated with soy or peanut allergy. Respimat: 1 inhalation four times per day, max 6 inhalations/day. [Trade only: MDI: 90 mcg albuterol/18 mcg ipratropium per actuation, 200/ canister. Respimat: 100 mcg albuterol/20 mcg ipratropium per inhalation, 120/canister.] ▶L ♀C ▶? $$$$

DULERA (mometasone—inhaled + formoterol, ✦Zenhale) Chronic asthma: 2 puffs two times per day (all strengths). [Trade only: MDI 100/5, 200/5 mcg mometasone/formoterol per actuation; 120 doses/canister.] ▶L - ♀C ▶? $$$$$ ■

DUONEB (albuterol + ipratropium, ✦Combivent inhalation soln) 1 unit dose four times per day. [Generic/Trade: Unit dose: 2.5 mg albuterol/0.5 mg ipratropium per 3 mL vial, premixed; 30, 60 vials/carton.] ▶L ♀C ▶? $$$$$

SYMBICORT (budesonide + formoterol) Asthma: 2 puffs two times per day (both strengths). COPD: 2 puffs two times per day (160/4.5). [Trade only: MDI: 80/4.5, 160/4.5 mcg budesonide/formoterol per actuation; 120 doses/ canister.] ▶L ♀C ▶? $$$$ ■

Inhaled Steroids

NOTE: *See Endocrine—Corticosteroids when oral steroids necessary.*

BECLOMETHASONE—INHALED (*QVAR*) 1 to 4 puffs two times per day (40 mcg). 1 to 2 puffs two times per day (80 mcg). [Trade only: HFA MDI: 40, 80 mcg/actuation, 7.3 g 100 actuations/canister.] ▶L ♀C ▶? $$$

BUDESONIDE—INHALED (*Pulmicort Respules, Pulmicort Flexhaler*) 1 to 2 puffs daily up to 4 puffs two times per day. Respules: 0.5 to 1 mg daily or divided two times per day. [Trade only: DPI (Flexhaler) 90, 180 mcg powder/ actuation 60, 120 doses respectively/canister, Respules 1 mg/2 mL unit dose. Generic/Trade: Respules 0.25, 0.5 mg/2 mL unit dose.] ▶L ♀B ▶? $$$$

CICLESONIDE—INHALED (*Alvesco*) 80 mcg/puff: 1 to 4 puffs two times per day. 160 mcg/puff: 1 to 2 puffs two times per day. [Trade only: 80 mcg/actuation, 60 per canister. 160 mcg/actuation, 60, 120 per canister.] ▶L ♀C ▶? $$$$

FLUNISOLIDE—INHALED (*AeroBid, AeroBid-M, Aerospan*) 2 to 4 puffs two times per day. [Trade only: MDI: 250 mcg/actuation, 100 metered doses/ canister. AeroBid-M (AeroBid + menthol flavor). Aerospan HFA MDI: 80 mcg/ actuation, 60, 120 metered doses/canister.] ▶L ♀C ▶? $$$

FLUTICASONE—INHALED (*Flovent HFA, Flovent Diskus*) 2 to 4 puffs two times per day. [Trade only: HFA MDI: 44, 110, 220 mcg/actuation 120/ canister. DPI (Diskus): 50, 100, 250 mcg/actuation delivering 44, 88, 220 mcg respectively.] ▶L ♀C ▶? $$$$

MOMETASONE—INHALED (*Asmanex Twisthaler*) 1 to 2 puffs in the evening or 1 puff two times per day. If prior oral corticosteroid therapy: 2 puffs two times per day. [Trade only: DPI: 110 mcg/actuation with #30 dosage units, 220 mcg/actuation with #30, 60, 120 dosage units.] ▶L ♀C ▶? $$$$

TRIAMCINOLONE—INHALED 2 puffs three to four times per day or 4 puffs two times per day; max dose 16 puffs/day. [Trade only: MDI: 75 mcg/actuation, 240/canister. Built-in spacer.] ▶L ♀C ▶? $$$$

Leukotriene Inhibitors

MONTELUKAST (*Singulair*) Adults: 10 mg PO daily in the evening. Chronic asthma, allergic rhinitis: Give 5 mg PO daily for age 6 to 14 yo, give 4 mg (chew tab or oral granules) PO daily for age 2 to 5 yo. Asthma age 12 to 23 mo: 4 mg (oral granules) PO daily. Allergic rhinitis age 6 to 23 mo: 4 mg (oral granules) PO daily. Prevention of exercise-induced bronchoconstriction: 10 mg PO 2 h before exercise. [Generic/Trade only: Tabs 10 mg. Oral granules 4 mg packet, 30/box. Chewable tabs (cherry flavored) 4, 5 mg.] ▶L ♀B ▶? $$$$
ZAFIRLUKAST (*Accolate*) 20 mg PO two times per day. Peds age 5 to 11 yo, 10 mg PO two times per day. Take at least 1 h before or 2 h after meals. Potentiates warfarin and theophylline. [Trade only: Tabs 10, 20 mg.] ▶L ♀B ▶– $$$$
ZILEUTON (*Zyflo CR*) 1200 mg PO two times per day. Take within 1 h after morning and evening meals. Hepatotoxicity, potentiates warfarin, theophylline, and propranolol. [Trade only: Tabs, extended-release 600 mg.] ▶L ♀C ▶? $$$$$

Other Pulmonary Medications

ACETYLCYSTEINE—INHALED (*Mucomyst*) Mucolytic: 3 to 5 mL of 20% or 6 to 10 mL of 10% soln nebulized three to four times per day. [Generic/Trade: Soln for inhalation 10, 20% in 4, 10, 30 mL vials.] ▶L ♀B ▶? $
ACLIDINIUM (*Tudorza*) COPD: Pressair: 400 mcg two times per day. [Trade only: Sealed aluminum pouches 400 mcg per actuation. To be used with "Pressair" device only. Packages of 60 with Pressair device.] ▶L – ♀C ▶? $$$$$
CROMOLYN—INHALED (*Intal, Gastrocrom, ✦Nalcrom*) Asthma: 2 to 4 puffs four times per day or 20 mg nebs four times per day. Prevention of exercise-induced bronchospasm: 2 puffs 10 to 15 min prior to exercise. Mastocytosis: Oral concentrate 200 mg PO four times per day for adults, 100 mg four times per day in children 2 to 12 yo. [Generic only: Soln for nebs: 20 mg/2 mL. Generic/Trade: Oral concentrate 100 mg/5 mL in individual amps.] ▶LK ♀B ▶? $
DORNASE ALFA (*Pulmozyme*) Cystic fibrosis: 2.5 mg nebulized one to two times per day. [Trade only: Soln for inhalation: 1 mg/mL in 2.5 mL vials.] ▶L ♀B ▶? $$$$$
EPINEPHRINE RACEMIC (*S-2*) Severe croup: 0.05 mL/kg/dose diluted to 3 mL w/NS. Max dose 0.5 mL. [Trade only: Soln for inhalation: 2.25% epinephrine in 15, 30 mL.] ▶Plasma ♀C ▶– $
IPRATROPIUM—INHALED (*Atrovent, Atrovent HFA*) 2 puffs four times per day, or one 500 mcg vial neb three to four times per day. Contraindicated with soy or peanut allergy (Atrovent MDI only). [Trade only: Atrovent HFA MDI: 17 mcg/actuation, 200/canister. Generic/Trade: Soln for nebulization: 0.02% (500 mcg/vial) in unit dose vials.] ▶Lung ♀B ▶? $$$$

INHALER COLORS (Body then cap—Generics may differ)

Inhaler	Colors	Inhaler	Colors
Advair	purple	Maxair Autohaler	white/white
Advair HFA	purple/light purple	ProAir HFA	red/white
AeroBid-M	grey/green	Proventil HFA	yellow/orange
Aerospan	purple/grey		
Alupent	clear/blue	Pulmicort	white/brown
Alvesco		QVAR	
80 mcg	brown/red	40 mcg	beige/grey
160 mcg	red/red	80 mcg	mauve/grey
Asmanex	white/pink	Serevent Diskus	green
Atrovent HFA	clear/green		
Combivent	clear/orange	Spiriva	grey
Flovent HFA	orange/peach	Ventolin HFA	light blue/navy
Foradil	grey/beige	Xopenex HFA	blue/red

KETOTIFEN (✦ *Zaditen*) Canada only. For age 6 mo to 3 yo: Give 0.05 mg/kg PO two times per day. Age older than 3 yo: Give 1 mg PO two times per day. [Generic/Trade: Tabs 1 mg. Syrup 1 mg/5 mL.] ▶L ♀C ▶– $$

ROFLUMILAST (*Daliresp*, ✦ *Daxas*) Severe COPD due to chronic bronchitis: 500 mcg PO daily with or without food. [Trade: Tabs 500 mcg.] ▶L – ♀C ▶– $$$$

THEOPHYLLINE (*Elixophyllin, Uniphyl, Theo-24, T-Phyl,* ✦ *Theo ER, Theolair*) 5 to 13 mg/kg/day PO in divided doses. Max dose 900 mg/day. Peds dosing variable. [Generic/Trade: Elixir 80 mg/15 mL. Trade only: Caps: Theo-24: 100, 200, 300, 400 mg. T-Phyl: 12-h SR tabs 200 mg. Theolair: Tabs 125, 250 mg. Generic only: 12-h tabs 100, 200, 300, 450 mg, 12-h caps 125, 200, 300 mg.] ▶L ♀C ▶+ $

TIOTROPIUM (*Spiriva*) COPD: Handihaler: 18 mcg inhaled daily. [Trade only: Caps for oral inhalation 18 mcg. To be used with "Handihaler" device only. Packages of 5, 30, 90 caps with Handihaler device.] ▶K ♀C ▶– $$$$

TOXICOLOGY

Toxicology

ACETYLCYSTEINE (*N-acetylcysteine, Mucomyst, Acetadote,* ✦ *Parvolex*) Contrast nephropathy prophylaxis: 600 mg PO two times per day on the day before and on the day of contrast. Acetaminophen toxicity: Mucomyst (Oral): Loading dose 140 mg/kg PO or NG, then 70 mg/kg q 4 h for 17 doses. May be mixed in water or soft drink diluted to a 5% soln. Acetadote (IV): Loading

(cont.)

dose 150 mg/kg in 200 mL of D5W infused over 60 min; maintenance dose 50 mg/kg in 500 mL of D5W infused over 4 h followed by 100 mg/kg in 1000 mL of D5W infused over 16 h. [Generic/Trade: Soln 10%, 20%. Intravenous (Acetadote).] ▶L ♀B ▶? $$$$

CHARCOAL (activated charcoal, *Actidose-Aqua, CharcoAid, EZ-Char, ✦ Charcodate*) 25 to 100 g (1 to 2 g/kg) PO or NG as soon as possible. May repeat q 1 to 4 h prn at doses equivalent to 12.5 g/h. When sorbitol is coadministered, use only with the first dose if repeated doses are to be given. [OTC/Generic/Trade: Powder 15, 30, 40, 120, 240 g. Soln 12.5 g/60 mL, 15 g/75 mL, 15 g/120 mL, 25 g/120 mL, 30 g/120 mL, 50 g/240 mL. Susp 15 g/120 mL, 25 g/120 mL, 30 g/150 mL, 50 g/240 mL. Granules 15 g/120 mL.] ▶Not absorbed ♀+ ▶+ $

DEFEROXAMINE (*Desferal*) Chronic iron overload: 500 to 1000 mg IM daily and 2 g IV infusion (no faster than 15 mg/kg/h) with each unit of blood or 1 to 2 g SC daily (20 to 40 mg/kg/day) over 8 to 24 h via continuous infusion pump. Acute iron toxicity: IV infusion up to 15 mg/kg/h (consult poison center). ▶K ♀C ▶? $$$$$

FLUMAZENIL (*Romazicon*) Benzodiazepine sedation reversal: 0.2 mg IV over 15 sec, then 0.2 mg q 1 min prn up to 1 mg total dose. Overdose reversal: 0.2 mg IV over 30 sec, then 0.3 to 0.5 mg q 30 sec prn up to 3 mg total dose. Contraindicated in mixed drug overdose or chronic benzodiazepine use. ▶LK ♀C ▶? $$$$

HYDROXOCOBALAMIN (*Cyanokit*) Cyanide poisoning: 5 g IV over 15 min; may repeat prn. ▶K ♀C ▶? $$$$$

IPECAC SYRUP Emesis: 30 mL PO for adults, 15 mL age 1 to 12 yo. [OTC Generic only: Syrup 30 mL.] ▶Gut ♀C ▶? $

METHYLENE BLUE (*Urolene blue*) Methemoglobinemia: 1 to 2 mg/kg IV over 5 min. Dysuria: 65 to 130 mg PO three times per day after meals with liberal water. May turn urine/contact lenses blue. [Trade only: Tabs 65 mg.] ▶K ♀C ▶? $

ANTIDOTES

Toxin	Antidote/Treatment
acetaminophen	N-acetylcysteine
TCAs	sodium bicarbonate
arsenic, mercury	dimercaprol (BAL)
benzodiazepine	flumazenil
beta-blockers	glucagon
calcium channel blockers	calcium chloride, glucagon
cyanide	cyanide antidote kit, Cyanokit (hydroxocobalamin)

Toxin	Antidote/Treatment
digoxin	dig immune Fab
ethylene glycol	fomepizole
heparin	protamine
iron	deferoxamine
lead	BAL, EDTA, succimer
methanol	fomepizole
methemoglobin	methylene blue
opioids/opiates	naloxone
organophosphates	atropine + pralidoxime
warfarin	vitamin K, FFP

PRALIDOXIME (*Protopam, 2-PAM*) Organophosphate poisoning: Consult poison center: 1 to 2 g IV infusion over 15 to 30 min or slow IV injection over 5 min or longer (max rate 200 mg/min). May repeat dose after 1 h if muscle weakness persists. High-dose regimen (unapproved): 2 g over 30 min, followed by 1 g/h for 48 h, then 1 g/h q 4 h until improved. Peds: 20 to 50 mg/kg/dose IV over 15 to 30 min. ▶K ♀C ▶? $$$$

SUCCIMER (*Chemet*) Lead toxicity in children 1 yo or older: Start 10 mg/kg PO or 350 mg/m^2 q 8 h for 5 days, then reduce the frequency to q 12 h for 2 weeks. [Trade only: Caps 100 mg.] ▶K ♀C ▶? $$$$$

UROLOGY

Benign Prostatic Hyperplasia

ALFUZOSIN (*UroXatral*, ✦*Xatral*) 10 mg PO daily after a meal. [Generic/Trade: Tabs, extended-release 10 mg.] ▶KL ♀B ▶– $

DUTASTERIDE (*Avodart*) 0.5 mg PO daily. [Trade only: Caps 0.5 mg.] ▶L ♀X ▶– $$$$

FINASTERIDE (*Proscar, Propecia*) To reduce the risk of symptomatic progression of BPH: Proscar: 5 mg PO daily alone or in combination with doxazosin. Androgenetic alopecia in men: Propecia: 1 mg PO daily. [Generic/Trade: Tabs 1 mg (Propecia), 5 mg (Proscar).] ▶L ♀X ▶– $$$

JALYN (dutasteride + tamsulosin) 0.5 mg dutasteride + 0.4 mg tamsulosin daily 30 minutes after a meal. [Trade only: Caps 0.5 mg dutasteride + 0.4 mg tamsulosin.] ▶LK – ♀X ▶– $$$$

SILODOSIN (*RAPAFLO*) 8 mg PO daily with a meal. [Trade: Caps 8 mg.] ▶LK – ♀B ▶– $$$$

TAMSULOSIN (*Flomax*) 0.4 mg PO daily, 30 min after a meal. Maximum 0.8 mg/day. [Generic/Trade: Caps 0.4 mg.] ▶LK ♀B ▶– $$$$

Bladder Agents—Anticholinergics and Combinations

DARIFENACIN (*Enablex*) Overactive bladder with symptoms of urinary urgency, frequency, and urge incontinence: 7.5 mg PO daily. May increase to max dose 15 mg PO daily in 2 weeks. Max dose 7.5 mg PO daily with moderate liver impairment or when coadministered with potent CYP3A4 inhibitors (ketoconazole, itraconazole, ritonavir, nelfinavir, clarithromycin, and nefazodone). [Trade only: Tabs, extended-release 7.5, 15 mg.] ▶LK ♀C ▶– $$$$

FESOTERODINE (*Toviaz*) Overactive bladder: 4 to 8 mg PO daily. [Trade only: Tabs, extended-release 4, 8 mg.] ▶plasma ♀C ▶– $$$$

OXYBUTYNIN (*Ditropan, Ditropan XL, Gelnique, Oxytrol*, ✦*Oxybutyn, Uromax*) Bladder instability: 2.5 to 5 mg PO two to three times per day, max 5 mg PO four times per day. Extended-release tabs: 5 to 10 mg PO daily, increase 5 mg/day q week to 30 mg/day. Oxytrol: 1 patch twice a week on

(cont.)

abdomen, hips, or buttocks. Gelnique: Apply gel once daily to abdomen, upper arms/shoulders, or thighs. [Generic/Trade: Tabs 5 mg. Syrup 5 mg/5 mL. Tabs, extended-release 5, 10, 15 mg. Trade only: Transdermal patch (Oxytrol) 3.9 mg/day. Gelnique 3%, 10% gel, 1 g unit dose.] ▶LK ♀B ▶? $$

PROSED/DS (methenamine + phenyl salicylate + methylene blue + benzoic acid + hyoscyamine) Bladder spasm: 1 tab PO four times per day with liberal fluids. May turn urine/contact lenses blue. [Trade only: Tabs (methenamine 81.6 mg/phenyl salicylate 36.2 mg/methylene blue 10.8 mg/benzoic acid 9.0 mg/hyoscyamine sulfate 0.12 mg).] ▶KL ♀C ▶? $$

SOLIFENACIN (*VESIcare*) Overactive bladder with symptoms of urinary urgency, frequency, or urge incontinence: 5 mg PO daily. Max dose: 10 mg daily (5 mg daily if CrCl less than 30 mL/min, moderate hepatic impairment, or concurrent ketoconazole or other potent CYP3A4 inhibitors). [Trade only: Tabs 5, 10 mg.] ▶LK ♀C ▶– $$$$

TOLTERODINE (*Detrol, Detrol LA*) Overactive bladder: 1 to 2 mg PO two times per day (Detrol) or 2 to 4 mg PO daily (Detrol LA). [Generic/Trade: Tabs 1, 2 mg. Trade only: Caps, extended-release 2, 4 mg.] ▶L ♀C ▶– $$$$$

TROSPIUM (*Sanctura, Sanctura XR, ✦ Trosec*) Overactive bladder with urge incontinence: 20 mg PO two times per day; give 20 mg at bedtime if CrCl less than 30 mL/min. If age 75 yo or older may taper down to 20 mg daily. Extended-release: 60 mg PO q am, 1 h before food. [Generic/Trade: Tabs 20 mg, Caps, extended-release 60 mg.] ▶LK ♀C ▶? $$$$

URISED (methenamine + phenyl salicylate + atropine + hyoscyamine + benzoic acid + methylene blue) Dysuria: 2 tabs PO four times per day. May turn urine/contact lenses blue. Do not use with sulfa. [Trade only: Tabs (methenamine 40.8 mg/phenyl salicylate 18.1 mg/atropine 0.03 mg/hyoscyamine 0.03 mg/4.5 mg benzoic acid/5.4 mg methylene blue).] ▶K ♀C ▶? $

UTA (methenamine + sodium phosphate + phenyl salicylate + methylene blue + hyoscyamine) Bladder spasm: 1 cap PO four times per day with liberal fluids. [Trade only: Caps (methenamine 120 mg/sodium phosphate 40.8 mg/phenyl salicylate 36 mg/methylene blue 10 mg/hyoscyamine 0.12 mg).] ▶KL ♀C ▶? $$

UTIRA-C (methenamine + sodium phosphate + phenyl salicylate + methylene blue + hyoscyamine) Bladder spasm: 1 cap PO four times per day with liberal fluids. [Trade only: Tabs (methenamine 81.6 mg/sodium phosphate 40.8 mg/phenyl salicylate 36.2 mg/methylene blue 10.8 mg/hyoscyamine 0.12 mg).] ▶KL ♀C ▶? $$

Bladder Agents—Other

BETHANECHOL (*Urecholine, Duvoid*) Urinary retention: 10 to 50 mg PO three to four times per day. [Generic/Trade: Tabs 5, 10, 25, 50 mg.] ▶L ♀C ▶? $$$$

MIRABEGRON (*Myrbetriq*) Overactive bladder with symptoms of urge urinary incontinence, urgency, and urinary frequency: 25 mg PO daily. May increase to 50 mg unless severe renal impairment or moderate hepatic impairment. [Trade only: Extended-release tabs: 25, 50 mg.] ▶LK – ♀C ▶?

PHENAZOPYRIDINE (*Pyridium, Azo-Standard, Urogesic, Prodium, Pyridiate, Urodol, Baridium, UTI Relief*) Dysuria: 200 mg PO three times per day for 2 days. May turn urine/contact lenses orange. [OTC Generic/Trade: Tabs 95, 97.2 mg. Rx Generic/Trade: Tabs 100, 200 mg.] ▶K ♀B ▶? $

Erectile Dysfunction

ALPROSTADIL (*Muse, Caverject, Caverject Impulse, Edex, Prostin VR Pediatric*, prostaglandin E1, ✦ *Prostin VR*) 1 intraurethral pellet (Muse) or intracavernosal injection (Caverject, Edex) at lowest dose that will produce erection. Onset of effect is 5 to 20 min. [Trade only: Syringe system (Edex) 10, 20, 40 mcg. (Caverject) 5, 10, 20, 40 mcg. (Caverject Impulse) 10, 20 mcg. Pellet (Muse) 125, 250, 500, 1000 mcg. Intracorporeal injection of locally compounded combination agents (many variations): "Bi-mix" can be 30 mg/mL papaverine + 0.5 to 1 mg/mL phentolamine, or 30 mg/mL papaverine + 20 mcg/mL alprostadil in 10 mL vials. "Tri-mix" can be 30 mg/mL papaverine + 1 mg/mL phentolamine + 10 mcg/mL alprostadil in 5, 10, or 20 mL vials.] ▶L ♀- $$$$

AVANAFIL (*Stendra*) Start 100 mg PO 30 minutes prior to sexual activity. Max 1 dose/day. May increase to 200 mg or decrease to 50 mg prn. Contraindicated with nitrates and strong CYP3A4 inhibitors. Start at 50 mg if concurrent alpha blocker or moderate CYP3A4 inhibitor. [Trade only (Stendra): Tabs 50, 100, 200 mg.] ▶L – ♀C ▶? $$$$

SILDENAFIL (*Viagra*) Start 50 mg PO 0.5 to 4 h prior to intercourse. Max 1 dose/day. Usual effective range 25 to 100 mg. Start at 25 mg if age 65 yo or older or liver/renal impairment. Contraindicated with nitrates. [Trade only (Viagra): Tabs 25, 50, 100 mg. Unscored tab but can be cut in half.] ▶LK ♀B ▶- $$$$

TADALAFIL (*Cialis*) 2.5 to 5 mg PO daily without regard to timing of sexual activity. As-needed dosing: Start 10 mg PO at least 30 to 45 min prior to sexual activity. May increase to 20 mg or decrease to 5 mg prn. Max 1 dose/day. Start 5 mg (max 1 dose/day) if CrCl is 31 to 50 mL/min. Max 5 mg/day if CrCl < 30 mL/min, including patients on dialysis. Start 10 mg/day if mild to moderate hepatic impairment; avoid in severe hepatic impairment. Max 10 mg once in 72 h if concurrent potent CYP3A4 inhibitors. BPH with or without erectile dysfunction: 5 mg PO daily. Contraindicated with nitrates and alpha-blockers (except tamsulosin 0.4 mg daily). Not FDA approved for women. [Trade only (Cialis): Tabs 2.5, 5, 10, 20 mg.] ▶L ♀B ▶- $$$$

VARDENAFIL (*Levitra, Staxyn*) Start 10 mg PO 1 h before sexual activity. Usual effective dose range 5 to 20 mg. Max 1 dose/day. Use lower dose (5 mg) if age 65 yo or older or moderate hepatic impairment (max 10 mg). Contraindicated with nitrates and alpha-blockers. Not FDA approved in women. [Trade only: Tabs 2.5, 5, 10, 20 mg. Orally disintegrating tabs 10 mg (Staxyn).] ▶LK ♀B ▶- $$$$$

YOHIMBINE (*Yocon, Yohimex*) 5.4 mg PO three times per day. Not FDA approved. [Generic/Trade: Tabs 5.4 mg.] ▶L ♀- ▶- $

Nephrolithiasis

CITRATE (*Polycitra-K,   Urocit-K,   Bicitra,   Oracit,   Polycitra, Polycitra-LC*) Urinary alkalinization: 1 packet in water/juice PO three to four times per day. [Generic/Trade: Polycitra-K packet 3300 mg potassium citrate/ea, Polycitra-K oral soln (1100 mg potassium citrate/5 mL, 480 mL). Oracit oral soln (490 mg sodium citrate/5 mL, 15, 30, 480 mL). Bicitra oral soln (500 mg sodium citrate/5 mL, 480 mL). Urocit-K wax (potassium citrate) Tabs 5, 10 mEq. Polycitra-LC oral soln (550 mg potassium citrate/500 mg sodium citrate per 5 mL, 480 mL). Polycitra oral syrup (550 mg potassium citrate/500 mg sodium citrate per 5 mL, 480 mL.] ▶K ♀C ▶? $$$

INDEX

A

A-200 77
abacavir 21–23
ABC 22–23
abciximab 62
Abelcet 16
Abenol 12
Abilify 168
Abilify Discmelt 168
Abilify Maintena 168
abobotulinumtoxin
    A 144
Abreva 79
Absorica 74
Abstral 7
acamprosate 173
Acanya 73
acarbose 86
Accolate 180
AccuNeb 177
Accu-Prep 116
Accupril 47, 48
accuretic 60
Accutane
    Roche 74
acebutolol 63
acemannan 126
Aceon 47, 48
Acetadote 181–182
acetaminophen 3,
    9–12, 153, 182
acetazolamide 67
acetic acid 106
acetylcysteine—
    181–182
acetylcysteine—
    inhaled 180
acetylsalicylic acid—
    2–4, 10, 11, 48,
    62, 111
Acidophilus ... 129–130
AcipHex 114
acitretin 78
Aclasta 84–85
aclidinium 181
ActHIB 131
Acticin 78
Actidose-Aqua 182

Actifed Cold & Allergy
    104
Actifed Cold & Sinus ..
    104
Actigall 120
Actiq 7
Activase 70
Activase rt-PA 70
activated charcoal 182
Activella 147
Actonel 84
Actoplus Met 87
Actoplus Met XR 87
Actos 93
Actron 5
Acular 161
Acular LS 161
Acuvail 161
acyclovir ... 20, 35, 36,
    153
acyclovir—topical ... 79
Aczone 18
Adacel 131
Adalat 65–66
Adalat CC 65–66
Adalat PA 65–66
Adalat XL 65–66
adalimumab 1
adapalene 73, 74
Adcirca 70
Adderall 174
Adderall XR 174
adefovir 30
Adenocard 49
adenosine 49–50
ADH 102
Adipex-P 176
Adoxa 44
adrenalin 69
Advagraf 135
Advair 178, 181
Advair HFA ... 178, 181
Advicor 56
Advil 6
Aerius 103
AeroBid 179
AeroBid-M ... 179, 181
Aerospan 179, 181
Aesculus
    hippocastanum .. 129

Afeditab CR 65–66
aflibercept 161
Afluria 132
African plum tree . 130
Afrin 108
Aggrastat 63
Aggrenox 62
Agrylin 125
AK Tracin 157
Akarpine 160
AK-Con 155
AK-Dilate 161
Akineton 142
AK-Mycin 157
AK-Pentolate 161
Akten 162
Akurza 74
Alamast 156
Alavert 103
Alavert D-12 104
Albalon 155
albendazole 18
Albenza 18
albumin 71
Albuminar 71
albuterol ... 177, 179
alcaftadine 155
Alcaine 162
alclometasone
    dipropionate 80
Aldactazide 48
Aldactone 48
Aldara 79
Aldomet 59
Aldoril 60
alefacept 1
alendronate 84
Alertec 176
Aleve 6
alfuzosin 50, 183
Align 129–130
Alinia 19
aliskiren 60–61
alitretinoin 81
Alka-Seltzer 1
All Clear 155
Allegra 103

Allegra-D 12-h 104
Allegra-D 24-h 104
Aller-Chlor 103
Allerdryl 103
Allerfrim 104
Allermax 103
AllerNaze 108
Aller-Relief 103
Alli 120
Allium sativum 128
allopurinol 94
Alluna 131
Almora 96
almotriptan 140
Alocril 156
aloe vera 126
alogliptin 88
Alomide 156
Aloprim 94
Alora 146
alosetron 118
Aloxi 110
alpha lipoic acid .. 126
alpha-
    galactosidase 119
Alphagan 160
Alphagan P 160
alprazolam 172
alprostadil 185
Alrex 159
Alsuma 140
Altabax 76
Altace 47, 48
Altafrin 161
altavera 148
alteplase 70
Alternagel 112
Altoprev 57
Alu-Cap 112
aluminum
    acetate 106
aluminum
    chloride 81
aluminum hydroxide...
    2, 112
Alupent 177, 181
Alu-Tab 112
Alvesco 179, 181
alvimopan 119
alyacen 149

amantadine...... 28, 50
Amaryl.................. 92
Amatine................ 70
Ambien................ 173
Ambien CR.......... 173
AmBisome........... 16
amcinonide......... 80
Amerge............... 140
Amevive.............. 78
Amicar................ 125
Amidate.............. 13
Amigesic............... 4
amikacin............. 14
amiloride............ 61
aminocaproic
    acid................ 125
amiodarone..... 50–51
Amitiza.............. 117
amitriptyline........ 4
AmLactin............ 82
amlexanox.......... 107
amlodipine..... 56–57,
    60–61, 65
Amnesteem........ 74
amoxicillin.... 34, 39,
    40, 113
amoxicillin-
    clavulanate ... 39, 41
amphetamine..... 174
Amphojel............ 112
Amphotec............ 16
amphotericin B
    deoxycholate.... 16
amphotericin B lipid
    formulations..... 16
ampicillin....... 40, 41
ampicillin-
    sulbactam........ 41
Ampyra.............. 141
Amrix................. 12
Amturnide.......... 60
Anacin................. 4
Anafranil............ 162
anagrelide.......... 125
anakinra............... 1
Anaprox............... 6
Anaspaz.............. 115
Ancobon.............. 16
Andriol......... 83–84
Androderm.... 83–84
AndroGel...... 83–84
Anectine............. 14

Anexsia................. 9
Angeliq.............. 147
Angiomax... 120–121
angiotensin
    receptor blocker.. 60
anhydrous glycerins ...
    106
anidulafungin 15
Ansaid.................. 5
Antabuse............ 173
antacids............. 153
Antara.......... 54–55
antazoline........... 155
Anthemis nobilis—
    Roman
    chamomile 126
Anthraforte......... 78
anthralin............. 78
Anthranol............ 78
Anthrascalp......... 78
antipyrine........... 106
antivenin—
    crotalidae immune
    FAB ovine
    polyvalent........ 133
Antivert............. 105
Anzemet............. 109
Aphthasol........... 107
Apidra........... 91, 92
Aplenzin..... 165–166
Aplisol............... 135
Apokyn............... 142
apomorphine....... 142
Apprilon............. 44
aprepitant........... 110
Apresazide.......... 60
Apresoline.......... 62
Apriso................ 118
Aprodine............ 104
Aptivus.............. 28
AquaMephyton.... 100
Aquasol E........... 101
Aralen................ 17
aranelle.............. 149
Aranesp.............. 124
Arava................... 1
Arcapta.............. 176
Aredia................ 84
arformoterol...... 176
argatroban.......... 120
Aricept.............. 159
aripiprazole ... 168, 169
Aristospan.......... 86
Arixtra............... 121
armodafinil........ 175
arsenic............... 182

arsenic trioxide...... 50
Artane................ 142
artemether........... 17
Arthrotec.............. 4
articaine............... 13
artichoke leaf extract ..
    126
artificial tears 162
Asacol................ 118
Asaphen................ 4
Ascriptin.............. 2
asceorbic acid.. 99, 100
asenapine ... 168, 169
Aslera................ 127
Asmanex............ 181
Asmanex
    Twisthale........ 179
A-spaz................ 115
Aspirin................ 4
Aspir-Mox............ 2
Astelin............... 108
Astepro.............. 108
astragalus........... 126
Astragalus
    membranaceus . 126
Atacand.............. 49
Atacand HCT....... 60
Atacand Plus....... 60
Atarax............... 105
Atasol................ 12
Atasol
    (-8,-15,-30)........ 11
atazanavir... 24, 50
Atelvia............... 84
atenolol......... 61, 63
Atgam............... 133
Ativan................ 172
atomoxetine....... 175
atorvastatin... 56–57,
    60
atovaquone ... 17, 19
Atripla................ 21
AtroPen............... 51
atropine.... 51, 109,
    114, 182, 184
Atropine
    Care
    160–161
atropine—ophthalmic
    160–161
atrovastatin........ 57
Atrovent............. 180
Atrovent
    HFA..... 180, 181
Atrovent Nasal
    Spray............. 108
A/T/S.................. 74

ATV..................... 24
Augmentin...... 39, 41
Augmentin
    ES-600...... 39, 41
Augmentin XR . 39, 41
Auralgan........... 106
Auvi-Q................ 69
Avage................. 75
Avalide............... 60
Avamys............. 108
avanafil............. 185
Avandamet.......... 87
Avandaryl........... 87
Avandia.............. 93
Avapro............... 49
Avaxim.............. 131
Aveeno................ 82
Avelox................ 42
Aventyl.............. 163
Aviane............... 148
Avinza............. 8–9
Avodart............. 183
Avonex.............. 141
Axert................. 140
Axid................. 112
Axid AR............. 112
Axiron.......... 83–84
Aygestin............ 151
Azactam.............. 44
Azasan................. 1
Azasite.............. 157
azathioprine......... 1
azelaic acid......... 73
azelastine—
    nasal............. 108
azelastine—
    ophthalmic...... 155
Azelex................ 73
Azilect............... 144
azilsartan..... 49, 60
azithromycin.... 35,
    37–38, 50, 153
azithromycin—
    ophthalmic...... 157
Azopt................ 159
Azor.................. 60
Azo-Standard..... 185
AZT.................... 23
aztreonam........... 44
Azulfidine.......... 118
Azulfidine EN-tabs 118
azurette............. 148

B

BabyBIG............ 133
Bacid........... 129–130

bacitracin.............. 75, 76, 157
bacitracin—
ophthalmic 157
baclofen 2
Bactrim 42–43
Bactroban 76
BAL 182
balsalazide 118
balziva 148
banana bag 98
Banophen 103
Banzel 139
Baraclude 30
Baridium 185
barium
sulfate.......... 73
Basaljel............. 112
basiliximab 134
Bayer................. 4
Baygam 133
BayTet 133
BCG vaccine 131
B-D Glucose 93
Beano 119
becaplermin 81
beclomethasone
107, 153
beclomethasone
HFA MDI 178
beclomethasone—
inhaled............ 179
Beconase AQ 107
bedaquiline 50
belatacept 134
Belviq 119
Benadryl 103
Benadryl Allergy/
Cold.............. 104
Benadryl-D Allergy/
Sinus Tablets 104
benazepril 47, 61
bendroflume-
thiazide 60
Benicar.............. 49
Benicar HCT 60
Benoquin 82
Bentyl 114
Bentylol 114
Benylin 105
Benzac 74
Benzaclin 74
Benzagel 10% 74
Benzamycin 74
benzathine
penicillin 36, 38
benzocaine 106, 108

benzodiazepines.....
171–172, 176
benzoic acid 184
benzonatate 105
benzoyl peroxide
73–74, 153
benztropine
mesylate 142
benzyl alcohol...... 78
bepotastine 155
Bepreve............ 155
besifloxacin 156
Besivance 156
beta-blockers. 60, 182
Betagan 159
Betaject 85
Betaloc............. 64
betamethasone
78, 81, 85
betamethasone
dipropionate....... 80
betamethasone
valerate 80
Betapace............ 53
Betapace AF 53
Betaseron 141
betaxolol—
ophthalmic 159
bethanechol 184
Bethkis 14
Betimol............. 159
Betoptic 159
Betoptic S......... 159
beyaz 148
bezafibrate 54
Bezalip SR 54
Biaxin 38
Biaxin XL 38
bicarbonate.. 111, 114
Bicillin C-R......... 38
Bicillin L-A 38
Bicitra 186
BIDIL 71
Bifantis 129–130
Bifidobacteria......
129–130
bile acid
sequestrants 53
Biltricide 19
bimatoprost 160
Binosto............. 84
Bionect 82
BioRab 87
biotin......... 99, 100
biperiden 142
Biphentin 176
bisacodyl 117, 153

*Bisacodyl Tablet
Kit* 116
bismuth subcitrate
potassium 113
bismuth
subsalicylate.... 109,
113
bisoprolol 61, 63
bivalirudin 120
Bleph-10.......... 157
Blephamide........ 157
Bloxiverz 13, 14
boceprevir 30
Bonamine 105
Bonine 105
Boniva 84
Boostrix........... 131
boric acid 152
Botox............. 145
Botox Cosmetic.... 145
botulism immune
globulin 133
Breo ellipt....... 179
Brevibloc.......... 64
brevicon 148
Brevital 13
briellyn 148
Brilinta 63
brimonidine 160
brinzolamide 159, 160
bromazepam 171
Bromday 161
bromfenac—
ophthalmic 161
Bromfenex 105
bromocriptine 101
Brovana 176
buckeye 129
budesonide. 119, 153,
178, 179
budesonide DPI ... 178
budesonide—
inhaled............ 179
budesonide—
nasal 107
Bufferin............ 3
bumetanide 67
Bumex 67
Buminate 67
bupivacaine 13
Buprenex 6
buprenorphine.. 6, 8,
174
Buproban 165–166
bupropion 153,
165–166
Burinex 67

burn plant 126
Buscopan 114
BuSpar 172
buspirone ... 153, 172
butalbital 3, 10
butamben 108
butenafine 76
butoconazole .. 35, 152
butorphanol 7, 8
Butrans 6
butterbur 126
Bydureon 89
Byetta 89
Bystolic 65

C

cabergoline 101
Caduet 56–57, 60
Cafcit 175
Cafergot 141
Caffedrine 175
caffeine ... 3, 10, 11,
141, 175
calamine 81
Calan 66–67
Calciferol 99
Calcijex 99
Calcimar 101
calcipotriene 78
calcitonin 101
calcitriol 99
calcium acetate 94
calcium carbonate .. 2,
3, 94–95, 112, 113
calcium channel
blockers....... 60, 182
calcium chloride.... 95
calcium citrate 95
calcium gluconate.. 95
Caldolor............. 5
CalMist 99
Caltine 101
Caltrate 94–95
Cambia 4–5
Camellia sinensis...
128–129
Camila 148, 151
Campral 173
canagliflozin 93
Canasa 118

Cancidas................. 16
candesartan... 49, 60
CanesOral 14–15
Canesten..................
14, 77, 152
Cankermelt............ 129
Capital with Codeine
suspension 86
Capoten.................. 47
Capozide................ 60
capsaicin 81
captopril.... 47, 60
Carac 115
Carafate.............. 115
carbamazepine.... 136
Carbatrol 136
carbidopa 144
carbidopa/
levodopa 142
Carbocaine 13
carboprost........... 151
Cardene................ 65
Cardene SR 65
Cardizem.............. 66
Cardizem CD 66
Cardizem LA......... 66
Cardura................ 59
Cardura XL............ 59
Carimune 133
carisoprodol .. 2, 3, 11
Carnitor 98
carteolol—
ophthalmic 159
Cartia XT............. 66
carvedilol 64
cascara 117
caspofungin 16
castor oil 117
Cataflam.......... 4–5
Catapres.............. 59
Catapres-TTS 59
Cathflo 70
Caverject.......... 185
Caverject
Impulse 185
Cayston 44
caziant 149
Ceclor................. 32
Cedax 33
cefaclor................ 32
cefadroxil 32
cefazolin 32

cefdinir............. 33, 34
cefditoren 33
cefepime 37
cefixime 33, 35
cefotaxime............
33, 35, 40
cefoxitin 32, 36
cefpodoxime ....
33, 34, 40
cefprozil 32
ceftaroline.......... 37
ceftazidime 33
ceftibuten 33
ceftizoxime 33, 35
ceftriaxone ....
33–36, 40
cefuroxime....32–34
Cefzil..................... 32
Celebrex 4
celecoxib 4, 5
Celestone 85
Celestone
Soluspan........... 85
Celexa 164
Cellcept 134
Celsentri 20–21
Cena-K............... 97
Cenestin 147
cephalexin 32
cephalosporins 153
Cerebyx............. 137
Cervidil............. 150
Cesamet 111
Cetacaine 108
cetirizine 103
Cetraxal............ 106
cevimeline........ 107
chamomile 126
Champix 174
Chantix.............. 174
CharcoAid......... 182
Charcocaps 182
Charcodote 182
chasteberry 126
Chemet.............. 183
ChiRhoStim 120
chloramphenicol.... 144
chlordiazepoxide ... 171
chlordiazepoxide—
clidinium 119
Chlordrine
SR 104

chlorhexidine
gluconate 107
chlorophyllin
copper complex ... 83
chloroquine ... 17, 50
chlorpheniramine 103,
153
chlorpromazine.... 50,
167, 169
chlorthalidone......
60, 61, 68
Chlor-Trimeton 103
chlorzoxazone 2
cholecalciferol.... 101
cholesterol absorption
inhibitor 55
cholestyramine.... 55
choline magnesium
trisalicylate 4
chondroitin 126
Chrysanthemum
parthenium 127
Cialis................. 185
ciclesonide 107
ciclesonide—
inhaled 179
ciclopirox 76
cidofovir 19
cilazapril 47, 61
cilostazol 72
Ciloxan............. 106
cimetidine 112, 153
Cimzia 119
Cipralex 164
Cipro 42
Cipro HC Otic 106
Cipro XR 42
Ciprodex Otic...... 106
ciprofloxacin ......
35, 42, 106
ciprofloxacin—
ophthalmic 156
cisapride 50
cisatracurium...... 14
citalopram.... 50, 164
Citracal 95
citrate 111, 186
citric acid 116
Citrucel 117
Ci-wu-jia 128
Claforan 33
Claravis.............. 74
Clarinex............ 103
Clarinex-D 24-h.... 104
Claripel 82
clarithromycin ......
38, 50, 113

Claritin................. 103
Claritin Hives
Relief................ 103
Claritin-D 12-h..... 104
Claritin-D 24-h..... 104
Clarus................... 74
Clavulin...... 39, 41
Clear Eyes 155
Clearasil.............. 74
Clearasil Cleanser.. 74
clemastine 103
Clenia 74
Cleocin 44, 152
Cleocin T............. 74
clevidipine 65
Cleviprex............. 65
Climara 146
Climara Pro........ 147
Clindagel............. 74
ClindaMax............ 74
clindamycin....34–36,
40, 44, 73–75, 153
clindamycin—
topical............. 74
clindamycin—
vaginal............ 152
Clindesse 152
Clindoxyl..... 73, 74
Clinoleic 98
Clinoril 6
clobazam 136
clobetasol........... 80
clocortolone
pivalate............ 80
Clomid............... 150
clomiphene 150
clomipramine 162
Clonapam 171
clonazepam 171
clonidine 59, 60
clorazepate........ 171
Clorpres............... 60
Clotrimaderm .. 14, 77,
152
clotrimazole.. 14, 81,
153
clotrimazole—
topical............. 77
clotrimazole—
vaginal............ 152
clozapine 50,
168, 169
Clozaril 168
coal tar.............. 104
Coartem 17
coarteemether........ 17

cobicistat 21
codeine.... 7, 8, 10, 11, 153
coenzyme Q10, ... 127
Cogentin 142
Colace 117
Colazal 118
Colbenemid 94
colchicine 94
Colcrys 94
Cold-fX 128
colesevelam 53
Colestid 53
Colestid Flavored 53
colestipol 53
Colyte 116
Combantrin 94
Combigan 160
Combipatch 147
Combivent 170, 181
Combivent
  inhalation soln ... 179
Combivent
  Respimat 179
Combivir 21
Combunox 10
Commit 174
Compazine 111
Complera 21
Comtan 142
Comvax 131
Concerta 176
Condyline 79
Condylox 79
cone flower 127
Congest 147
Conray 73
Conzip 12
Copegus 31
CoQ-10 127
Cordarone 50
Coreg 64
Coreg CR 64
Corgard 64
Corlopam 61
Correctol 117
Cortef 86
Cortenema 86
cortisone 86
Cortisporin 81
Cortisporin Otic .. 106
Cortisporin TC
  Otic 106
Cortisporin—
  ophthalmic 158
Cortone 85
Cortrosyn 94

Corvert 52
Corzide 60
Cosamin DS 128
Cosopt 160
cosyntropin 94
Cotazym 120
cotrimoxazole .. 42–43
Coumadin 123
Covera-HS 66–67
Coversyl 48
Cozaar 49
Cranactin 127
cranberry 127
Crataegus
  laevigata 129
creatine 127
Creon 120
Crestor 58
Crinone 151
CroFab 133
crofelemer 119
Crolom 156
cromolyn 153
cromolyn—inhaled ...
  180
cromolyn—nasal . 108
cromolyn—
  ophthalmic 156
crotamiton 78
cryselle 148
Cubicin 45
Culturelle 129–130
Cutar 82
Cuvposa 119
cyanide 182
cyanocobalamin .. 99,
  100, 153
Cyanokit 182
cyclamate 148, 149
Cyclessa 149
cyclobenzaprine 2
Cyclogyl 161
Cyclomen 153
cyclopentolate 161
Cycloset 101
cyclosporine 134
cyclosporine—
  ophthalmic 158
Cyestra-35 74
Cymbalta 165
Cynara scolymus .. 126
cyproheptadine ... 103
cyproterone 74
Cystaran 162
cysteamine 162
Cystografin 73
Cystospaz 115

Cytomel 98
Cytotec 115, 150
Cytovene 19

D

dabigatran 121
daclizumab 134
Dalacin 152
Dalacin C 44
Dalacin T 74
dalfampridine 2
dalfopristin 45
Daliresp 181
Dalmane 171
dalteparin ... 121–122
danazol 153
Danocrine 153
Dantrium 2
dantrolene 2
dapsone 18
Daptacel 131
daptomycin 45
darbepoetin 124
darifenacin 183
darunavir 24–25
dasetta 148, 149
Daxas 181
Daypro 6
daysee 149
Daytrana 176
DDAVP 102
DDI 22
DDrops 101
Debacterol 107
Debrox 106
Decadron 85–86
Deconamine 104
Deconamine SR ... 104
Deconsal I 104
deferasirox 125
deferoxamine 182
dehydroepiand-
  rosterone 127
Delatestryl 83–84
Delestrogen 146
Delsym 105
Delzicol 118
Demadex 67
demeclocycline 44
Demerol 2
Denavir 79
denosumab 101
Denticare 107
Depacon 139–140
Depade 173

Depakene 139–140
Depakote ....
  139–140, 167
Depakote ER ..
  139–140, 167
DepoDur 8
Depo-Estradiol ... 146
Depo-Medrol 86
Depo-Provera 151
depo-subQ
  provera 104 151
Depo-Testosterone ..
  83–84
DermOtic 106
Desferal 182
desipramine . 153, 163
desirudin 121
desloratadine 103
desmopressin 102
desogen 148
desogestrel 148
desonide 80
desoximetasone 80
Desquam 74
desvenlafaxine 165
Desyrel 166
Detrol 184
Detrol LA 184
devil's claw 127
Dex-4 93
DexAlone 105
dexamethasone ....
  85–86, 103
dexamethasone—
  ophthalmic 158
Dexasone 85–86
dexchlorpheniramine ..
  103
Dexedrine 175
DexFerrum 96
Dexiron 96
dexmedetomidine .. 13
dexmethylphenidate ..
  175
Dexpak 85–86
dextran 71
dextroamphetamine ..
  174, 175
dextromethorphan ....
  105, 153
dextromethorphan/
  quinidine 144

dextrose.................. 93
D.H.E. 45................ 141
DHEA.................... 127
DiaBeta.................. 92
Diamicron.............. 92
Diamicron MR........ 92
Diamox.................. 67
Diamox Sequels...... 67
Diane-35................ 74
Diar-eze................ 171
Diastat.................. 171
Diastat AcuDial...... 171
diatrizoate............. 73
Diazemuls............. 171
diazepam.............. 171
dibucaine.............. 84
Diclegis................ 110
diclofenac............ 4–5
diclofenac—
  ophthalmic........ 161
diclofenac—
  topical.............. 75
dicloxacillin........... 39
dicyclomine.......... 114
didanosine............ 23
Didronel............... 84
dienogest.............. 149
difenoxin.............. 109
Differin................. 73
Dificid.................. 38
diflorasone
  diacetate........... 80
Diflucan......... 14–15
diflunisal.......... 4, 5
difluprednate........ 158
dig immune Fab.... 182
Digibind................ 51
DigiFab................. 51
Digitek................. 51
digoxin........... 51, 182
digoxin immune
  Fab.................. 51
dihydrocodeine...... 11
dihydroergotamine
  141
Dilacor XR............ 66
Dilantin.......... 138–139
Dilatrate-SR.......... 68
Dilaudid................ 4
Diltia XT................ 66
diltiazem.............. 66

Diltiazem CD........ 66
Diltzac................. 66
dimenhydrinate..... 110
dimercaprol.......... 182
Dimetane-DX....... 104
Dimetapp Cold &
  Allergy Elixir...... 104
Dimetapp
  Decongestant
  Infant Drops.....
  105–106
Dimetapp DM Cold &
  Cough.............. 104
dimethyl
  fumarate........... 141
dinoprostone........ 150
Diocarpine........... 160
Diogent................ 156
Diopred................ 159
Diovan.................. 49
Diovan HCT.......... 60
Dipentum............ 118
Diphen................ 103
Diphenhist.......... 103
diphenhydramine
  103, 107, 153
diphenoxylate...... 109
diphtheria, tetanus
  and acellular
  pertussis
  vaccine.... 131, 132
diphtheria-tetanus
  toxoid.............. 131
Diprivan.............. 13
dipyridamole........ 62
direct renin
  inhibitor........... 60
Disalcid................ 4
Diskets.................. 8
disopyramide.... 50, 51
disulfiram............ 173
Ditropan........ 183–184
Ditropan XL..183–184
divalproex.... 139–140,
  167
Divigel................ 146
Dixarit................ 59
dobutamine......... 69
docosanol............ 79
Docu-Liquid......... 117
docusate...... 117–118,
  153
Docu-Soft........... 117
docusate sodium
  117
dofetilide....... 50, 51
DOK.................... 117
dolasetron..... 50, 109
Dolobid................ 4

Dolophine............. 8
Doloral.............. 8–9
Doloteffin........... 127
Domeboro
  Otic................. 106
domperidone....... 110
Dona.................. 128
donepezil............ 135
Donnatal............. 114
dopamine............ 69
Doribax............... 32
doripenem........... 32
dornase alfa........ 180
Doryx.................. 44
dorzolamide.. 159, 160
Dostinex............. 101
Dovobet............... 78
Dovonex.............. 78
doxazosin............ 59
doxepin...... 153, 163
doxepin—
  topical.............. 82
doxercalciferol...... 99
Doxycin............... 44
doxycycline
  35, 36, 40, 44
doxylamine
  10, 110, 153
Dramamine......... 110
Drisdol................ 99
Dristan 12 Hr
  Nasal............... 108
Drithocreme......... 78
Drixoral Cold &
  Allergy............. 104
dronabinol........... 111
dronedarone...50–52
droperidol..... 50, 111
drospirenone
  147, 148
Droxia................ 125
DRV.............. 24–25
Dry Eyes............. 162
Drysol.................. 81
DT...................... 131
DTaP.................. 131
Duac................... 74
Duetact................ 87
Dulcolax............. 117
Dulera................ 179
duloxetine........... 165
Duodopa............. 142
Duolube.............. 162
Duoneb............... 179
Duragesic............. 8
Duratuss............ 104
Duratuss HD...... 104

Durela................. 12
Durezol............... 158
dutasteride......... 183
Dutoprol.............. 60
Duvoid................ 184
Dyazide............... 60
Dymista.............. 108
DynaCirc............. 65
DynaCirc CR........ 65
Dysport.............. 144
Dytan................. 103

E
E. angustifolia...... 127
E. pallida............ 127
E. purpurea........ 127
Ebixa................. 136
Echinacea........... 127
Echinacin
  Madaus........... 127
EchinaGuard...... 127
EC-Naprosyn........ 6
econazole............ 77
Econopred Plus.... 159
Ecotrin................. 4
ED Spaz.............. 115
Edarbi................. 49
Edarbyclor........... 60
Edecrin................ 67
Edex.................. 185
Edluar................ 173
edrophonium
  141–142
EDTA................. 182
Edurant............... 22
EEMT................. 147
EEMT H.S........... 150
EES.................... 38
efavirenz...... 21, 22
Effer-K................ 97
Effexor.............. 165
Effexor XR.......... 165
Effient........... 62–63
Efidac/24.....105–106
eflornithine.......... 82
Efudex................ 75
EFV.................... 22
EGb 761............ 128
Elavil................. 162
Eldepryl............. 144
elderberry.......... 127
Eldopaque............ 82
Eldoquin............. 82
Eldoquin Forte..... 82
Electropeg.......... 116
Elestat............... 155

Elestrin.............. 146
eletriptan 140
Eleutherococcus
    senticosus 128
Elidel................... 79
Elimite.................. 78
elinest 148
Eliphos 94
Eliquis 121
Elixophyllin 181
Ella....................... 146
Eltroxin 98
elvitegravir 21
Emadine 155
emedastine 155
Emend 110
Emetrol 111
EMLA 77
emoquette 148
Empirin 4
Empirin with
    Codeine 10
Emsam 163
emtricitabine... 21, 23
Emtriva 23
Enablex 183
enalapril 47, 61
enalaprilat 47
Enbrel 1
Enca 44
Endantadine 28
Endocet 11
Endocodone 9
Endodan 11
Endometrin 151
Enemeez 117
Enemol 116
Energix-B 131
Enjuvia 147
Enlon 141–142
enoxaparin 122
enpresse 149
entacapone .. 142, 144
entecavir 30
Entereg 119
Entex PSE 104
Entocort EC 119
Entrophen 4
Entsol 108
Enulose 115–116
Epaxal 131
Epiduo 77
epinastine 155
epinephrine 69
epinephrine racemic...
    180
EpiPen 69

EpiPen Jr 69
EpiQuin Micro......... 82
Epitol 136
Epivir 23
Epivir-HBV 23
eplerenone 48
epoetin alfa 124
Epogen 124
Eprex 124
eprosartan 49, 61
eptifibatide 62
Epzicom 21
Equalactin 115
Equetro 136
ER niacin 55
Eraxis 23
ergocalciferol 99
ergotamine 141
eribulin 50
Errin 148, 151
Ertaczo 77
ertapenem 32
Eryc 38
Erycette 74
Eryderm 74
Erygel 74
EryPed 38
Erysol 74
Ery-Tab 38
Erythrocin IV 38
erythromycin... 35, 36,
    50, 153
erythromycin base
    38, 74
erythromycin
    lactobionate 38
erythromycin—
    ophthalmic 157
erythromycins 153
erythromycin—
    topical 74
erythropoietin
    alpha 124
escitalopram .. 50, 164
Esgic 3
Eskalith 166–167
Eskalith CR
    166–167
esmolol 64
esomeprazole 113
Esoterica 82
Estalis 147
estazolam 172
esterified estrogens...
    146, 147, 150
Estrace 146–147

estradiol..... 146–147,
    150
estradiol
    acetate 146
estradiol acetate
    vaginal ring 146
estradiol cypionate
    146
estradiol gel 146
estradiol topical
    emulsion 146
estradiol transdermal
    patch 146
estradiol transdermal
    spray 146
estradiol vaginal
    ring 146
estradiol vaginal
    tab 146
estradiol valerate......
    146, 149
Estradot 146
Estrasorb 146
Estring 146
Estrogel 146
estrogen vaginal
    cream 146–147
estrogens conjugated.
    147, 150
estrogens synthetic
    conjugated A 147
estrogens synthetic
    conjugated B ... 147
estropipate 147
Estrostep Fe 149
eszopiclone 172
etanercept 1
ethacrynic acid....... 67
ethambutol............ 32
ethinyl estradiol .. 74,
    148–150
ethinyl estradiol
    transdermal 145
ethinyl estradiol
    vaginal ring 145
ethosuximide....... 136
ethylene glycol...... 182
Etibi 23
etidronate............. 84
etodolac 5
etomidate 112
etonogestrel 145
ETR....................... 22
etravirine 22
Euglucon 92
Eurax 78
Euthyrox 98

Evamist................ 146
everolimus 134
Evista 151
Evoclin 74
Evoxac 107
Evra 145
Exalgo 7
Excedrin Migraine.... 3
Exelon 135–136
Exelon Patch
    135–136
exenatide.............. 89
Exforge 60
Exforge HCT......... 60
Exjade 125
Ex-Lax 117
Exsel 83
Extina 77
Eylea 161
EZ-Char 182
ezetimibe... 55, 57–58
Ezetrol 58
ezogabine 137

F

Factive 42
falmina 148
famciclovir 20, 35, 36,
    153
famotidine.... 50, 112,
    153
Fampyra 141
Famvir 20
Fanapt 168
fat emulsion......... 98
FazaClo ODT 168
febuxostat 94
Feen-a-Mint 117
felbamate.... 50, 137
Felbatol 137
Feldene 6
felodipine 61, 65
Femaprin 126
Femcon Fe 148
femhrt................. 150
Femizol-M........... 152
Femring 146
Femtrace 146
fenofibrate..... 54–55

fenofibric acid 56
Fenoglide 54–55
fenoldopam 61
fentanyl 7, 8
transdermal 9
Fentora 9
fenugreek 127
Feosol 95
Feraheme 95
Fergon 95
Feridex 72
Fer-in-Sol 95
Ferodan 95
Ferrex 150 96
ferric gluconate
complex 95
Ferrlecit 95
ferrous gluconate ... 95
ferrous sulfate 95
ferumoxides 72
ferumoxsil 73
ferumoxytol 95
fesoterodine 183
feverfew 127
Fexicam 6
Fexmid 132
fexofenadine 103
FFP 182
Fiberall 115
FiberCon 115
fibrates 54
Fibricor 55
fidaxomicin 38
Fidelin 73
15-methyl-
prostaglandin F2
alpha 151
filgrastim 125
Finacea 73
finasteride 183
Finevin 73
fingolimod 50, 141
Fioricet 3
Fioricet with
Codeine 10
Fiorinal 10
Fiorinal C-1/2 10
Fiorinal C-1/4 10
Fiorinal with
Codeine 10
fish oil 95
5-Aspirin 118

5-FU 75
FK 506 135
Flagyl 45
Flagyl ER 45
Flamazine 76
Flarex 159
flavocoxid 127
Flebogamma 133
flecainide 50, 52
Flector 4–5
Fleet 115, 117
Fleet enema 116
Fleet EZ-Prep 116
Fleet Mineral Oil
Enema 116
Fleet Pain Relief 81
Fleet Phospho-Soda....
116
Fleet Sof-Lax 117
Fletcher's Castoria 117
Flexeril 2
Flomax 183
Flonase 108
Flo-Pred 86
Florastor 129–130
Florazole ER 45
Florinef 86
Floxin Otic 106
Fluarix 132
fluconazole 14–15, 35
flucytosine 16
fludrocortisone 85, 86
FluLaval 132
Flumadine 28
flumazenil 182
FluMist 132
flunarizine 141
flunisolide 107
flunisolide HFA MDI
178
flunisolide—
inhaled 179
fluocinolone 80, 83
fluocinolone—otic 106
fluocinonide 80
Fluor-A-Day 95
fluoride 95
fluorometholone ... 159
Fluoroplex 75
fluoroquinolones ... 35
fluorouracil—topical...
75
fluoxetine 164, 173
fluphenazine ...
167, 169

flurandrenolide 80
flurazepam 171
flurbiprofen 5
fluticasone DPI 178
fluticasone HFA
MDI 178
fluticasone
propionate—inhaled.
178–179
fluticasone—
nasal 108
fluvastatin 57
fluvastatin XL 57
Fluviral 132
Fluvirin 132
fluvoxamine 164
Fluzone 132
FML 159
FML Forte 159
FML-S Liquifilm ... 158
Focalin 175
Focalin XR 175
folate 99
folic acid ....
99, 100, 153
Folvite 99
fomepizole 182
fondaparinux 21
Foradil 176, 181
Forfivo XL 165–166
formoterol 176, 179
Fortamet 93
Fortaz 33
Forteo 101
Fortical 101
Fosamax 84
Fosamax Plus D 84
fosamprenavir 25
fosaprepitant 110
Fosavance 84
foscarnet 19, 50
Foscavir 19
fosfomycin 45
fosinopril 47, 50
fosphenytoin ... 50, 137
Fosrenol 98
FPV 25
Fragmin 121–122
Frisium 136
Froben 5
Froben SR 5
Frova 140
frovatriptan 140
FTC 23
Fucidin H 81
Fulvicin 16

Fulyzaq 119
Furadantin 45
furosemide 67
fusidic acid 81
fusidic acid—
topical 76

G

G115 128
gabapentin 137
Gabitril 139
Gadavist 72
gadobenate 72
gadobutrol 72
gadodiamide 72
gadopentetate 72
gadoteridol 72
gadoversetamide ... 72
galantamine 135
Galzin 97
Gamastan 133
gamma
hydroxybutyrate . 145
Gammagard 133
Gammaplex 133
Gamunex 133
ganciclovir 19, 157
Garamycin 76, 156
Gardasil 132
garlic
supplements 128
Gastrocrom 180
Gastrografin 73
GastroMARK 73
Gas-X 115
gatifloxacin 50
gatifloxacin—
ophthalmic 156
Gattex 120
Gaviscon 112
G-CSF 125
Gelclair 107
Gelnique
183–184
gemfibrozil 56
gemifloxacin ... 42, 50
Generess Fe 148
Gengraf 134
Genisoy 130
gen-K 97
Genoptic 156
Genotropin 102
Gentak 156
gentamicin 14, 36,
158

gentamicin—
  ophthalmic 156
gentamicin—
  topical 76
GenTeal 162
Gentran 71
Geodon 171
GHB 145
GI cocktail 114
Giazo 111
Gildagia 148
Gildess Fe 148
Gilenya 141
ginger 128
ginkgo
  biloba 128
Ginkgold 128
Ginkoba 128
Ginsana 128
ginseng—
  American 128
ginseng—
  Asian 128
ginseng—
  Siberian 128
glatiramer 141
gliclazide 92
glimepiride 87, 92
glipizide 88, 92
GlucaGen 93
glucagon 93
Glucobay 86
Gluconorm 92
Glucophage 93
Glucophage
  XR 93
glucosamine 128
Glucotrol 92
Glucotrol XL 92
Glucovance 87
Glumetza 92
Glutose 93
glyburide 87, 92
glycerin 115
GlycoLax 116
glycopyrrolate 119
Glycyrrhiza
  glabra 129
Glycyrrhiza
  uralensis 129
Glynase
  PresTab 92
Glyquin 82
Glyset 86
GM-CSF 125
Golimumab 1
GoLytely 116

Goody's Extra
  Strength Headache
  Powder 3
Gralise 137
gramicidin 157
granisetron 50, 110
Gravol 110
green goddess 114
green tea 128–129
Grifulvin V 16
griseofulvin 16
guaifenesin .. 105, 153
Guiatuss 105
Guiatuss PE 104
Gynazole 152
Gyne-Lotrimin 152
Gynodiol 146

H

Habitrol 174
Haemophilus B
  vaccine 131, 132
halcinonide 80
Halcion 172
Haldol 167
Halflytely 116
Halfprin 4
halobetasol
  propionate 80
halofantrine 50
haloperidol 50, 167,
  169
Harpadol 127
Harpagophytum
  procumbens 127
Havrix 131
hawthorn 129
H-BIG 133
HCE50 129
HCTZ 60–61, 68
Healthy
  Woman 130
HeartCare 129
Heather 148, 151
Hectorol 99
Helidac 113
Hemabate 151
HepaGam B 133
heparin 123, 153,
  182
hepatitis A
  vaccine 131, 132

hepatitis B immune
  globulin 133
hepatitis B
  vaccine 131, 132
Hepsera 30
Heptovir 23
Hespan 71
hetastarch 71
Hexabrix 73
Hextend 71
Hiberix 131
Histussin D 104
Histussin HC 104
Hizentra 133
homatropine 161
honey 129
Horizant 137
horse chestnut
  seed extract 129
HP-Pac 6
huang qi. 126
Humalog 91, 92
Humalog Mix
  50/50 .... 89, 91
Humalog Mix
  75/25 .... 89, 91
human growth
  hormone 102
human papillomavirus
  recombinant
  vaccine 132
Humatin 19
Humatrope 102
Humibid DM 104
Humira 1
Humulin 70/30 .. 89–91
Humulin N 91
Humulin R 91, 92
hyaluronic
  acid 82
Hycotuss 104
hydralazine 60, 62,
  71, 153
HydraSense 108
Hydrea 125
hydrochlorothiazide 68
Hydrocil 115
hydrocodone 8–12
hydrocortisone—
  80, 81, 83, 85,
  86, 106
hydrocortisone
  acetate 80
hydrocortisone
  butyrate 80
hydrocortisone
  valerate 80

195
Index

hydrocortisone—
  ophthalmic 158
Hydromorph Contin... 7
hydromorphone 7, 8
hydroquinone... 82, 83
hydroxocobalamin
  182
hydroxychloroquine ... 1
hydroxyprogesterone
  caproate 153
hydroxypropyl
  cellulose 162
hydroxyurea 125
hydroxyzine 105
hymenoptera
  venom 135
hyoscine 114
hyoscyamine.........
  114, 115, 184
Hyosol 115
Hyospaz 115
Hypaque 73
HyperHep B 133
Hypericum
  perforatum 130
HyperRAB S/D. 133
HyperRHO S/D. 153
Hypocol 130
Hypotears 162
Hytrin 63
Hytuss 105
Hyzaar 61

I

ibandronate 84
Ibudone 10
ibuprofen 5, 10, 11
ibutilide 50, 52
icosapent
  ethyl 58
Ilevro 161
iloperidone 50, 168,
  169
Ilotycin 157
Imdur 68
imipenem-cilastatin...
  32
imipramine 163
imiquimod 79
Imitrex 140
Immucyst 131

immune globulin—
  intramuscular ... 133
immune globulin—
  intravenous ... 133
immune globulin—
  subcutaneous ... 133
Imodium ... 109
Imodium AD ... 109
Imodium multi-
  symptom relief .. 109
Imogam Rabies-HT...
  133
Imovane ... 173
Imovax Rabies ... 132
Imuran ... 1
Inapsine ... 111
Incivek ... 31–32
incobotulinumtoxin
  A ... 144
indacaterol ... 176
indapamide ... 50, 68
Inderal ... 65
Inderal LA ... 65
Inderide ... 61
Indocid-P.D.A. ... 5
Indocin ... 5
Indocin IV ... 5
Indocin SR ... 5
indomethacin ... 5
Infanrix ... 131
InFed ... 96
Inflamase
  Forte ... 159
infliximab ... 1
influenza vaccine—
  inactivated
  injection ... 132
influenza vaccine—
  live intranasal .. 132
Infufer ... 96
ingenol ... 75
INH ... 18
Inhibace ... 47
Inhibace Plus ... 61
InnoPran XL ... 65
Inspra ... 48
Insta-Glucose ... 93
insulin ... 153
insulin aspart ... 91
insulin aspart
  protamine ... 91

insulin detemir ... 91
insulin glargine ... 91
insulin glulisine ... 91
insulin lispro ... 91
insulin lispro prot-
  amine ... 91
insulin—injectable
  combinations
  89, 91
insulin—injectable
  intermediate-/
  long-acting ... 91
insulin—injectable
  short-/rapid-
  acting ... 92
Intal ... 180
Integrilin ... 62
Intelence ... 22
interferon alfa-2B .. 30
interferon beta-1B 141
Intermezzo ... 173
Intestinex ... 129–130
Intralipid ... 98
intravaginal
  clotrimazole ... 35
Intron A ... 30
intravale ... 149
Intuniv ... 175
Invanz ... 32
Invega ... 170
Invega Sustenna .. 170
Invirase ... 28
Invokana ... 93
iodixanol ... 73
iohexol ... 73
Ionamin ... 176
iopamidol ... 73
iopromide ... 73
iothalamate ... 73
ioversol ... 73
ioxaglate ... 73
ioxilan ... 73
IPOL ... 132
ipratropium ... 179
ipratropium—
  inhaled ... 180
ipratropium—
  nasal ... 108
Iprivask ... 121
Iquix ... 156
irbesartan ... 49, 60
iron ... 182
iron dextran ... 96
iron polysaccharide 96
iron sucrose ... 96
Isentress ... 21
ISMO ... 68

isocarboxazid ... 163
isoniazid ... 18
isopropyl alcohol .. 106
isoproterenol ... 52
Isopto SR ... 66–67
Isopto Atropine
  160–161
Isopto Carpine .. 160
Isopto
  Homatropine ... 161
Isordil ... 68
isosorbide
  dinitrate ... 68, 71
isosorbide
  mononitrate ... 68
Isotamine ... 18
isotretinoin ... 74
Isovue ... 73
isradipine ... 50, 65
Istalol ... 159
Isuprel ... 52
itraconazole ... 15
ivermectin ... 19, 78
Ixiaro ... 132

J

Jalyn ... 183
Jantoven ... 123
Janumet ... 87–88
Janumet XR ... 87–88
Januvia ... 89
japanese encephalitis
  vaccine ... 132
jencycla ... 148
Jentadueto ... 88
Jetrea ... 162
JE-Vax ... 132
Jin Fu Kang ... 126
Jolivette ... 148, 151
junel ... 148
Junel Fe ... 148
Jurnista ... 7
Juvisync ... 88

K

K+8 ... 97
K+10 ... 97
Kabikinase ... 70
Kadian ... 8–9
Kaletra ... 25
Kaochlor ... 97
Kaochlor 10% ... 97
Kaochlor S-F ... 97
Kaon ... 97

Kaon Cl ... 97
Kaopectate ... 109
Kapvay ... 59
kariva ... 148
Kay Ciel ... 97
Kayexalate ... 102
Kaylixir ... 97
Kazano ... 88
K+Care ... 97
K+Care ET ... 97
K-Dur ... 97
K-Dur 10 ... 97
K-Dur 20 ... 97
Keflex ... 32
kelnor ... 148
Kenalog ... 86
Keppra ... 138
Keppra XR ... 138
Ketalar ... 13
ketamine ... 13
Ketek ... 45
ketoconazole—
  topical ... 77
Ketoderm ... 77
ketoprofen ... 5
ketorolac ... 5
ketorolac—
  ophthalmic ... 161
ketotifen ... 181
ketotifen—ophthal-
  mic ... 155
K-G Elixir ... 97
Kineret ... 1
Kinlytic ... 71
Kira ... 130
Kivexa ... 21
Klaron ... 75
Klean-Prep ... 116
K-Lease ... 97
Klonopin ... 171
Klonopin Wafer ... 171
K-Lor ... 97
Klor-con ... 97
Klor-Con 8 ... 97
Klor-Con M20 ... 97
Klor-Con M10
  Klotrix ... 97
Klor-Con/EF ... 97
Klorvess
  Effervescent ... 97
Klotrix ... 97
K-Lyte ... 97
K-Lyte Cl ... 97
K-Lyte DS ... 97
K-Lyte/Cl ... 97
K-Norm ... 97
Kolyum ... 97

Kombiglyze XR 88
kombiglyze 88
Kondremul 118
Konsyl 115
Konsyl Fiber 115
Korean red ginseng ....
128
K-Phos 96–97
Kristalose 115–116
Krystexxa 94
K-Tab 97
kurvelo 148
Ku-Zyme HP 113
K-vescent 97
Kwai 128
Kwellada-P 78
Kyolic 128
Kytril 110

L

labetalol 64, 153
Lac-Hydrin 82
lacosamide 137
Lacrilube 162
Lacrisert 162
Lactaid 119
lactase 119
lactic acid 82
Lactobacillus ....
129–131
lactulose 115–116,
153
Lamictal 137–138,
166
Lamictal CD 137–138,
166
Lamictal ODT ....
137–138, 166
Lamictal XR 137–138,
166
Lamisil 16, 77
Lamisil AT 77
lamivudine 21, 23
lamotrigine .. 137–138,
166
Lanoxin 51
lansoprazole. 113, 114
lanthanum
carbonate 91
Lantus 91
lapatinib 50
Lariam 17
Lasix 67
Lastacaft 155
latanoprost 160
Latisse 160

Latuda 168
Lazanda 7
lead 182
Lectopam 171
leflunomide 1
Legalon 129
Lescol 57
Lescol XL 57
lessina 148
Leukine 125
levalbuterol 177
Levaquin 42
Levbid 115
Levemir 91
levetiracetam 138
Levitra 185
levobunolol 159
levocabastine—
nasal 108
levocabastine—oph-
thalmic 155
levocarnitine 98
levocetirizine 105
levodopa 144
Levo-Dromoran 7
levofloxacin 35,
40, 42, 50
levofloxacin—oph-
thalmic 156
levonest 149
levonorgestrel .. 145,
147, 148–149
levonorgestrel 1S. 145
Levophed 70
levora 148
levorphanol 7, 8
Levothroid 98
levothyroxine . 98, 153
Levoxyl 98
Levsin 115
Levsinex 115
Lexapro 164
Lexiva 25
LI-160 130
Lialda 118
Librax 119
Librium 171
licorice 129
lidocaine 52, 82
lidocaine—local
anesthetic 13
lidocaine—ophthal-
mic 162
lidocaine—
topical 82, 83
lidocaine—viscous ....
107

Lidoderm 82
Limbrel 127
linaclotide 119
linagliptin 88
lindane 78
linezolid 45
Linzess 119
Lioresal 2
Lioresal D.S. 2
liothyronine . 98, 153
Lipidil EZ 54–55
Lipidil Micro .. 54–55
Lipidil Supra .. 54–55
Lipitor 56
Lipofen 54–55
Liposyn 98
Liptruzet 57
Liqui-Doss 118
liraglutide 89
lisdexamfetamine ......
175
lisinopril ... 47, 48, 61
lisinopril HCTZ 61
Lithane 166–167
lithium ... 50, 166–167
Lithobid 166–167
Livalo 57
Livostin ... 108, 155
LMX 82
Lo Loestrin Fe 148
Lo Minastrin Fe ... 148
LoCHOLEST 53
LoCHOLEST Light ... 53
Lodalis 53
lodoxamide 156
Loestrin 148
Loestrin Fe 148
Lofibra 148
Lomotil 109
lo/ovral 148
Loperacap 109
loperamide .. 109, 153
Lopid 56
lopinavir-ritonavir .. 25
Lopressor 64
Loprox 76
Loprox TS 76
loratadine 105
lorazepam 172
lorcaserin 119
Lorcet 10
Lortab 10
loryna 148
Lorzone 2
losartan 49, 61
LoSeasonique ....
147, 149

Lotemax 159
Lotensin 47
Lotensin HCT 61
loteprednol . 158, 159
Lotrel 61
Lotriderm 81
Lotrimin AF 77
Lotrimin Ultra 76
Lotrisone 81
Lotronex 118
lovastatin 55–57
Lovaza 59
Lovenox 122
Low-Ogestrel 148
loxapine 169
Lozide 68
Lozol 68
LPV/r 25
lubiprostone 117
lumefantrine 17
Lumigan 160
Luminal 138
Lunesta 172
lurasidone 168
Luride 95
Lustra 82
lutera 148
Luvox 164
Luvox CR 164
lybrel 149
lymphocyte immune
globulin 133
Lyrica 139

M

Maalox 112
Macrobid 45
Macrodantin 45
Macrodex 71
mafenide 76
Mag-200 96
magaldrate 112
Maganate 96
Magic
mouthwash 10
Maglucate 96
magnesiu
oxide 116
magnesium
carbonate 3, 112

magnesium
  chloride 96
magnesium
  citrate 116
magnesium
  gluconate 96
magnesium
  hydroxide 2,
  112, 116
magnesium
  oxide 3, 96
magnesium
  sulfate 96, 117
Magnevist 72
Mag-Ox 400 3
Magtrate 96
Makena 153
Malarone 17
malathion 78
maltodextrin 107
mangafodipir 73
mannitol 145
Mantoux 135
maraviroc 20–21
Marcaine 13
Marinol 111
marlissa 148
Marplan 163
Matricaria
  recutita—German
  chamomile 126
Mavik 47, 48
Maxair Autohaler .. 177,
  181
Maxalt 140
Maxalt MLT 140
Maxeran 111
Maxidone 10
Maxilene 82
Maximum Strength
  Pepcid AC 112
Maxipime 37
Maxitrol 158
MD-Gastroview 73
measles mumps &
  rubella
  vaccine 132
Meclicot 105
meclizine 105, 153
meclofenamate .. 5, 6
Medihoney 129
Medispaz 115

Medivert 105
Medrol 86
medroxyprogesterone..
  150
medroxyprog-
  esterone—inject-
  able 151
mefenamic acid 6
mefloquine 17
Megace 151
Megace ES 151
megestrol 151
Melaleuca
  alternifolia 131
melaleuca oil 131
Melanex 82
melatonin 129
Mellaril 167
meloxicam 5, 6
memantine 136
Menactra 132
Menest 146
Meni-D 105
meningococcal
  vaccine 132
Menjugate 132
Menomune-
  A/C/Y/W-135 .. 132
Menostar 146
Mentax 76
Mentha x perita
  oil 129
Menveo 132
meperidine 8, 153
Mephyton 100
mepivacaine 13
Mepron 19
mequinol 83
mercury 176
meropenem 32
Merrem IV 32
Mersyndol with
  Codeine 10
mesalamine 118
Mesasal 118
M-Eslon 8–9
Mestinon 142
Mestinon
  Timespan 142
mestranol 148
Metadate CD 176
Metadate ER 176
Metadol 8
Metaglip 88
Metamucil 115
metaproterenol 177
metaxalone 2

metformin .. 87–88, 93
methadone . 8, 50, 153
Methadose 8
methanol 182
methazolamide 160
methemoglobin 182
methenamine 184
Methergine 151
methimazole 98
methocarbamol 2
methohexital 13
methotrexate—
  rheumatology 1
methyaminol-
  evulinate 75
methylcellulose ... 115
methyldopa 59,
  60, 153
methylene blue .. 182,
  184
methylergonovine . 151
Methylin 176
Methylin ER 176
methylnaltrexone.. 119
methylphenidate .. 176
methylprednis 85
methylprednisolone—
  86
methyltestosterone—
  147, 150
metipranolol 159
metoclopramide ...
  111, 153
metolazone 68
metoprolol 61, 64
metoprolol
  succinate 60
Metozolv ODT.... 111
MetroCream 76
MetroGel 76
MetroGel-Vaginal . 152
MetroLotion 76
metronidazole ....
  35–37, 43, 45,
  113, 153
metronidazole—
  topical 76
metronidazole—
  vaginal 152
Metvix 75
Metvixia 75
Mevacor 57
mexiletine 52
Mexitil 52
Mezavant 118
Miacalcin 101
micafungin 16

Micardis 49
Micardis HCT 61
micardis plus 61
Micatin 77
miconazole 35, 152
miconazole—
  buccal 15
miconazole—
  topical 77, 83
Micozole 152
MICRhoGAM 153
microgestin 148
Microgestin Fe .. 148
Micro-K 97
Micro-K 10 97
Micro-K LS 97
Micronor 148, 151
Microzide 68
midazolam 13
midodrine 70
Midol Teen
  Formula 12
Mifeprex 153
mifepristone 153
miglitol 86
MigraLief 127
Migranal 141
Milk of Magnesia . 116
milk thistle 126
milnacipran 145
milrinone 70
Minastrin 24 Fe .. 148
mineral oil 118
Minipress 59
Minirin 102
Minitran 69
Minivelle 146
Minocin 44
minocycline 44
Minoxidil for Men.. 82
minoxidil—topical. 82
mirabegron 184
MiraLax 115
Mirapex 142–143
Mirapex ER.. 142–143
Mircette 148
mirtazapine .. 50, 166
misoprostol 4, 115
misoprostol—OB . 150
M-M-R II 132
MMRV 132
Mobic 6
Mobicox 6
modafinil 176
Modecate 167
Modicon 148
Moduret 61

Moduretic 61
moexipril ... 47, 48, 61
moexipril/HCTZ 50
molindone 169
mometasone DPI .. 178
mometasone
  furoate 80
mometasone—
  inhaled 179
mometasone—
  nasal 108
Monascus
  purpureus 130
Monazole 152
Monistat 152
Monistat 1-Day ... 152
monobenzone 82
Monocor 63
Monodox 44
monogyna 129
Monoket 68
mono-linyah 148
Monopril 47
Monopril HCT 61
montelukast . 153, 180
Monurol 45
Morinda citrifolia . 129
morphine 8–9
M.O.S. 8–9
Motofen 109
Motrin 5
Moviprep 116
Moxatag 39
Moxeza 156
moxifloxacin 40,
  42, 50
moxifloxacin—oph-
  thalmic 156
MS Contin 8–9
MSIR 8–9
Mucaine 112
Mucinex 105
Mucinex-DM
  Extended-Release ....
  104
Mucomyst 180,
  181–182
Multaq 51–52
MultiHance 72
multivitamins 99
mupirocin 76
Murine Ear 106
Muse 185
MVC 20–21
MVI 99
Myambutol 18
Mycamine 16

Mycelex 77
Mycelex-3 152
Mycelex 7 152
Mycobutin 18
Mycolog II 81
mycophenolate
  mofetil 134
Mycostatin 77, 152
Mydfrin 161
Mydriacyl 161
Myfortic 134
Mylanta 107, 112
Mylanta Children's ....
  94–95
Mylicon 115
Myorisan 74
Myrbetriq 184
Mysoline 139
Mytussin DM 104
myzila 149
M-Zole 152

N

NABI-HB 133
nabilone 111
nabumetone 5, 6
N-acetylcysteine ....
  181–182
N-acetyl-5-
  methoxytryptamine..
  129
nadolol 60, 64
nafcillin 39
naftifine 77
Naftin 77
nalbuphine 7
Nalcrom 180
naloxone . 12, 174, 182
naltrexone 173
Namenda 136
Namenda XR 136
naphazoline 155
Naphcon 155
naphcon-A 155
Naprelan 163
Naprosyn 5
naproxen .. 5, 6, 140
naratriptan 140
Narcan 12
Nardil 163
Nasacort AQ 108
Nasacort HFA 108
NaSal 108
nasal cromolyn ... 153
nasal steroids 153
NasalCrom 108

Nasalide 107
Nascobal 99
Nascom 108
Natazia 149
nateglinide 92
Natrecor 72
Natroba 78
nebivolol 65
necon 148, 149
nedocromil 153
nedocromil—
  ophthalmic 156
Nembutal 13
Neo-Fradin 119
neomycin . 76, 81, 106,
  157–158
neomycin—oral ... 119
NeoProfen 5
Neoral 134
Neosporin cream .. 76
Neosporin ointment 76
Neosporin ointment—
  ophthalmic 157
Neosporin solution—
  ophthalmic 157
neostigmine .. 13, 14
Neo-Synephrine .. 108
nepafenac 161
Nephrocap 99
Nephrovite 100
Nesina 88
nesiritide 72
NESP 124
Neulasta 125
Neumega 125
Neupogen 125
Neupro 144
Neurontin 137
Neutra-Phos .. 96–97
Nevanac 161
nevirapine 22
Nexium 113
Next Choice 145
Next Choice One-Step..
  145
niacin .. 55, 56, 58, 99,
  100
Niacor 100
Niaspan 100
nicardipine .. 50, 65
NicoDerm CQ 174
Nicolar 100
Nicorette 174
Nicorette DS 174
Nicorette inhaler.. 174
nicotine gum 174

nicotine inhalation
  system 174
nicotine
  lozenge 174
nicotine nasal spray..
  174
nicotine patches... 174
nicotinic acid 100
Nicotrol 174
Nicotrol Inhaler... 174
Nicotrol NS 174
Nidazol 45
nifedipine
  65–66, 153
Niferex 96
Niferex-150 96
nilotinib 50
Nimbex 14
nimodipine 145
Nimotop 145
Niravam 172
nisoldipine 66
nitazoxanide 19
Nitoman 145
Nitro-BID 68
Nitro-Dur 68
nitrofurantoin. 45, 153
nitroglycerin 120
nitroglycerin
  intravenous
  infusion 68
nitroglycerin
  ointment 68
nitroglycerin spray.. 69
nitroglycerin
  sublingual 69
nitroglycerin
  transdermal 69
Nitrolingual 69
NitroMist 69
Nitropress 62
nitroprusside 62
NitroQuick 69
Nitrostat 69
Nix 78
nizatidine .. 112, 153
Nizoral 77
Nizoral AD 77
NoDoz 175
Nolvadex 151
noni 129
Nora-BE.... 148, 151

Norco............... 10
Norcuron............... 14
Nordette............ 148
Norditropin............ 102
Norditropin NordiFlex..
102
norelgestromin 145
norepinephrine 70
norethin............. 145
norethindrone 147,
148-149, 150
Norflex............... 2
norfloxacin............. 42
Norgesic............... 3
norgestimate 149, 150
norgestrel............. 148
Norinyl............ 148
Noritate............... 76
Noroxin............. 42
Norpace............... 51
Norpace CR 51
Norpramin 162
Norvasc............... 65
Norvir........ 25, 28
Nostrilla............. 108
Novasen............. 4
Novasoy............ 130
Novolin 70/30.. 89, 91
Novolin N........... 91
Novolin R 91, 92
NovoLog........ 91, 92
Novolog Mix 70/30...
89, 91
NovoRapid........... 92
Noxafil............... 15
Nubain............... 7
Nucynta............. 12
Nucynta CR 12
Nucynta ER....... 12
Nucynta IR...... 12
Nuedexta 144
Nu-Iron 150 96
NuLev............. 115
Nulojix............. 134
NuLytely........... 116
Numby Stuff.......... 82
Nupercainal............ 81
Nuprin............... 5

Nutropin............... 102
Nutropin AQ..... 102
Nutropin Depot.... 102
NuvaRing............. 145
Nuvigil............... 175
NVP............... 22
Nyaderm.... 77, 152
Nymalize............. 145
nystatin .. 16, 35, 81,
153
nystatin—topical... 77
nystatin—
vaginal............. 152
Nytol............... 103

O

oatmeal............... 82
Ocean............... 3
ocriplasmin 162
Octagam............ 133
octreotide 117
Octycine............ 117
Ocuflox............. 156
Ocupress......... 159
Oesclim......... 146
Ofirmev............. 12
ofloxacin .. 35, 42, 50
ofloxacin—
ophthalmic 156
ofloxacin—otic... 106
Ogen............... 147
Ogestrel............. 148
olanzapine...... 50,
168-170, 173
Oleptro............. 166
Olestyr............. 59
olmesartan. 49, 60, 61
Olmetec............. 49
olone............... 85
olopatadine 155
olopatadine—
nasal............. 108
olsalazine......... 118
omega 3 fatty
acids 55, 59
omega-3-acid ethyl
esters............. 59
omeprazole 114
Omnaris............ 107
Omnipaque..... 73
Omniscan 72
Omnitrope 102
onabotulinum toxin
type A 145

Onbrez............. 176
Oncotice........... 131
ondansetron 50,
110, 153
ONFI............... 136
Onglyza 88
Onmel............. 15
Onsolis............ 7
Opana............. 9
Opana ER 9
Ophthaine 162
Ophthetic 162
opioids/opiates.... 182
opium............. 109
opium tincture.... 109
oprelvekin........... 125
Opticrom 156
OptiMARK 72
Optipranolol 159
Optiray............. 73
Optivar 155
Oracea............. 44
Oracit 186
OraDisc A 107
Oramorph SR 8-9
Orap............... 167
Orapred............. 86
Orapred ODT....... 86
Oravig............. 15
Orazinc............. 98
Oretic............... 68
organophosphates 182
orlistat............. 120
Orphenace 2
orphenadrine 2, 3
orsythia............. 148
Ortho Evra 145
Ortho Tri-Cyclen.... 149
Ortho Tri-Cyclen
Lo............. 149
Ortho-Cept 148
Ortho-Cyclen 148
Ortho-Est....... 147
Ortho-Novum ....
148, 149
Orudis............. 5
Orudis KT........... 5
Oruvail............ 5
Os-Cal............94-95
oseltamivir ... 28, 29
Oseni............. 88
Osmitrol 145
Osmoprep......... 116
ospemifene....... 151
Osphena 151
Ovcon-35............. 148
Ovcon-50,......... 148

Ovide............... 78
oxacillin............. 39
oxaprozin 5, 6
oxazepam 172
oxcarbazepine 138
Oxecta............. 9
Oxeze Turbuhaler... 176
oxiconazole 77
Oxilan............. 73
Oxistat............. 77
Oxizole............. 77
Oxtellar XR 138
oxyacantha 129
oxybate............. 145
Oxybutyn.... 183-184
oxybutynin 183
Oxycocet 11
Oxycodan 11
oxycodone...9-11, 153
OxyContin 9
OxyFAST 9
OxyIR............... 9
oxymetazoline 108
oxymorphone 9
OxyNEO 9
oxytocin 50, 150
Oxytrol.... 183-184
Oyst-Cal............94-95

P

Pacerone 50-51
paliperidone ......
50, 169, 170
palivizumab 30
palonosetron 110
pamabrom 12
Pamelor............. 163
pamidronate........ 84
Panadol............ 12
Panafil............. 83
Panax ginseng...... 128
Panax quinquefolius
L............. 128
Pancrease 120
pancreatin....... 120
Pancreaze....... 120
Pancrecarb....... 120
pancrelipase 120
Panretin............ 81
Pantoloc 114
pantoprazole 114
pantothenic acid ....
99, 100
papain............. 83
paracetamol 12
Parafon Forte DSC.... 2

Parcopa 142
paregoric 109
paricalcitol 100
Pariet 114
Parlodel 101
Parnate 163
paromomycin 19
paroxetine 164–165
Parvolex 181–182
Pataday 155
Patanase 108
Patanol 155
Paxil 164–165
Paxil CR 164–165
P.C.E. 38
pecac syrup 182
PediaCare Infants'
    Decongestant Drops
    105–106
Pediapred 86
Pediarix 132
Pediatrix 12
Pediotic 106
PedvaxHIB 131
Pegasys 30–31
pegfilgrastim 125
peginterferon alfa-2A,
    30–31
peginterferon
    alfa-2B 31
PEG-Intron 31
pegloticase 94
Peg-Lyte 116
pemirolast 156
penciclovir 79
penicillin 153
penicillin G 36, 38
penicillin V 38, 39
Penlac 76
Pennsaid 4–5, 75
pentamidine 50
Pentasa 118
pentazocine 7, 11
pentobarbital 13
Pentolair 161
pentoxifylline 72
Pepcid 112
Pepcid AC 112
Pepcid complete ... 112
peppermint oil 129
Peptic Relief 113
Pepto-Bismol 109
Percocet 11
Percocet-demi 11
Percodan 11
Percolone 9

perflutren lipid
    microspheres 50
Performist 176
Periactin 103
Peri-Colace 118
Peridex 107
perindopril 47, 48
Periogard 107
Periostat 44
perphenazine 155
    167, 169
Persantine 62
Petadolex 126
Petasites
    hybridus 126
pethidine 8
petrolatum 162
Pexeva 164–165
PGE1 .... 115, 150
PGE2 150
Phazyme 115
phenazopyridine 185
phenelzine 163
Phenergan 111
Phenergan VC 104
Phenergan VC w/
    codeine ©V 104
Phenergan/
    Dextromethorphan—
    104
pheniramine 155
phenobarbital 114,
    138
phenothiazines 50
phentermine . 120, 176
phentolamine 62
phenyl salicylate ... 184
phenylephrine 105
phenylephrine—
    intravenous 71
phenylephrine—
    nasal 108
phenylephrine—
    ophthalmic 161
Phenytek 138–139
phenytoin 138–139
philith 148
Phoslax 116
PhosLo 94
Phoslyra 94
phosphorated
    carbohydrates 182
phosphorus 96–97
Phrenilin 3
phytonadione 100

Phytosoya 130
Picato 75
pilocarpine 107
pilocarpine—
    ophthalmic 160
Pilopine HS 160
pimecrolimus 79
pimozide ......
    50, 167, 169
pinaverium 120
Pinworm 19
Pin-X 19
pioglitazone ....
    87, 88, 93
piperacillin-
    tazobactam 41
piperonyl butoxide ...
    77, 78
pirbuterol 177
pirmella 148
piroxicam 5, 6
pitavastatin 57
Pitocin 150
Pitressin 102
plague vaccine 132
Plan B 145
Plan B One-Step 145
Plaquenil 1
Plasbumin 71
plasma protein
    fraction 71
Plavix 62
Plendil 65
Pletal 72
Pliagis 82
Pneumo 23 132
pneumococcal
    13-valent conjugate
    vaccine 132
pneumococcal
    23-valent
    vaccine 132
Pneumovax 132
Podocon-25 79
Podofilm 79
podofilox 79
Podofin 79
podophyllin 79
Polaramine 103
polio vaccine 132
Polocaine 13
polycarbophil 115
Polycitra 186
Polycitra-K 186
Polycitra-LC 186
polyethylene
    glycol 116

polyethylene
    glycol with
    electrolytes 116
polymyxin 76,
    81, 106, 157–158
Polyphenon E ...
    128–129
Polysporin 76
Polysporin—
    ophthalmic 157
Polytar 82
polythiazide 61
Polytopic 76
Polytrim—
    ophthalmic 157
Ponstan 6
Ponstel 6
Pontocaine 162
portia 148
posaconazole 15
Posanol 15
Potasalan 97
potassium 97
potassium
    sulfate 117
Potiga 137
Power-Dophilus
    129–130
PPD 135
Pradaxa 121
pralidoxime . 182, 183
pramipexole . 142–143
pramlintide 93
Pramosone 83
Pramox HC 83
pramoxine 81, 83
Prandimet 88
Prandin 92
Prasterone 127
prasugrel 62–63
Pravachol 57
pravastatin 57
praziquantel 19
prazosin 59, 61
Precedex 13
Precose 86
Pred
    Forte 159
Pred G 158
Pred Mild 159
prednisolone ... 85, 86

prednisolone—
  ophthalmic..............
  157–159
prednisone ....
  85, 86, 153
Prednisone
  Intensol 86
Prefest 150
pregabalin 139
Prelone 86
Premarin ...146–147
Premesis-Rx 153
Premphase 150
Premplus 150
Prempro 150
Prepidil 150
Prepopik 116
Pressyn AR 102
Pretz 108
Prevacid 114
Prevacid NapraPac... 6
Prevalite 53
previfem 148
Prevnar 13 132
Prevpac 113
Prezista 24–25
Priftin 18
prilocaine 82
Prilosec 114
Primacor 70
Primadophilus ...
  129–130
Primalev 11
primaquine 17
Primaxin 32
primella 149
primidone 139
Primsol 46
Prinivil 47, 48
Priorix 132
Pristiq 165
Privigen 133
ProAir HFA ... 177, 181
Pro-Banthine 115
probenecid 94
probiotics ...129–130
procainamide 50,
  52–53
procaine
  penicillin 38, 39
Procan SR...52–53

Procardia.......65–66
Procardia XL....65–66
Procentra.......... 175
Prochieve 151
prochlorperazine... 111
Procrit 124
ProctoFoam NS ... 81
Prodium 185
progesterone gel... 151
progesterone
  micronized 151
progesterone
  vaginal insert .. 151
Prograf 135
proguanil 17
Prohance 72
Prolensa 161
Prolia 101
Prolixin 167
Promensil 130
promethazine 111
Prometrium 151
Pronestyl 52
propafenone 53
propantheline 115
proparacaine 162
propofol 13
propoxyphene 11
propranolol ... 61, 65
Propecia 183
Proquad 132
Proscar 183
Prosed/ds 184
ProSom 172
prostaglandin E1.. 185
Prostin E2......... 150
Prostin VR 185
Prostin VR
  Pediatric 185
protamine ... 125, 182
Protonix 114
Protopam 183
Protopic 79
protriptyline 163
Protropin 102
Proventil HFA ... 177,
  181
Provera 150
Provigil 176
Prozac 164
Prozac
  Weekly 164

pseudoephedrine.....
  105–106
Pseudofrin... 105–106
psyllium ... 115, 153
PTU 98
Pulmicort 181
Pulmicort
  Flexhaler 179
Pulmicort
  Respules 179
Pulmozyme 180
Pygeum
  africanum 130
Pylera 113
pyrantel 19
pyrazinamide 18
pyrethrins 77, 78
Pyridiate 185
Pyridium 185
pyridostigmine ... 142
pyridoxine ....
  99, 100, 110, 153
PZA 18

Q

Qnas 107
Qsymia 120
Qualaquin 17
quartette 149
quasense 149
Quelicin 14
Questran 53
Questran Light 53
quetiapine ... 50, 169,
  170
Quick-Pep......... 175
Quillivant XR 176
quinapril ... 47, 48, 60
quinidine 50, 53
quinine 17
quinupristin 45
Quixin 156
Qutenza 81
QVAR 179, 181

R

RabAvert 132
rabeprazole 114
rabies immune
  globulin human. 133
rabies vaccine 132
Rabies Vaccine
  Adsorbed 132

RAL 21
Ralivia 12
raloxifene 151
raltegravir 21
ramelteon 172
ramipril 47, 48
Ranexa 72
ranitidine ... 113, 153
ranolazine 50, 72
RAPAFLO 183
Rapamune 135
rasagiline 144
Rasilez 61
rasilez HCT 61
Rayos 85
Razadyne 135
Razadyne ER 135
R&C 77
Reactine 103
Rebetol 31
Rebif 141
Reclast 84–85
Recombivax HB .. 131
Rectiv 120
red clover 130
red clover
  isoflavone
  extract 130
red yeast rice 130
Redoxon 99
Refresh 161
Refresh PM 162
Refresh Tears 162
Regitine 62
Reglan 111
Regonol 142
Regranex 81
Rejuva-A 75
Relafen 6
Relenza 29, 30
Relistor 119
Relpax 140
Remeron 166
Remeron SolTab... 166
Remicade 1
Reminyl 135
Remular-S............ 2
Renagel 98
Renedil 65
Reno-60 73
RenoCal 73
Reno-DIP 73
Renografin 73
Renova 75
Renvela 98
ReoPro 62
repaglinide ... 88, 92
Requip 143

Requip XL 143
Rescula 160
Resectisol 145
RespiGam 133
Restasis 162
Restoril 172
Restylane 82
retapamulin 76
Retavase 70
reteplase 70
Retin-A 75
Retin-A Micro 75
Retisol-A 75
Retrovir 23
Revatio 70
ReVia 173
Reyataz 24
Rheomacrodex 71
Rheumatrex 1
Rhinalar 107
Rhinocort Aqua 107
RHO immune
    globulin 153
RhoGAM 153
Rhophylac 153
Ribasphere 31
ribavirin—oral 31
riboflavin 99, 100
RID 78
rifabutin 18
Rifadin 18
Rifamate 18
rifampin 18
rifapentine 18
Rifater 18
rifaximin 45
rilpivirine 21, 22
Rilutek 145
riluzole 145
rimantadine 28, 30
rimexolone 159
Riomet 93
Riopan 112
risedronate 84
Risperdal 170–171
Risperdal
    Consta 170–171
Risperdal M-Tab ...
    170–171
risperidone 50, 169,
    170–171
Ritalin 176
Ritalin LA 176
Ritalin SR 176
ritonavir 25, 28
rivaroxaban 121
rivastigmine ... 135–136

Rivotril 171
rizatriptan 140
Robaxin 2
Robaxin-750 2
Robinul 119
Robinul Forte 119
Robitussin 105
Robitussin AC 104
Robitussin CF 104
Robitussin Cough 105
Robitussin
    DAC 104
Robitussin DM 104
Robitussin PE 104
Rocaltrol 99
Rocephin 33–34
rocuronium 14
Rofact 18
roflumilast 181
Rogaine 82
Rogaine
    Extra Strength .. 82
Rogitine 62
Rolaids 112
Romazicon 182
Rondec DM Oral
    Drops 104
Rondec DM
    Syrup 104
Rondec Oral
    Drops 104
Rondec Syrup 104
ropinirole 143
rosiglitazone .. 87, 93
Rosula 74
rosuvastatin .. 57, 58
Rotarix 132
RotaTeq 132
rotavirus vaccine . 132
rotigotine 144
Rowasa 118
Roxanol 8–9
Roxicet 11
Roxicodone 9
Rozerem 172
RPT 18
RPV 22
RSV immune
    globulin 133
RTV 25, 28
RU-486 153
Rubini 127
Rufen 4
rufinamide 139
Rum-K 97
Rybix ODT 12
Rylosol 53

Rynatan 104
Rynatan-P
    Pediatric 104
Rythmodan 51
Rythmodan-LA 51
Rythmol 53
Rythmol SR 53
Ryzolt 12

S

S-2, 180
Saccharomyces
    boulardii 129–130
s-adenosylmethionine
    130
safyral 153
Saint John's wort . 130
Saizen 102
Salagen 107
Salazopyrin
    EN-tabs 118
salbutamol 177
Salofalk 118
salicin 131
Salicis cortex 131
salicylic acid 74
saline nasal
    spray 108
Salix alba 131
salmeterol 176, 178
salsalate 4, 5
Sambucol 127
Sambucus nigra ... 127
SAM-e 130
Sanctura 184
Sanctura XR 184
Sancuso 110
Sandimmune 134
Sandostatin 119
Sandostatin LAR .. 119
Saphris 168
saquinavir 28, 50
Sarafem 150
sargramostim 125
Savella 145
saxagliptin 88
Scopace 111
scopolamine 111, 114
SeaMist 108
Seasonale 149
Seasonique 149
Sebivo 32
SecreFlo 120
secretin 120
Sectral 63

Sedapap 3
selegiline 144
selegiline—transder-
    mal 163
selenium sulfide .. 83
Selsun 83
Selzentry 20–21
Semprex-D 104
senna 117, 118
sennosides 118
Senokot 117
Senokot-S 118
SenokotXTRA 117
Sensorcaine 13
Septocaine 13
Septra 42–43
Serax 172
Serevent Diskus .. 176,
    181
Serophene 150
Seroquel 170
Seroquel XR 170
Serostim 102
Serostim LQ 102
sertaconazole 77
sertraline 165
sevelamer 98
sevoflurane 50
Silace 117
Siladryl 104
sildenafil 70, 185
Silenor 163
silodosin 183
Silvadene 76
silver sulfadiazine . 76
Silybum
    marianum 129
silymarin 129
Simbrinza 160
Simcor 58
simethicone 109,
    112, 115, 153
Simponi 1
Simulect 134
simvastatin 55,
    57, 58, 88
sinecatechins 79
Sinemet 142
Sinemet CR 142
Sinequan 163
Singulair 180

Sinupret 127
sirolimus 135
sitagliptin 87–89
Sitavig 20
Skelaxin 2
Sklice 78
SI 97
Slo-Niacin 100
Slow-Fe 95
Slow-K 97
Slow-Mag 96
sodium
    bicarbonate. 53, 182
sodium
    phosphate. 116, 184
sodium
    picosulfate 116
sodium polystyrene
    sulfonate 102
sodium sulfate 117
sodium valproate ....
    139–140
Solage 83
Solaquin 82
Solaraze 75
solifenacin 184
Solodyn 44
Soltamox 151
Solu-Cortef 86
Solu-Medrol 86
Soma 2
Soma Compound 3
Soma Compound with
    Codeine 3
somatropin 102
Sominex 103
Sonata 173
sorbitol 116
Soriatane 78
Sorilux 78
sotalol 50, 53
Sotret 74
soy 130
Spacol 115
Spasdel 115
Spectracef 33
spinosad 78
Spiriva 181
spironolactone.. 48, 60
Sporanox 52
sprintec 148
SQV 28
sronyx 148
Stadol 7
Stadol NS 7
Stalevo 144
standardized
    extract WS
    1442-Crataegutt
    novo 129
starch 81
Starlix 92
Statex 8–9
statins 55
Stavzor 139–140,
    167
Staxyn 185
Stay Awake 175
Stelara 179
Stelazine 168
Stemetil 169
Stendra 185
Stieprox shampoo ... 76
Stieva-A 74
Stimate 102
Strattera 175
Streptase 70
streptokinase 70
streptomycin 14
Striant 83–84
Stribild 21
Stridex Pads 74
Stromectol 19
Sublimaze 7
Sublinox 173
Suboxone 174
Subsys 7
Subutex 6
succimer ... 182, 183
succinylcholine 14
Suclear 116
sucralfate ... 107, 115
Sudafed 105–106
Sudafed 12 Hour ......
    105–106
Sudafed PE 105
Sular 66
Sulcrate 115
Sulfamylon 76
Sulf-10 157
sulfacetamide. 74, 75,
    157–158
sulfacetamide—oph-
    thalmic 157
sulfacetamide—topi-
    cal 74
Sulfacet-R ... 74, 75
Sulfamylon 76
sulfasalazine 118
Sulfatrim 42–43
sulfonated phenolics ..
    107
sulfur 74, 75
sulfuric acid 107
sulindac 5, 6
sumatriptan 140
Sumavel 140
sunitinib 50
Supeudol 9
Suprax 33
Suprenza 176
Suprep 116
Supro 130
Surpass 94–95
Sustiva 22
Swim-Ear 106
syeda 148
Symax 115
Symbicort 179
Symbyax 173
Symlin 93
Symlinpen 93
Symmetrel 28
Synacthen Depot 30
Synagis 30
Synalgos-DC 11
Synera 83
Synercid 45
Synthroid 98
Systane 162

T

T3 98
T4 98
Taclonex 78
tacrolimus.. 50, 135
tacrolimus—
    topical 79
Tactuo 74
tadalafil ... 70, 185
tafluprost 160
Tagamet 112
Tagamet HB 112
Talacen 11
Talwin NX 7
Tambocor 52
Tamiflu ... 28, 29
Tamone 151
tamoxifen ... 50, 151
tamsulosin 183
Tanacetum
    parthenium L.... 127
Tanafed 104
Tapazole 98
tapentadol 12
Targin 9
Tarka 61
Tarsum 82
Tavist-1 103
Tavist ND 103
tazarotene 75
Tazicef 33
Tazocin 41
Tazorac 75
Taztia XT 66
TCAs 170
Td 131
Tdap 131
TDF 23
tea tree oil 131
Tears Naturale 162
Tebrazid 18
Tecfidera 141
Tecta 114
teduglutide 120
Teflaro 37
Tegretol 136
Tegretol XR 136
Tegrin 82
Tekamlo 61
Tekturna 61
Tekturna HCT 61
telaprevir 31–32
telavancin 45
telbivudine 32
telithromycin .. 45, 50
telmisartan ... 49, 61
Telzir 25
temazepam 172
Tempra 12
tenecteplase 71
tenofovir ... 21, 23
Tenoretic 61
Tenormin 63
Tensilon 141–142
Terazol 152
teriparatide 102
Teslascan 73
Tessalon 105
Tessalon Perles 105
Testim 83–84
Testopel 83–84
testosterone 83–84
Testro AQ 83–84
tetanus 131
tetanus immune
    globulin 133
tetanus toxoid 132

tetrabenazine 145
tetracaine 83, 108
tetracaine—ophthalmic 162
tetracycline 113
Teveten 49
Teveten HCT 61
Tev-Tropin 102
Thalitone 68
Theo-24 181
Theo ER 181
Theolair 181
theophylline ... 153, 181
thiamine 99, 100
thioridazine 50, 167, 169
thiothixene ... 168, 169
Thisylin 129
thonzonium 106
Thorazine 167
3TC 23
tiagabine 139
Tiazac 66
ticagrelor 63
ticarcillin-clavulanate 41
Ticlid 63
ticlopidine 63
Tigan 111
tigecycline 46
Tikosyn 51
Timentin 41
timolol 160
timolol—ophthalmic 159
Timoptic 159
Timoptic Ocudose .159
Timoptic XE 159
Tinactin 77
Tindamax 19
tinidazole 19, 37
tioconazole ... 35, 152
tiotropium 181
tipranavir 28
tirofiban 63
Tirosint 98
tizanidine 2, 50
TNKase 71
Tobi 14
Tobradex 158
Tobradex ST 158
tobramycin ... 14, 158
tobramycin—ophthalmic 156
Tobrex 156
tocopherol 101
Toctino 81

Tofranil 163
Tofranil PM 163
Tolectin 6
tolmetin 5, 6
tolnaftate 77
Toloxin 51
tolterodine ... 50, 184
Topamax 139, 167
topiramate ... 120, 139, 167
Toprol-XL 64
Toradol 7
torsemide 67
Toviaz 183
tpa 70
t-PA 70
T-Phyl 181
TPV 28
Tradjenta 88
Trajenta 88
Tramacet 3
tramadol 3, 12
Trandate 64
trandolapril 47, 48, 61
Transderm-Nitro 69
Transderm-Scop .. 111
Transderm-V 111
Tranxene 171
tranylcypromine .. 163
Travatan Z 160
travoprost 160
trazodone 166
trefoil 130
Trental 72
tretinoin 75, 83
tretinoin—topical .. 75
Trexall 1
Treximet 140
triamcinolone .. 80, 81, 85, 86
triamcinolone—inhaled 180
triamcinolone—nasal 108
Triaminic Cold &
Allergy 104
Triaminic Oral Infant
Drops 105–106
triamterene ... 60, 61
Trianal 3
Trianal C-1/2 10
Trianal C-1/4 10
Triazide 61
triazolam 172

Tribenzor 61
TriCor 54–55
Tridural 12
tri-estarylla 149
trifluoperazine ... 168, 169
trifluridine 157
Trifolium pratense 130
Triglide 54–55
Trigonella foenum-graecum 127
trihexyphenidyl ... 142
Trihibit 132
Tri-K 97
Trikacide 45
tri-legest 149
Tri-Legest Fe 149
Trileptal 138
tri-linya 149
TriLipix 56
Trilisate 4, 5
Tri-Luma 83
TriLyte 116
trimethobenzamide 111, 153
trimethoprim .. 46, 157
trimethoprim-sulfamethoxazole 42–43
Tri-Nasal 108
Trinipatch 69
Tri-Norinyl 149
Trinovin 130
Triostat 98
Tripacel 131
Tripedia 131
tri-previfem 149
tri-sprintec 149
Trivaris 86
Trivora-28 149
Trizivir 21
Tropicacyl 161
tropicamide 161
Trosec 184
trospium 184
Trusopt 159
Truvada 21
tuberculin PPD ... 135
Tubersol 135
Tucks 81
Tucks Hemorrhoidal
Ointment 81
Tucks
Suppositories .. 81
Tudorza 180
Tums 94–95
Tussionex 104

Twin-K 97
Twinrix 132
2-PAM 183
Twynsta 61
Tygacil 46
Tylenol 12
Tylenol #1 11
Tylenol # 2 11
Tylenol # 3 11
Tylenol # 4 11
Tylenol with
Codeine 11
Tylox 11
Typherix 133
Typhim Vi 133
typhoid vaccine—inactivated
injection 133
typhoid vaccine—live
oral 133
Tyzeka 32

U

ubiquinone 127
Uceris 119
Ulesfia 78
uliprista
acetate 146
Uloric 94
Ultracet 3
Ultram 12
Ultram ER 12
Ultraquin 82
Ultravist 73
Ultresa 120
Unasyn 41
Uniphyl 181
Uniretic 61
Unisom Nighttime
Sleep Aid 110
Unithroid 98
Univasc 47, 48
unoprostone 160
UP446 127
urea 83
urecholine 184
Urised 184
Urocit-K 186
Urodol 185
Urogesic 185

urokinase 71
Urolene blue 182
Uromax 183–184
UroXatral 183
URSO 120
URSO Forte 120
ursodiol 120
ustekinumab 101
UTA 184
UTI Relief 185
Utira-C 184

V

Vaccinium
  macrocarpon 127
Vagifem 146
Vagistat-1, 152
valacyclovir ... 20, 35,
  36, 153
Valcyte 19–20
valerian 131
Valeriana officinalis ...
  131
valganciclovir ... 19–20
Valium 171
valproic acid—neuro.
  139–140
valproic acid—psych.
  167
valsartan 49, 60
Valtrex 20
Valtropin 102
Vancenase 107
Vancocin 46
vancomycin ... 43, 46
Vandazole 152
Vaniqa 82
Vanspar 172
Vaqta 133
vardenafil 50, 185
varenicline 174
varicella
  vaccine 133
varicella-zoster
  immune
  globulin 133
Varilrix 133

Varivax 133
VariZIG 133
Vascepa 58
Vaseretic 61
Vasocidin 158
vasocon-A 155
vasopressin 102
Vasotec 47
Vaxigrip 132
vecuronium 14
velvet 149
Veltin 79
Venastat 129
venlafaxine ... 50, 165
Venofer 96
Ventolin HFA .. 177, 181
Veramyst 108
verapamil .. 61, 66–67
Veregen 79
Verelan 66–67
Verelan PM 66–67
Versed 13
Versel 83
VESIcare 184
Vexol 159
Vfend 15
Viactiv 94–95
Viagra 185
Vibativ 45
Vibramycin 44
Vibra-Tabs 44
Vicks Sinex 108
Vicks Sinex
  12 Hr 108
Vicodin 11
Vicoprofen 11
Victoza 89
Victrelis 30
Videx 22
Videx EC 22
Vigamox 156
Viibryd 163
vilanterol 179
vilazodone 163
vimpat 137
Viokace 120
Viokase 120
viorele 148
Viracept 22
Viramune 22
Viramune
  XR 22
Viread 23
Viroptic 157
Visicol 116

visine-A 155
Visipaque 73
Vistaril 105
Vistide 19
vitamin A 100
Vitamin A Acid
  Cream 75
vitamin B1 100
vitamin B2 100
vitamin B3 100
vitamin B6 100
vitamin B12 99
vitamin C 99
vitamin D2 99
vitamin D3 101
vitamin E 101
vitamin K 100, 182
Vitex agnus castus
  fruit extract 126
Vivactil 163
Vivaglobulin 133
Vivarin 175
Vivelle Dot 146
Vivitrol 173
Vivotif Berna 133
Voltaren .. 4–5, 75, 161
Voltaren
  Emulgel 4–5
Voltaren Ophtha .. 4–5,
  161
Voltaren Rapide .. 4–5
Voltaren SR 4–5
Voltaren XR 4–5
voriconazole .. 15, 50
Vosol HC 106
VoSpire ER 177
VSL#3 129–130
Vusion 83
Vyloma 79
Vytorin 58
Vyvanse 175
VZIG 133

W

warfarin 123, 182
Wartec 79
Welchol 53
Wellbutrin ... 165–166
Wellbutrin
  SR 165–166
Wellbutrin
  XL 165–166
white petrolatum 83

willow bark
  extract 131
Winpred 86
WinRho SDF 153
witch hazel 81
Women's
  Rogaine 82
Wygesic 11

X

Xalatan 160
Xanax 172
Xanax XR 172
Xarelto 121
Xatral 183
Xenazine 145
Xenical 120
Xeomin 144
Xgeva 101
Xifaxan 45
Xodol 11
Xolegel 77
Xopenex 177
Xopenex
  HFA 177, 181
Xuezhikang 130
Xylocaine ... 13, 52,
  82, 107
Xylocard 52
Xyrem 145
Xyzal 105

Y

Yasmin 148
Yaz 148
yellow fever
  vaccine 133
YF-Vax 133
Yocon 185
yohimbine 185
Yohimex 185

Z

Zaditen 181
Zaditor 155
zafirlukast 180
zaleplon 173
Zanaflex 2
zanamivir 29, 30
Zantac 113

Zantac 75............ 113
Zantac 150.......... 113
Zantac Efferdose.. 113
Zarontin 136
Zaroxolyn 68
ZDV 23
ZeaSorb AF 77
Zebeta 63
Zecuity 140
Zegerid 114
Zelapar.............. 144
Zeldox................ 171
Zemplar.............. 100
Zemuron 14
Zenapax 134
Zenatane.............. 74
Zenhale 179
Zenpep 120
Zenzedi.............. 175
zestoretic............. 61
Zestril........... 47, 48
Zetia................... 58
Zetonna.............. 107

Zhibituo 130
ziac 61
Ziagen.............22–23
Ziana.................... 75
zidovudine 21, 23
zileuton 180
Zinacef............32–33
zinc acetate......... 97
zinc oxide 83
zinc sulfate 98
Zincate................ 98
Zingiber
    officinale 128
Zingo.................... 82
Zioptan.............. 160
ziprasidone... 50, 169,
    171
Zipsor................4–5
Zirgan 157
Zithromax........37–38
Zmax 37–38
Zocor.................... 58
Zofran 110

zoledronic acid.84–85
zolmitriptan....... 141
Zoloft................ 165
zolpidem............ 173
Zolpimist............ 173
Zometa............84–85
Zomig................ 141
Zomig ZMT....... 141
Zonalon............... 82
Zonegran........... 140
zonisamide........ 140
zopiclone........... 173
Zorbtive............ 102
Zorcaine 13
ZORprin................ 4
Zortress............ 134
Zostavax............ 133
zoster
    vaccine—live..... 133
Zostrix................ 81
Zostrix-HP........... 81
Zosyn.................. 41
Zovia................ 148

Zovirax......... 20, 79
Zyban 165–166
Zyclara................ 79
Zydone................ 12
Zyflo CR............ 180
Zylet................ 158
Zyloprim.............. 94
Zymar................ 156
Zymaxid............ 156
Zyprexa 168–170
Zyprexa
    Relprevv... 168–170
Zyprexa
    Zydis 168–170
Zyrtec................ 103
Zytram XL............ 12
Zyvox................. 45
Zyvoxam.............. 45

APPENDIX

ADULT EMERGENCY DRUGS (selected)

ALLERGY	diphenhydramine (*Benadryl*): 25 to 50 mg IV/IM/PO. epinephrine: 0.1 to 0.5 mg IM/SC (1:1000 solution), may repeat after 20 minutes. methylprednisolone (*Solu-Medrol*): 125 mg IV/IM.
HYPERTENSION	esmolol (*Brevibloc*): 500 mcg/kg IV over 1 minute, then titrate 50 to 200 mcg/kg/min. fenoldopam (*Corlopam.*): Start 0.1 mcg/kg/min, titrate up to 1.6 mcg/kg/min. labetalol: Start 20 mg slow IV, then 40 to 80 mg IV q10 min prn up to 300 mg total cumulative dose. nitroglycerin: Start 10 to 20 mcg/min IV infusion, then titrate prn up to 100 mcg/min. nitroprusside (*Nipress*): Start 0.3 mcg/kg/min IV infusion, then titrate prn up to 10 mcg/kg/min.
DYSRHYTHMIAS / ARREST	adenosine (*Adenocard*): PSVT (not A-fib): 6 mg rapid IV & flush, preferably through a central line or proximal IV. If no response after 1-2 minutes, then 12 mg. A third dose of 12mg may be given prn. amiodarone: V-fib or pulseless V-tach: 300 mg IV/IO; may repeat 150 mg just once. Life-threatening ventricular arrhythmia: Load 150 mg IV over 10 min, then 1 mg/min × 6 h, then 0.5 mg/min × 18 h. atropine: 0.5 to 1 mg IV, may repeat q 3-5 minutes prn to maximum of 3 mg. diltiazem (*Cardizem*): Rapid A-fib: bolus 0.25 mg/kg or 20 mg IV over 2 min. May repeat 0.35 mg/kg or 25 mg 15 min after 1st dose. Infusion 5-15 mg/h. epinephrine: 1 mg IV/IO q 3-5 minutes for cardiac arrest. [1:10,000 solution]. lidocaine (*Xylocaine*): Load 1 mg/kg IV, then 0.5 mg/kg q 8-10 min prn to max 3 mg/kg. Maintenance 2 g in 250 mL D5W (8 mg/mL) at 1 to 4 mg/min (2-4 mL/min). magnesium sulfate: 1-2 g in 250 mL D5W (7-30 mL/h).
PRESSORS	dobutamine: 2 to 20 mcg/kg/min. 70 kg: 5 mcg/kg/min with 1 mg/mL concentration (eg, 250 mg in 250 mL D5W) = 21 mL/h. dopamine: Pressor: Start at 5 mcg/kg/min, increase prn by 5 to 10 mcg/kg/min increments at 10 min intervals, max 50 mcg/kg/min. 70 kg: 5 mcg/kg/min with 1600 mcg/mL concentration (eg, 400 mg in 250 mL D5W) = 13 mL/h. Doses in mcg/kg/min: 2-4 = (traditional renal dose, apparently ineffective) dopaminergic receptors; 5-10= (cardiac dose) dopaminergic and beta1 receptors; >10 = dopaminergic, beta1, and alpha1 receptors. norepinephrine (*Levophed*): 4 mg in 500 mL D5W (8 mcg/mL), start 8 to 12 mcg/min (1 to 1.5 mL/h), usual dose once BP is stabilized 2 to 4 mcg/min. 22.5 mL/h = 3 mcg/min. phenylephrine: 20 mg in 250 mL D5W (80 mcg/mL), start 100 to 180 mcg/min (75 to 135 mL/h), usual dose once BP is stabilized 40 to 60 mcg/min (30 to 45 mL/h).
INTUBATION	etomidate (*Amidate*): 0.3 mg/kg IV. methohexital (*Brevital*): 1 to 1.5 mg/kg IV. propofol (*Diprivan*): 2.0 to 2.5 mg/kg IV. rocuronium (*Zemuron*): 0.6 to 1.2 mg/kg IV. succinylcholine (*Anectine, Quelicin*): 0.6 to 1.1 mg/kg IV. Peds (<5 yo): 2 mg/kg IV. thiopental: 3 to 5 mg/kg IV.
SEIZURES	diazepam (*Valium*): 5 to 10 mg IV, or 0.2 to 0.5 mg/kg rectal gel up to 20 mg PR. fosphenytoin (*Cerebyx*): Load 15 to 20 mg "phenytoin equivalents" (PE)/ kg IV, no faster than 100 to 150 mg PE/min. lorazepam (*Ativan*): Status epilepticus: 4 mg IV over 2 min, may repeat in 10-15 min. Anxiolytic/sedation: 0.04 to 0.05 mg/kg IV/IM; usual dose 2 mg, max 4 mg. phenobarbital: Status epilepticus: 15 to 20 mg/kg IV load; may give additional 5 mg/kg doses q 15-30 mins to max total dose of 30 mg/kg. phenytoin (*Dilantin*): 15 to 20 mg/kg IV up to 1000mg IV no faster than 50 mg/min.

CARDIAC DYSRHYTHMIA PROTOCOLS (for adults and adolescents)

Chest compressions ~100/min. Ventilations 8-10/min if intubated; otherwise 30:2 compression/ventilation ratio. Drugs that can be administered down ET tube (use 2–2.5 × usual dose): epinephrine, atropine, lidocaine, naloxone, vasopressin*.

V-Fib, Pulseless V-Tach
Airway, oxygen, CPR until defibrillator ready
Defibrillate 360 J (old monophasic), 120–200 J (biphasic), or with AED
Resume CPR × 2 min (5 cycles)
Repeat defibrillation if no response
Vasopressor during CPR:
- Epinephrine 1 mg IV/IO q 3–5 minutes, or
- Vasopressin* 40 units IV to replace 1st or 2nd dose of epinephrine
Rhythm/pulse check every ~2 minutes
Consider antiarrhythmic during CPR:
- Amiodarone 300 mg IV/IO; may repeat 150 mg just once
- Lidocaine 1.0–1.5 mg/kg IV/IO, then repeat 0.5–0.75 mg/kg to max 3 doses or 3 mg/kg
- Magnesium sulfate 1–2 g IV/IO if suspect torsades de pointes

Asystole or Pulseless Electrical Activity (PEA)
Airway, oxygen, CPR
Vasopressor (when IV/IO access):
- Epinephrine 1 mg IV/IO q 3–5 min, or
- Vasopressin* 40 units IV/IO to replace 1st or 2nd dose of epinephrine
Consider atropine 1 mg IV/IO for asystole or slow PEA. Repeat q 3–5 min up to 3 doses.
Rhythm/pulse check every ~2 minutes
Consider 6 H's: hypovolemia, hypoxia, H+acidosis, hyper/ hypokalemia, hypoglycemia, hypothermia
Consider 5 T's: Toxins, tamponade-cardiac, tension pneumothorax, thrombosis (coronary or pulmonary), trauma

Bradycardia, <60 bpm and Inadequate Perfusion
Airway, oxygen, IV
Prepare for transcutaneous pacing; don't delay if advanced heart block
Consider atropine 0.5 mg IV; may repeat q 3–5 min to max 3 mg
Consider epinephrine (2–10 mcg/min) or dopamine(2–10 mcg/kg/min)
Prepare for transvenous pacing

Tachycardia with Pulses
Airway, oxygen, IV
If unstable and heart rate >150 bpm, then synchronized cardioversion
If stable narrow-QRS (<120 ms):
- Regular: Attempt vagal maneuvers, If no success, adenosine 6 mg IV, then 12 mg prn (may repeat x 1),
- Irregular: Control rate with diltiazem or beta blocker (caution in CHF or severe obstructive disease).
If stable wide-QRS (>120 ms):
- Regular and suspect V-tach: Amiodarone 150 mg IV over 10 min; repeat prn to max 2.2 g/24 h. Prepare for elective synchronized cardioversion.
- Regular and suspect SVT with aberrancy: adenosine as per narrow-QRS above.
- Irregular and A-fib: Control rate with diltiazem or beta blocker (caution in CHF/ severe obstructive pulmonary disease).
- Irregular and A-fib with pre-excitation (WPW): Avoid AV nodal blocking agents; consider amiodarone 150 mg IV over 10 min.
- Irregular and torsades de pointes: magnesium 1–2 g IV load over 5–60 min, then infusion.

bpm=beats per minute; CPR=cardiopulmonary resuscitation; ET=endotracheal; IO=intraosseous; J=Joules; ms=milliseconds; WPW=Wolff-Parkinson-White. Sources: Circulation 2005; 112, suppl IV; *NEJM 2008;359:21–30 (demonstrated no benefit over epinephrine and worse long-term neurological outcomes).